Essential Drug Data
for Rational Therapy
in Veterinary Practice

T0225834

Essential Drug Data for Rational Therapy in Veterinary Practice

KINGSLEY EGHIANRUWA

authorHOUSE®

AuthorHouse™ UK Ltd.
1663 Liberty Drive
Bloomington, IN 47403 USA
www.authorhouse.co.uk
Phone: 0800.197.4150

Published by AuthorHouse 01/24/2014

ISBN: 978-1-4918-0000-3 (sc)
ISBN: 978-1-4918-0010-2 (e)

CONTENTS

FOREWORD

This book, Essential Drug Data for Rational Therapy in Veterinary Practice provides drug data needed by practicing veterinarians, veterinary students, other professionals and animal owners who must use veterinary drugs safely, rationally and effectively. Proficient drug therapy requires knowledge and judgment, among others, rather than tagging a drug name to that of a disease. The chemical and pharmacological classifications, sources, pharmacokinetic, pharmacodynamic and pharmaceutical data which are presented in the book give knowledge. The information on drug interactions, precautions, management of toxicity/overdose and contraindications contribute to the formation of judgment.

Professor S. M. Anika.
July 2013

PREFACE

Drugs, whether in humans or animals, can do both good and harm. The veterinary practitioner has the professional and ethical obligation to use drugs in proper manner to treat, protect or alleviate disease conditions without causing death or iatrogenic diseases. Evidence-based drug therapy demands adequate knowledge of the pharmacokinetics and pharmacodynamics of the drugs. This book, Essential Drug Data for Rational Therapy in Veterinary Practice, presents the much sought after drug information by practicing veterinarians. Drug information has become paramount to effective veterinary practice. The rate at which new drugs are developed and made available for clinical use has increased tremendously. To keep pace with this rate the veterinary practitioner requires the help of pharmacologist to assemble the information which he needs for effective animal care in one volume. This is exactly what this book is out to achieve. The book presents vital drug information including chemical and pharmacological classifications, sources, pharmacokinetic, pharmacodynamic and pharmaceutical data for drugs used in veterinary practice.

K. I. Eghianruwa
July 2013

NOTICE

Every effort has been made to ensure that the information provided in this book, Essential Drug Data for Rational Therapy in Veterinary Practice is accurate, up-to-date and generally in accord with the standards accepted at the time of publication. The book is not intended to cover all possible uses, directions, precautions, warnings, drug interactions, allergic reactions, or adverse effects of the drugs presented. The content of this book which has been compiled from sources believed to be reliable is an informational resource designed to assist licensed veterinary practitioners in caring for their patients. Readers other than veterinarians should bear in mind that the information contained in this book is not a substitute for the expertise, skill, knowledge and judgment of the veterinary practitioners. All readers should realize that drug information is time sensitive since new research and clinical experience broaden our knowledge requiring changes in treatment and drug therapy. The information contained herein is used entirely at the reader's discretion, and is made available on the express condition that no liability, expressed or implied, is accepted by the author or publisher for any undesirable result arising from the use of any drug contained in this book. In particular, all drug doses, indications, and contraindications should be confirmed from the drug package insert.

ACKNOWLEDGEMENT

The author is grateful to Professors S. M Anika and
Helen Nottindge for reviewing the manuscript.

ABAMECTIN

Synonyms—Avermectin B$_1$.

Proprietary Name—Avomec*.

Chemical Class—Macrocyclic lactone.

Pharmacological Class—Endectocide; Anthelmintic; Ectoparasiticide.

Source—Semi synthetic; obtained from a mixture of B$_{1a}$ and B$_{1b}$ avermectins, products of *Streptomyces avermitilis*.

Solubility, Stability and Storage—Abamectin is poorly soluble in water but soluble in most organic solvents.

Pharmacological Actions—Abamectin has nematocidal and ectoparasiticidal properties, hence it is also classified as endectocide. It is extremely potent being active in microgram level. Its spectrum of activity includes major gastrointestinal nematodes, lung nematodes, and ectoparasites of cattle. It is highly effective against adult and larval forms of *Ostertagia*, *Haemonchus*, *Cooperia*, *Oesophagostomum* and *Dictyocaulus* species. Adult forms of *Trichostrongylus* and *Chabertia* are susceptible. Abamectin protects cattle from sucking lice for up to 8 weeks. It reduces egg production in female ticks that survives treatment. Abamectin may also stop the development of larvae forms of dung-breeding flies.

Mechanism of Action—Abamectin, like other macrocyclic lactones, increases neuronal chloride conductance by opening glutamate-gated chloride channels and also by potentiating the release and binding of GABA at certain synapses in invertebrates. These actions result in hyperpolarization and reduced neuronal excitability thereby causing tonic paralysis of the peripheral musculature of susceptible parasites.

Mechanism of Selective Toxicity—High affinity avermectin receptors are absent in cestodes and trematodes. The sensitivity of avermectin receptors in nematodes and arthropods is 100-fold higher than those in mammals.

Indications—Control of endo—and ecto—parasites including adult and larval forms of gastrointestinal nematodes, lung worms, sucking lice, and ticks in cattle.

Dosages—200 mcg/kg.

Route(s) of Administration—Subcutaneous.

Distribution—Abamectin crosses the blood-brain-barrier (BBB) poorly presumably because of a P-glycoprotein efflux pump operative at the BBB.

Route(s) of Excretion—Excreted largely in feces as unchanged drug. The active drug in feces may affect developmental forms of dung-breeding flies for up to three weeks.

Dialysis Status—Unknown.

Toxicity and Adverse Effects—Abamectin is less tolerated than ivermectin. Abamectin causes tremor, depression, ataxia at low doses. Ataxia may become pronounced at high doses leading to paresis, recumbency, decreased lip and tongue tone, drooling of saliva, coma, and death.

Management of Overdose/Toxicity—Give symptomatic and supportive therapy. Hypersensitivity reaction may be controlled with corticosteroids.

Contraindications—Hypersensitivity reaction to abamectin or its formulation component; milk producing animals; pregnant dairy cow within 28 days to calving; animals less than 4 months of age.

Precautions—Avoid concurrent administration with drugs that cause CNS depression. Do not administer in cases where the integrity of the blood-brain–barrier may be compromised as in meningitis.

Drug Interactions—Picrotoxin, a GABA antagonist can reverse the actions of abamectin.

Pharmaceutical Formulations—Available as 1.0% sterile solution for injection.

ACEPROMAZINE

Acepromazine

Synonyms—Acetylpromazine; ACE; ACP.

Proprietary Names—Plegicil®, Notensil®, Atravet®.

Chemical Class—Phenothiazine derivative.

Pharmacological Class—Tranquilizer; Sedative-hypnotic, CNS depressant.

Source—Synthetic.

Stability and Storage—Protect acepromazine products from light. Do not freeze injection solutions.

Pharmacological Actions—Acepromazine causes sedation, inhibits spontaneous motor activity, and reduces aggressive behavior and hostility. It decreases spontaneous motor activity and causes catalepsy at high doses. It prevents and reverses the peripheral actions of epinephrine. For instance, ventricular fibrillation induced by epinephrine during use of halogenated inhalant anesthetics can be prevented to some extent by acepromazine. Acepromazine increases the plasma level of prolactin. It has hypothermic, anticonvulsive, skeletal muscle relaxant, weak anticholinergic, antihistaminic, and antispasmodic actions. Acepromazine causes splenic sequestration of erythrocytes resulting in reduced PCV. This is prominent in the horse and may last up to 12 hours. It has little effect on respiration except at high doses when respiration may be depressed. It reduces arterial pressure.

Mechanism of Action—Acepromazine antagonizes the actions of dopamine and other agonists of the dopamine excitatory (DAe) receptors such as amphetamine and apomorphine.

Indications—Acepromazine is used in preanaesthetic medication; to control intractable animals; alleviate cutaneous itching, control emesis due to motion sickness; and induce sedation prior to administration of local anesthetic agent in cattle.

Dosages—

Horse. 0.044-0.088 mg/kg parenterally;

Dog. 0.55-2.2 mg/kg PO or 0.55-1.1 mg/kg parenterally.

Cat. 1.1-2.2 mg/kg PO or parenterally;

Pig. 0.1-0.2 mg/kg parenterally, or 0.5 mg/kg IM followed in 30 minutes with ketamine (15 mg/kg) and atropine (0.044 mg/kg).

Cattle, Sheep, and Goat. 0.05-0.1 mg/kg.

Rabbit. 1 mg/kg IM.

Route(s) of Administration—Administered per os, intravenously, intramuscularly and subcutaneously.

Absorption—Acepromazine is well absorbed from the oral route.

Onset of Action—15 minutes (IV)

Peak Action—30 to 60 minutes (IV)

Distribution—Vd = 6.6 L/kg (horse)

Plasma Protein Binding—>99% (horse).

Metabolism—Acepromazine is metabolized in the liver to inactive products.

Plasma Half-life—3 hours

Route(s) of Excretion—Urine

Toxicity and Adverse Effects—Extrapyramidal symptoms characterized by rigidity, tremor and catalepsy are prominent side effects at high doses. Acepromazine causes priapism (penile prolapse) in the stallion. ACP has been observed to produce excitement occasionally.

Management of Overdose/Toxicity—Doxapram effectively reverses ACP's CNS sedation.

Contraindications—Administration of epinephrine; Epidural anesthetic procedures; pregnancy; history of seizure; hypovolemia; circulatory shock; tetanus; strychnine poisoning.

Precautions—Use cautiously in equine colic; weak, debilitated, aged animals and in those with cardiac disease. Reduce the dose in animals with hepatic and cardiac impairment. Do not mix phenothiazines in the same syringe with glycopyrrolate or diazepam. Give IV injections slowly. In the dog, use acepromazine in conjunction with atropine (0.044 mg/kg) prior to induction of anesthesia to prevent bradycardia or sinoatrial arrest.

Drug Interactions—ACP and other phenothiazine derivatives block the α-adrenergic receptor activity of epinephrine leaving the β—component active. This may then cause vasodilatation, arteriolar hypotension and shock. Acepromazine is physically incompatible with diazepam and glycopyrrolate. Organophosphates enhance the toxicity of phenothiazines. The use of acepromazine with other CNS depressants produces additive effect. Similarly, quinidine may produce additive cardiac depression if used with phenothiazines. Antidiarrheal mixture and antacids may reduce the absorption of ACP. The blood levels of ACP and propranolol may increase when both drugs are administered concomitantly. Phenothiazines may enhance procaine activity and depress phenytoin metabolism.

Pharmaceutical Formulations—ACP is available as acepromazine maleate in 10 mg/ml solution for injection, and 5 mg, 10 mg and 25 mg tablets.

ACETAZOLAMIDE

Proprietary Names—Diamox*; AK-Zol*.
Chemical Class—A sulfonamide derivative.
Pharmacological Class—Diuretic; carbonic anhydrase inhibitor.
Source—Synthetic.

$$CH_3CONH \quad \overset{S}{\diagup} \quad SO_2NH_2$$

Acetazolamide

Solubility, Stability and Storage—The drug is slightly soluble in water and alcohol. Acetazolamide tablets and acetazolamide sodium sterile powder should be stored at room temperature. Store acetazolamide extended-release capsules at 20–25°C.

Pharmacological Actions—Acetazolamide is a weak diuretic which causes alkaline urine and reduction in total body bicarbonate stores. It reduces the rate of aqueous humor production and intra ocular pressure.

Mechanism of Action—Acetazolamide inhibits carbonic anhydrase, an enzyme that catalyzes the synthesis of carbonic acid from CO_2 and H_2O. Carbonic acid dissociates in renal cells to provide H^+ ion necessary for the reabsorption of bicarbonate from renal luminal fluid. Inhibition of the enzyme causes decreased secretion of both H^+ ions and reabsorption of bicarbonate. Decreasing bicarbonate reabsorption also reduces Na reabsorption because H^+ ion secretion and bicarbonate reabsorption are coupled to sodium reabsorption through sodium-hydrogen ion counter transport mechanism. Potassium ion secretion and excretion is enhanced because H^+ ions and K^+ ions compete with each other and with Na^+ ions.

Indications—Used in the treatment of chronic glaucoma.

Dosages—1-3 mg/kg/24 hours orally or 1 mg / kg /24 hours IM.

Route(s) of Administration—Administered orally and intramuscularly. The intramuscular route is associated with pain.

Absorption—Acetazolamide is readily absorbed from the GIT. Peak plasma concentration is attained within two hours.

Onset of Action—2 minutes (IV); 2 hours (extended release capsule).

Peak Action—Varies with the dosage form. Peak action is usually 15 minutes (IV), 1-4 hours (tablet) and 3-6 hours (extended release capsule).

Duration of Action—Varies with dosage form. It may be 4-5 hours (IV); 8-12 hours (tablet); 18-24 hours (extended release capsule).

Distribution—Acetazolamide is widely distributed. It crosses the blood-brain barrier and placenta; distributes into erythrocytes, kidneys and milk.

Plasma Protein Binding—95%.

Metabolism—Acetazolamide is not metabolized.

Plasma Half—Life—2.4-5.8 hours.

Route(s) of Excretion—Urine; acetazolamide is completely excreted within 24 hours in humans.

Dialysis Status—20-50 % dialyzable.

Toxicity and Adverse Effects—Acetazolamide causes metabolic acidosis. Drowsiness and paraesthesia appear at high doses. It may cause disorientation in patients with hepatic cirrhosis. Teratogenic effects have been demonstrated in animals. It may cause the formation of renal stones.

Contraindications—Renal hyper-chloremic acidosis; hepatic cirrhosis; depressed sodium or potassium levels; pregnancy (in animals); hypersensitivity to acetazolamide or sulfonamide derivatives.

Precautions—Coma may result in patients with impaired hepatic function. Avoid use of acetazolamide if clearance is less than 10 ml/minute. The drug loses efficiency within days due to accumulation of H^+ ions. Potassium supplements may be required.

Drug Interactions—Agents which cause metabolic alkalosis enhance the effects of acetazolamide. Simultaneous use of acetazolamide with phenytoin may cause drug-induced osteomalacia. Acetazolamide interferes with the action of methenamine as a urinary antiseptic. It alters the excretion of other drugs such as amphetamines, quinidine, lithium, salicylates, and phenobarbital due to alkalization of urine. The drug may increase the plasma concentration of cyclosporine.

Pharmaceutical Formulations—Acetazolamide is available as 125 mg or 250 mg tablets; 500 mg extended release capsules and as acetazolamide sodium in 500 mg vials for parenteral injection.

ACETYLSALICYLIC ACID

Synonyms—Aspirin, ASA.

Proprietary Names—Aspirin®, Bufferin˚, Anacin˚.

Chemical Class—Salicylate.

Pharmacological Class—Nonsteroidal anti-inflammatory drug (NSAID; Simple analgesic; Non-narcotic analgesic; Analgesic-antipyretic.

Source—Synthetic.

Acetylsalicilic acid

Pharmacological Actions—ASA reduces the intensity of pain, inflammation, and abnormally high body temperature.

Mechanism of Action—Aspirin nonselectively inhibits cyclooxygenase-1 and—2 (Cox-1 and Cox-2) and prevents the synthesis of prostaglandins and thromboxanes. It also acts on the heat regulating center in the hypothalamus to reduce fever.

Indications—Treatment of arthritis and related disorders such as immune mediated arthritis and osteoarthritis; treatment of bursitis and laminitis.

Dosage—10-40mg/kg daily or every 8-12 hours in dogs and cats.

Route(s) of Administration—Per os.

Absorption—ASA is rapidly absorbed from the stomach and small intestine. Peak serum concentration is attained in 1-2 hours.

Bioavailability—63±3%.

Distribution. Vd = 0.15 ± 0.03 L/kg. ASA distributes readily to most body fluids and tissues.

Plasma Protein Binding—49% (reduced in uremia).

Metabolism—Hydrolyzed to acetic acid and salicylic acid (an active by-product).

Plasma Half-Life—0.25-0.3 hours in man; 1 hour in herbivores; and 36 hours in cats. Plasma half-life for the active metabolite, salicylic acid is dose-dependent and ranges from 3 to 10 hours in humans.

Clearance—9.3±1.1 ml/min/kg.

Route(s) of Excretion—Excreted in urine with 1.4±1.2 as unchanged drug. Excretion is more rapid in equines.

Dialysis Status—Dialyzable.

Toxicity and Adverse Effects—Gastric or intestinal ulceration, hypersensitivity reactions and prolonged bleeding time are common.

Management of Overdose—Induce emesis or perform gastric lavage followed by oral activated charcoal, and symptomatic treatment.

Contraindications. Acute peptic ulcer; hypersensitivity to salicylates, their components or other NSAIDs.

Precautions—Use cautiously in patients with impaired renal function and in cats. ASA is not conjugated in cats. Administer with meals, water or antacids. Avoid use of ASA one week prior to surgery.

Pharmaceutical Formulations—Available in regular or enteric coated tablets ranging from 65-975 mg alone or in combination with other NSAIDs.

ACTIVATED CHARCOAL

Synonyms—Activated carbon; Active carbon; Active charcoal; Amorphous carbon; Medicinal charcoal; Adsorbent charcoal; Decolorizing carbon.

Proprietary Names—Ultra carbon®; Toxiban®.

Chemical Class—Porous carbon compound.

Pharmacological Class—Adsorbent; Antidote.

Source—Made by burning organic materials such as wood pulp followed by further treatment to enhance its absorptive capacity.

Solubility, Stability and Storage—Activated charcoal is insoluble in water or alcohol. It should be stored in tightly-closed glass or metal containers.

Pharmacological Actions—Activated charcoal is highly effective against both natural and synthetic toxins. It is effective in removing various mycotoxins, such as aflatoxin, fumonisins, ochratoxin A, trichothenes, and zearalenone. Natural toxins from plants are also removed or their actions are attenuated by activated charcoal. It can also remove synthetic pesticides from animals that might contaminate milk or meat. Treatment with activated carbon when using certain parasiticides can help reduce the residual levels in flesh and fatty tissue. Activated charcoal has an extraordinarily large surface area and pore volume that gives it a unique adsorptive capacity. Commercially available activated charcoal products differ in their adsorptive properties. To meet USP standards, one gram must adsorb 100 mg of strychnine sulfate in 50 ml of water. Adsorption capacity depends on five factors namely (a) physical and chemical characteristics of the adsorbent; (b) physical and chemical characteristics of the adsorbate; (c) concentration of the adsorbate in liquid solution; (d) characteristics of the liquid phase (e.g. pH, temperature); and (e) amount of time the adsorbate is in contact with the adsorbent (residence time).

Mechanism of Action—The specific mode of action is extremely complex, and has been the subject of much study and debate. However, it binds with certain poisons and drugs in the digestive tract and allows these poisons and drugs to safely pass through the GI track of the animal without being absorbed by the body. Adsorption can be either physical or chemical in nature, and frequently involves both. Physical adsorption involves the attraction by electrical charge differences between the adsorbent and the adsorbate. Chemical adsorption is the product of a reaction between the adsorbent and the adsorbate.

Indications—Treatment (GI decontamination) of most oral poisoning and drug over dosage; treatment of flatulence, diarrhea, and stomach ulcer pain. It is ineffective in poisoning caused by mineral acids, caustic alkali, boric acid, lithium, cyanides, malathion and petroleum products. Activated charcoal poorly adsorbs ethylene glycol, ethanol, methanol and iron salts.

Dosages—

Dog, cat	1-8 g/kg. Dissolve granules or powder in 50-200 ml of warm water; repeat every 3 hours for 72 hours in case of acute poisoning.
Ruminant	1-3 g/kg. Mix granule or powder with large volume (up to 4 litres) of warm water and administer via stomach tube. Leave in stomach for 20-30 minutes and then give a laxative to hasten removal of toxicants.
Horse	Minimum of 250 grams for foals and 750 grams for adult horses. Administer as in ruminants.

Activated charcoal is effective when given within 30 minutes to 1 hour after poisoning. Late administration may effectively remove drugs that undergo enterohepatic circulation. Repeated doses of activated charcoal may enhance the elimination of some drugs (e.g. theophylline, acetaminophen, digoxin, phenobarbital, and phenytoin) even after systemic absorption. Repeated administration is particularly beneficial if the ingested substance undergoes enterohepatic circulation and reabsorption.

Route(s) of Administration—Per os.

Absorption—Not absorbed.

Metabolism—Not metabolized.

Route of Excretion—Feces.

Toxicity and Adverse Effects—Activated carbon is generally considered non-toxic. However there could be a small risk (~ 4%) of aspiration pneumonia when administering activated charcoal to intubated patients. Very rapid GI administration can induce emesis. Charcoal can cause either constipation or diarrhea with black feces. Activated charcoal products containing sorbitol may cause loose stools and vomiting.

Contraindications—Poisoning caused by mineral acids, caustic alkali, boric acid, lithium, and petroleum products.

Precautions—Do not administer other therapeutic agents orally within 2-3 hours of the administration of activated charcoal except laxatives, drugs used for GI decontamination or antidotes for ingested toxins. If necessary, concomitant drug therapy can be given parenterally. Charcoal should not be administered with dairy products or mineral oil.

Drug Interactions—The adsorptive properties of activated charcoal are diminished by dairy products or mineral oils. Activated charcoal can decrease the absorption of and therapeutic response to other orally administered drugs.

Pharmaceutical Formulations—Activated charcoal for veterinary purposes is generally pharmaceutical (USP) grade. It is complexed with kaolin clay (bolus alba), propylene glycol, and various unspecified wetting and dispersing agents. Among the wetting agents and dispersants used are naphthalene sulfonates, alkyl aryl polymers, and triethanolamine. Alternative formulations may use other clays and mined minerals such as bentonite and gypsum; synthetically treated minerals such as dicalcium phosphate and silica gels; vegetable gums; synthetic vegetable derivatives such as sodium carboxymethylcellulose; solvents such as isopropanol as well as synthetic suspension polymers, such as, povidone. Activated charcoal is available in granules (containing 47.5% activated charcoal and 10% kaolin) and suspensions (containing 10.4% activated charcoal and 6.25% kaolin) for veterinary use. Human formulations include powder. The "universal antidote" (2 parts activated charcoal, 1 part magnesium oxide, and 1 part tannic acid) is inferior to activated charcoal alone.

ACYCLOVIR

Acyclovir

Synonyms—Aciclovir; ACV; Acycloquanosine.

Proprietary Names—Zovirax.

Chemical Class—Purine nucleoside analog.

Pharmacological Class—Antiviral drug.

Source—Synthetic.

Pharmacological Actions—Acyclovir has antiviral activity mainly against herpes viruses especially herpes simplex types 1 and 2. It enhances zidovudine inhibition of HIV-1. Varicella-zoster viruses are also susceptible. It is less active against cytomegalovirus, and Epstein-Barr virus.

Mechanism of Action—Acyclovir inhibits DNA synthesis and viral replication. Its phosphorylated product, acyclo-quanine triphosphate (acyclo-GTP) selectively inhibits viral DNA polymerase of susceptible viruses by competing with deoxyquanosine triphosphate. It also causes the termination of biosynthesis of viral DNA strand.

Indications—Treatment of herpes infection in psittacine birds; treatment of feline herpes virus 1 conjunctivitis and keratitis (trifluridine is the drug of choice in this condition).

Dosages—

Bird, 80 mg/kg orally or 40 mg/kg IM every 8 hours or 80 mg/kg orally once daily either as suspension or in drinking water for 7-14 days.

Cat, 200 mg orally four times daily.

Route(s) of Administration—Administered orally, intravenously (commonest in humans) and topically.

Absorption—Acyclovir is poorly (20%) absorbed from the GIT. Peak plasma concentration is attained within 1.5 hours following oral administration. Oral absorption is not significantly affected by the presence of food. Percutaneous absorption is poor but produces measurable plasma levels.

Bioavailability (Oral)—15-30 %.

Distribution—Vd = 0.69±0.19 liters/kg. Acyclovir is widely distributed. It reaches the brain, CSF, vagina, lung, liver, spleen, uterus and muscle.

Plasma Protein Binding. 9-33%.

Metabolism—Acyclovir is metabolized to an inactive 9-carboxymethoxy-methylquanine. Certain other metabolites are active.

Plasma Half-Life—2.5-3.6 hours (human adult); 4 hours (human neonates); 20 hours (in anuria).

Clearance (ml/min/kg). 3.37. Clearance is reduced in neonates.

Route(s) of Excretion—Urine (>70% appear as unchanged drug and 15% as active metabolite).

Dialysis Status—Partly (60%) dialyzable.

Toxicity and Adverse Effects—Topical acyclovir may cause local irritation. Intravenous acyclovir is well tolerated but it has been shown in humans to cause inflammation at injection site and encephalopathy in 1% of cases. Oral acyclovir causes occasional nausea, emesis and headache. Overdose may result in elevated serum creatinine and renal failure. Leukopenia and mild non-regenerative anemia has been observed in cats. The anemia is reversed following withdrawal of therapy.

Management of Toxicity/Overdose—Maintain sufficient urine flow and institute hemodialysis.

Contraindications—Hypersensitivity to acyclovir; dehydration.

Precautions—Use acyclovir cautiously in patients with renal dysfunction and in neurological, hepatic or electrolyte abnormalities. Also use with caution in patients concurrently receiving other nephrotoxic drugs.

Drug Interactions—Acyclovir decreases renal clearance of drugs that are normally eliminated by active tubular secretion (e.g. methotrexate, penicillin). Its CNS side effect is increased with zidovudine and probenecid.

Pharmaceutical Formulations—Available as acyclovir sodium in 200 mg capsules; 400 mg and 800 mg tablets; 5% ointment in polyethylene glycol base; 40 mg/ml oral suspension; and 500 mg (10 ml) or 1000 mg (20 ml) solution for injection.

ADRENALINE

Synonyms—Epinephrine; Levo-epinephrine, Racemic epinephrine; Epirenamine; Levorenin; Suprarenin.

Proprietary Names. Adrenalin®; EpiPen®.

Chemical Class—Catecholamine.

Pharmacological Class—Direct-acting sympathomimetic drug.

Source—Synthetic. Formerly obtained from the adrenal medullary extracts of animals.

Solubility, Stability and Storage—Adrenaline is sparingly soluble in water but practically insoluble in ethanol, chloroform, ether and light petroleum. Adrenaline readily forms water soluble salts (such as the hydrochloride and bitartrate) with acids. Solutions of adrenaline are unstable in alkaline medium or in the presence of oxidizing agents. It oxidizes readily to inactive product on exposure to light or heat. Oxidized solution turns pink and eventually becomes brown. Hence, solutions should be stored in tight containers and protected from light.

Adrenaline

Pharmacological Actions—The actions of adrenaline are complex due to its action on both α—and β—adrenergic receptors. The main effects of therapeutic parenteral doses of adrenaline are relaxation of smooth muscle of the bronchial tree, cardiac stimulation, and dilation of skeletal muscle vasculature. Adrenaline causes increase in blood pressure due to marked positive inotropic and chronotropic effects as well as vasoconstriction. Many vascular beds respond differently depending on the dose, route and rate of administration. The action of adrenaline on vascular bed results in redistribution of blood flow. In small doses, the effect of adrenaline on β-receptors may predominate, resulting in dilatation in certain peripheral blood vessels, especially in skeletal muscles. Peripheral blood flow may increase in those areas. In some areas, such as the skin, blood flow is markedly decreased due to vasoconstriction arising from the drug action on α-adrenergic receptors. Adrenaline causes relaxation of bronchial smooth muscle along with relaxation of the intestinal tract and stimulation of sphincters. The spleen and uterus of most animals contract to the action of adrenaline. Adrenaline dilates the pupils without loss of accommodation. Exocrine glands, apart from sweat glands are inhibited by adrenaline. The breakdown of glycogen (glycogenolysis) in tissues is enhanced by adrenaline. This causes increase in blood glucose and lactate.

Mechanism of Action—Adrenaline activates both α—and β-adrenergic receptors.

Indications—Control of bronchospasm, hypotension associated with shock, and various allergic conditions including anaphylaxis. Adrenaline is also used to control superficial bleeding on the skin, mucosa or eye during ophthalmology, and in cardiac resuscitation. The drug is also added to local anaesthetics to delay absorption and prolong their effect.

Dosages—200 to 500 mcg, subcutaneously or intramuscularly, as a single dose which may be repeated.

Route(s) of Administration—Adrenaline may be administered parenterally and topically. The intravenous route is strongly recommended if anaphylaxis is profound and life-threatening and vascular access is available.

Absorption—Adrenaline is not appreciably absorbed from the GIT. It is rapidly destroyed in the gastro-intestinal tract after oral administration. Absorption is slow after subcutaneous injection due to vasoconstriction. Absorption is faster following intramuscular injection.

Bioavailability (Oral)—Pharmacologically active concentrations are unachievable following oral administration.

Onset of Action—5-10 minutes following subcutaneous administration.

Distribution—Adrenaline is excluded from the CNS but its metabolites are detectable in the cerebrospinal fluid. It crosses the placenta and enters the mammary gland. It is rapidly taken up by the heart, spleen, several glandular tissues and adrenergic nerves.

Plasma Protein Binding—50%.

Metabolism—Adrenaline is rapidly conjugated and oxidized in the GI mucosa and liver following oral administration. Injected adrenaline is metabolized by monoamine oxidase (MAO) and catechol-o-methyl transferase (COMT) to inactive products.

Route(s) of Excretion—70 to 95% of an intravenous dose is excreted in the urine of which 80% exist as O-methyl metabolites, 2% as catechol metabolites, and only 1% as unchanged drug.

Toxicity and Adverse Effects—Adrenaline may cause disturbances of cardiac rhythm and rate which may result in palpitation and tachycardia. It can cause potentially fatal ventricular arrhythmias including fibrillation, especially in patients with organic heart disease or those receiving other drugs which sensitize the heart to arrhythmias. Adrenaline may cause nausea, vomiting, sweating, pallor, respiratory difficulty, or respiratory weakness and apnea. Overdose of adrenaline causes transient bradycardia followed by tachycardia, hypertension, circulatory collapse and respiratory arrest. Prolonged use can result in severe metabolic acidosis because of elevated blood concentrations of lactic acid.

Management of Toxicity/Overdose—This requires symptomatic and supportive treatment. The pressor effects of adrenaline may be counteracted by rapidly acting α-adrenergic blocking drugs such as phentolamine. Arrhythmias, if they occur, may be counteracted by a β-adrenergic blocking drug such as propranolol.

Contraindications—Cardiogenic shock (adrenaline increases myocardial oxygen demand); hemorrhagic or traumatic shock; coronary insufficiency; chloroform, trichloroethylene or cyclopropane induced general anesthesia; hypersensitivity to adrenaline. Parenteral use of adrenaline is contraindicated during labor.

Precautions—Expired, discolored or precipitated preparations should not be used. Use adrenaline cautiously, if at all, in hypertensive or hyperthyroid patients. Adrenaline should not be used in combination with halogenated hydrocarbon anesthetics such as halothane. If the combination is necessary, prophylactic administration of lidocaine or prophylactic IV administration of propranolol may be considered so as to protect against ventricular irritability. Adrenaline should also be used with caution in patients with diabetes mellitus, tachycardia, and myocardial infarction or in patients with history of sensitivity to sympathomimetic amines. Use adrenaline during pregnancy only if the potential benefits justify the possible risks to the fetus as it can cause anoxia in the fetus. Adrenaline should not be used to counteract circulatory collapse or hypotension caused by phenothiazines because adrenaline's pressor effects may be reversed leading to further lowering of blood pressure. Diabetic patients receiving adrenaline may require increased dose of insulin or oral hypoglycemic agents since adrenaline may cause hyperglycemia,

Drug Interactions—Concomitant administration with other sympathomimetic agents may cause additive effects and increased toxicity. β-adrenergic blocking drugs such as propranolol can antagonize the cardiac and bronchodilating effects of adrenaline while its vasoconstriction and hypertensive actions are antagonized by α-adrenergic blocking agents such as phentolamine. Ergot alkaloids can reverse the pressor response to adrenaline because of their α-adrenergic blocking properties. Cyclopropane or halogenated hydrocarbon general anesthetics sensitize the myocardium to adrenaline. Tricyclic antidepressants (e.g. imipramine), some antihistamines (especially diphenhydramine, tripelennamine, and dexchlorpheniramine), and thyroid hormones may potentiate the effects of adrenaline, especially on heart rhythm and rate. This may be due to inhibition of tissue uptake of adrenaline or by increased adrenoreceptor sensitivity to adrenaline.

Pharmaceutical Formulations—Available as Adrenaline hydrochloride and Adrenaline bitartrate in 0.01 mg/ml, 0.1 mg/ml and 1 mg/ml solution for injection. Formulations containing 1 mg/ml for topical application and 0.1%, 0.25% and 0.5% solution for ophthalmic application are available. Solution for oral inhalation and aerosol are available for human use.

ALBENDAZOLE

Albendazole

Proprietary Names—Albendazole®; Albidol®; Anizol®; Benezal®; Farbenda®; Sambezole®; Vermiprazol®; Worm Alba®; Zentel®.

Chemical Class—Benzimidazole.

Pharmacological Class—Anthelmintic.

Source—Synthetic.

Pharmacological Actions—Albendazole is lethal to the adult forms and larvae of *Bunostonum, Chabertia, Cooperia, Haemonchus, Nematodirus, Oesophagostomum, Ostertagia, Strongyloides* and *Trichostrongylus* species of sheep and cattle; *Strongyles* and *Oxyuris* in horses; and liver flukes in sheep and cattle.

Mechanism of Action—Albendazole inhibits microtubule polymerization in susceptible helminthes by binding to β-tubulin. Binding to parasite tubulin takes place at a lower concentration than does the binding to mammalian tubulin.

Indications—Treatment of threadworm, whipworm, pinworm, nodular worm, tapeworm and fluke infestations in horses, cattle, sheep and goats; treatment of capillariasis in dogs and cats.

Dosages—

　Horse, cattle, sheep and goat. 7.5 mg/kg; 15 mg/kg for liver fluke infection in horses and cattle.

　Pig. 5-10 mg/kg.

Dog and cat. 50 mg/kg for 21 days.

Route(s) of Administration—Per os.

Absorption Profile—Albendazole is poorly absorbed from the GIT. Peak plasma concentration which is about 1% of administered dose is achieved in 15-24 hours.

Bioavailability (Oral)—This appears to increase when the drug is administered with a fatty meal.

Metabolism—Albendazole is cleaved into an active albendazole sulfoxide and albendazole sulfone metabolites. It undergoes first pass metabolism.

Withdrawal Period—This varies with dosage form. With suspension, observe 10 days in sheep and 14 days in cattle before slaughter. With paste, withdrawal period is 27 days before slaughter in cattle.

Toxicity And Adverse Effects. Albendazole is well tolerated at therapeutic doses. Dogs may become anorectic while cats may become depressed, lethargic and anorectic following therapeutic doses. It is teratogenic in rats, rabbits and sheep during early pregnancy.

Contraindications—Lactating dairy cow; First 45 days of pregnancy; hypersensitivity to albendazole or any component.

Drug Interactions—Serum levels of albendazole are increased by dexamethasone and praziquantel.

Pharmaceutical Formulations. Albendazole is available in 250 mg boluses and 2.5% and 10% oral suspension.

ALBUTEROL

Proprietary Names—Ventolin®.

Synonyms—Salbutamol.

Chemical Class—Amine (it is a sympathomimetic amine).

Pharmacological Class—Sympathomimetic drug; Beta$_2$-selective bronchodilator.

Source—Synthetic.

Stability and Storage. Albuterol is sparingly soluble in water but soluble in alcohol. Albuterol sulfate is soluble in water but slightly soluble in ethanol. Albuterol and albuterol sulfate formulations should be stored in well-closed, light-resistant containers and at 2-30°C.

Albuterol sulphate

Pharmacological Actions—Albuterol dilates the bronchioles and improve airway conductance in obstructive pulmonary disorders such as bronchitis, emphysema, and asthma. It also relaxes uterine and vascular smooth muscles and causes temporary decrease in plasma potassium levels.

Mechanism of Action—Albuterol activates beta$_2$-adrenergic receptors by enhancing the production of cAMP (the intracellular messenger for beta-receptor activation) through activation of adenylate cyclase. Its action on potassium may be due to stimulation of Na^+-K^+-ATPase.

Indications—Relief of bronchospasm or cough in dogs and cats. It has potentials for use in horses for bronchodilation.

Dosages. Dogs. 50 mcg/kg orally every 8 hours. Horses. 8 mcg/kg orally every 12 hours.

Route(s) of Administration. Per os.

Absorption. Albuterol is rapidly and very well absorbed from the GIT. A peak plasma concentration is attained within 2-3 hours.

Onset of Action—30 minutes.

Peak Effect—2-3 hours—

Duration of Action—8 hours.

Distribution—**Albuterol** crosses the placenta. It does not enter the CNS significantly; it attains 5% of plasma concentration in the brain.

Metabolism—Albuterol is extensively metabolized in the liver into inactive albuterol 4'-O-sulfate.

Plasma Half—Life—2.7-5 hours (human).

Route(s) of Excretion—Urine (30% as unchanged drug).

Dialysis Status—Nondialyzable.

Toxicity and Adverse Effects—**Brief** tachycardia due to transient beta$_2$ vasodilatation and hypotension following systemic administration are common. Other adverse reactions include tremor, CNS excitement, nausea and vomiting. Albuterol is teratogenic in rodents at high doses and may delay pre-term labor since it may relax uterine smooth muscle through beta$_2$ adrenergic receptor activation. Overdose may cause cardiac stimulation characterized by increased heart rate.

Management of Overdose—Give general antidotal therapy.

Contraindications. Hypersensitivity to albuterol.

Precautions. Use albuterol cautiously with inhalation anesthetics, during pregnancy and in patients with diabetes, hyperthyroidism, and cardiovascular disorders.

Drug Interactions—Bronchodilation may be enhanced by concomitant administration of methylxanthine (e.g. aminophylline) in cases that have experienced receptor down regulation as a result of prolonged administration of albuterol. Albuterol antagonizes dinoprost (prostaglandin F$_2\alpha$) and oxytocin. Concomitant use with other sympathomimetic agents may increase the likelihood of cardiovascular adverse effects. Beta-adrenergic blockers may inhibit the action of albuterol. MAO inhibitors and tricyclic antidepressants may enhance its pressor effects. Administration of albuterol in animals under anesthesia induced by halogenated hydrocarbon anesthetic agents may enhance its potential to cause cardiac arrhythmias. Concurrent use with digitalis may induce cardiac arrhythmia.

Pharmaceutical Formulations—**Available** as albuterol sulfate in 2 mg and 4 mg tablets. Other formulations for human use are available.

ALLOPURINOL

Allopurinol

Proprietary Names. Zyloprim®, Milurit®, Mephanol®, Zyloric®, Uroquad®, Caplenal®, Apurin®, Allopurinol®.

Chemical Class—Hypozanthine analog.

Pharmacological Class—Xanthine oxidase inhibitor, Uric acid synthesis inhibitor.

Source—Synthetic.

Solubility, Stability and Storage—Slightly soluble in water and ethanol. Store allopurinol tablets at room temperature.

Pharmacological Actions—Allopurinol and its primary metabolite, alloxanthine (oxipurinol), inhibit the synthesis of uric acid and reduce its plasma concentration and urinary excretion. Uric acid is produced in the normal metabolism of purines. Normally, purines are converted to the water soluble and easily excreted allantoin through hypoxanthine, xanthine, and uric acid. The metabolic pathway is catalyzed by xanthine oxidase. Birds are naturally unable to produce allantoin. When uric acid is not converted to allantoin, it builds up and begins to form crystals which can show up as kidney stones (especially in human patients), bladder stones (canines especially in Dalmatians species and in dogs with liver shunts), joint deposits (birds or humans with gout) or other unpleasant places. The action of allopurinol causes accumulation of hypoxanthine and xanthine as they are not converted. Allopurinol and its active metabolite also prevent inflammatory reactions in re-perfused ischaemic tissues such as heart, kidney, brain, muscle and bowel.

Mechanism of Action—Allopurinol blocks the terminal steps in uric acid biosynthesis by inhibiting xanthine oxidase, thus delaying the inactivation of mercaptopurine.

Indications—Prophylaxis of recurrent urolithiasis resulting from excess uric acid and calcium oxalate in small animals; treatment
of gout in humans and pet birds.

Dosage—

Dog.	7-10 mg/kg orally three times daily.
Cat.	9 mg/kg orally per day.
Bird.	Dissolve 100 mg in 10 ml of water and then give one drop of the solution 4 times per day.

Route of Administration—Per os.

Absorption—Allopurinol is rapidly absorbed from the GIT in humans. Peak plasma concentration is attained within 30-60 minutes. Food does not influence the absorption profile.

Bioavailability (oral)—About 90%.

Distribution—Vd = 1.6 L/kg. It distributes into breast milk.

15

Plasma Protein Binding—Less than 5% for allopurinol and about 17% for oxipurinol.

Metabolism—Metabolized mainly to alloxanthine (oxipurinol), which is also a xanthine oxidase inhibitor but less potent than allopurinol.

Plasma Half-Life—0.5 to 2 hours for allopurinol and 12 to 40 hours for alloxanthine. Half-life is prolonged in patients with end stage renal disease.

Plasma Clearance (mL/min/kg)—About 11.

Route(s) of Excretion—Allopurinol is excreted in urine (with < 10% as unchanged drug and 40-60 % as the active metabolite, alloxanthine) and feces (it undergoes enterohepatic circulation).

Dialysis Status—Both allopurinol and alloxanthine are dialyzable.

Toxicity and Adverse Effects—Gastrointestinal distress, bone marrow depression and cutaneous hypersensitivity reactions appearing as rash, exfoliative or urticarial lesions may be observed in human cases. Prolonged use at high doses in dogs may cause xanthine urolithiasis.

Management of Overdose. Potential xanthine stone formation may be prevented by alkalization of urine and inducement of diuresis.

Contraindications. Acute gout, hypersensitivity to allopurinol.

Precautions—Diets low in purine are essential for dogs. The dose of allopurinol should be reduced with prolonged use and in patients with renal dysfunction. Treatment should be discontinued if signs of allergic rash appear. Liver function and blood picture should be monitored before and during therapy. Administer allopurinol with high fluid intake.

Drug Interactions—Thiazide diuretics may enhance the toxicity of allopurinol. The drug inhibits the metabolism of azathioprine and mercaptopurine; prolongs the half-life of oral anticoagulants; increases the concentration of 1-methylxanthine (an active metabolite of theophylline) when administered concurrently. Incidence of skin rash may increase if used with ampicillin or amoxicillin. Concurrent use of allopurinol and cyclophosphamide will have a greater tendency towards bone marrow suppression. Alcohol decreases its effects.

Pharmaceutical Formulations—Available in 100—and 300—mg tablets. No specific veterinary formulations are available.

AMIKACIN

Proprietary Names—Amikin* (human preparation); Amiglyde* (Veterinary preparation).

Chemical Class—An aminoglycosidic aminocyclitol.

Pharmacological Class—Aminoglycoside antibiotic; Antibacterial agent.

Source. Semisynthetic; amikacin is derived from kanamycin.

Solubility, Stability and Storage—Amikacin is sparingly soluble in water. It is heat resistant and stable in intravenous fluids. Amikacin products should be stored at room temperature. Its activity is enhanced in alkaline environment.

Pharmacological Action—Amikacin is rapidly bactericidal to most aerobic Gram-negative bacilli including most strains of *Serratia, Proteus,* and *Pseudomonas aeruginosa. Klebsiella Enterobacter, Mycobacterium tuberculosis* and *E. coli* are also susceptible. It is resistant to the aminoglycoside-inactivating enzymes.

Mechanism of Action—Amikacin binds to the 30s and 50s ribosomal subunit to interfere with the initiation of protein synthesis. This leads to accumulation of abnormal initiation complexes. It may also induce misreading of the RNA template resulting in incorrect amino acid incorporation into the growing polypeptide chains.

Indications—Treatment of aerobic Gram-negative infections which are resistant to gentamicin and tobramycin; also useful in the treatment of gram negative infection of the eye especially those caused by *Pseudomonas aeruginosa*.

Dosage—10 mg/kg every 8 hours in dogs, cats, and cattle; 7 mg/kg every 8 hours in horses.

Route(s) of Administration—Amikacin is administered parenterally (intramuscular, intravenous, and subcutaneous). The intrauterine route has been used in mares.

Absorption—Amikacin is poorly absorbed from the GIT or uterine site but rapidly absorbed from the intramuscular site. Peak plasma concentration is attained within 30-60 minutes following IM injection. It is appreciably absorbed from ocular site in cases of conjunctivitis.

Bioavailability—> 90% from IM or SC injections.

Distribution—Vd = 0.27±0.06 L/kg (humans; lower in obesity but higher in neonates]; 0.15-0.3 L/kg (cats and dogs); 0.26-0.58 L/kg (horses). Amikacin distributes into the ECF, crosses the placenta, and the blood-brain-barrier when the meninges are inflamed. It is sequestered in the inner ear and kidneys.

Plasma Protein Binding—4 ± 8% at serum concentration of 15 mcg/ml.

Metabolism—Amikacin is not metabolized.

Plasma Half-Life—2.3±0.4 hours (humans; higher in uremia but lower in cases of burn and cystic fibrosis); 1.14-2.3 hours (horses]; 2.2-2.7 hours (calves); 0.5-1.5 hours (dogs and cats).

Clearance—0.6 cl (cr.) ± 0.14 ml/ min/ kg. (Lower in obesity but higher in cystic fibrosis)

Route(s) of Excretion—Excreted in urine with 98% as unchanged drug.

Dialysis Status—Dialyzable.

Toxicity and Adverse Effects—Nephrotoxicity and ototoxicity manifesting most commonly as auditory defect are serious adverse effects caused by amikacin at therapeutic doses. At higher doses, neurotoxicity may appear as curare-like effect producing neuromuscular blockade and respiratory paralysis.

Management of Overdose/Toxicity—Discontinue treatment and initiate general antidotal therapy in case of overdose.

Contraindications—Hypersensitivity to amikacin or other aminoglycoside antibiotics, or their components.

Precautions—The doses or dosage interval should be modified in patients with renal impairment. Amikacin should be used with caution in pregnancy, working dogs, very young and very old animals and in patients with myasthenia gravis.

Drug Interactions—Indomethacin, amphotericin, loop diuretics, vancomycin, enflurane and methoxyflurane may increase the toxicity potential of amikacin. Amikacin may increase the toxicity of polypeptide antibiotics and neuromuscular blocking agents.

Pharmaceutical Formulations—Available as amikacin sulfate in 50 mg/ml solutions for injection. A 1% ophthalmic solution can be prepared from the injection solution by adding 3 ml of it to 12 ml of isotonic normal saline. Intrauterine solution containing 250 mg amikacin base per ml is available in some markets for use in horses. One gram amikacin base is equivalent to 1.3 gram of amikacin sulfate.

AMINOPHYLLINE

Proprietary Names—Amoline˙; Somophyllin˙; Aminophyllin˙; Phyllocontin˙; Truphylline˙.

Chemical Class—Alkaloid; Theophylline—ethylenediamine complex.

Pharmacological Class—Bronchodilator; Xanthine (theophylline) derivative.

Source—Synthetic; aminophylline contains theophylline and ethylenediamine in 2:1 ratio.

Aminophylline

Solubility, Stability and Storage—One gram of theophylline dissolves in 25 mL of water. It is insoluble in alcohol. Upon exposure to air, aminophylline gradually loses ethylenediamine and absorbs carbon dioxide with the liberation of free theophylline. Aminophylline products are better stored at room temperature away from excess heat, light and moisture.

Pharmacological Actions—Aminophylline causes bronchodilation. It is also a respiratory stimulant. It has mild diuretic properties, and positive chronotropic and positive inotropic effects (in large doses). It stimulates the secretion of both gastric acid and digestive enzymes.

Mechanism of Action—Aminophylline inhibits the intracellular enzyme, phosphodiesterase, which is responsible for the metabolism of cyclic AMP, the intracellular messenger for beta-adrenergic receptor activation. Inhibition of the enzymes leads to increased level of cAMP which mediates the resulting cellular reaction that culminates in beta adrenergic receptor activation.

Indications—To achieve bronchodilation associated with pulmonary edema, bronchial asthma and chronic obstructive pulmonary disease when sympathomimetics have been ineffective; also used in the treatment of heart failure.

Dosages—

Bird	10 mg/kg IV every 3 hours; administer orally after initial response.
Cat	10 mg/kg IM, IV every 8-12 hours: for IV use, dilute in 10-20 ml normal saline or 5% dextrose in water and inject slowly.
Dog	10 mg/kg IM, IV every 8-12 hours: for IV use, dilute in 10-20 ml normal saline or 5% dextrose in water and inject slowly.
NHP	25-100 mg/animal given orally twice a day.
Reptile	2-4 mg/kg IM as needed.

Route(s) of Administration—Per os, intramuscular, intravenous.

Absorption—Aminophylline is readily absorbed from oral route. The drug should be given 1 hour before or 2 hours after a meal.

Bioavailability (oral)—About 100% in dogs, cats and horses.

Onset of Action—Less than 15 minutes (IV).

Duration of Action—4 ½ hours.

Distribution—Vd = 0.82 L/kg (dog); 0.46 L/kg (cat); 0.85-1.02 L/kg (horse). Aminophylline is widely distributed throughout the ECF and body tissues. It crosses the placenta; attains 70% of serum level in milk.

Plasma Protein Binding—60% (human); 7-14% (dog).

Metabolism—Aminophylline is degraded mainly in the liver to 3-methylxanthine which is weakly active.

Plasma Half-life—7-9 hours (human); 5.7 hours (dog); 7.8 hours (cat); 11 hours (pig); 11.9-17 hours (horse).

Toxicity and Adverse Effects—Vomiting, diarrhea, central nervous system excitement, insomnia and increased hunger, thirst and urination are common adverse effects of aminophylline. These effects usually subside with dosage adjustments and/or continued therapy. Symptoms of overdose, which may be fatal, include tachycardia, arrhythmias, seizures and fever.

Management of Overdose/Toxicity—Initiate general antidotal therapy procedures.

Contraindications—Pregnancy; nursing animals; hypersensitivity to aminophylline or xanthines.

Precautions—Use aminophylline with caution in animals with seizure disorder, hypothyroidism, congestive heart failure, liver or kidney disease.

Drug Interactions—Beta blockers such as propranolol may antagonize aminophylline effects. Barbiturates and phenytoin may decrease theophylline levels. Cimetidine, erythromycin or quinolone antibiotics may increase aminophylline effects.

Pharmaceutical Formulations—Available as scored tablets and solution for injection. Each tablet contains 100mg Aminophylline. Injectable solution contains 25 mg/ml.

AMITRAZ

Proprietary Names—Mitaban®; Preventic®; Taktic®; Amitix®; Milbitrax®; Triatrix® and various generic brands.

Chemical Class—Formamidine.

Pharmacological Class—Acaricide; Insecticide; Pesticide.

Source—Synthetic.

Solubility, Stability and Storage—Amitraz is stable to heating; soluble in most organic solvents, and sparingly soluble in water. Store amitraz at room temperature.

Pharmacological Actions—Amitraz is rapidly lethal to mites and ticks. It has antipyretic and anti-inflammatory activity in vivo, and also has been shown to inhibit prostaglandin E_2 synthesis.

Mechanism of Action—The mechanism of action for amitraz is unknown. The drug may act on the central nervous system. *In vitro* housefly tests indicated that amitraz does not have significant cholinesterase inhibitory activity. Amitraz has been shown to have α_2-adrenergic agonist actions. The stimulation of α_2-receptors is in part responsible for neurotoxic and proconvulsant effects. Amitraz is also shown to activate octopamine receptors.

Amitraz

Indications—Treatment of generalized demodicosis (*Demodex canis*) in dogs; control of ticks and mites on dogs, cattle and sheep.

Dosages—10.6 ml per 10 litres of warm water (~250 ppm active drug). The entire dog should be thoroughly and completely wetted with the mixture, and then allowed to air dry. Prior to the initial treatment, all dogs should be bathed with a mild soap and water and towel dried. Three to six topical treatments (14 days apart) are recommended for generalized demodicosis.

Route(s) of Administration—Topical.

Metabolism—Amitraz is hydrolyzed ultimately to 4-amino-3-methylbenzoic acid.

Toxicity and Adverse Effects—The most frequently observed adverse reaction is transient sedation, which occurs in approximately 8% of treated patients within 2 to 6 hours post treatment. Transient pruritus, which may be an indirect effect due to inflammatory reaction associated with dead mites, occur in less than 3% of the generalized demodicosis patients within 24-48 hours post treatment. Other adverse effects include low incidence (less than 1%) of convulsions, ataxia, hyperexcitability, hypothermia, appetite stimulation, bloat, polyuria, vomiting, diarrhea, anorexia, edema, erythema and other varying degrees of skin irritation.

Management of Overdose/Toxicity—Give activated charcoal in order to reduce the amount of amitraz absorbed. Yohimbine reverses some of the sedative effects.

Contraindications—Hypersensitivity to amitraz; cats; dogs less than 4 months.

Precautions—Amitraz may alter the animal's ability to maintain homeostasis, hence treated animals should not be subjected to stress for a period of at least 24 hours post treatment. Use amitraz with caution in diabetic animals due to an effect on blood sugar. Diabetic humans should avoid contact with amitraz. Appropriate care should be taken to minimize exposure by the oral route both during and immediately after amitraz application.

Pharmaceutical Formulations—Available in liquid concentrate containing amitraz [19.9% (w/w] xylol, propylene oxide, a blend of alkyl benzene sulfonates and exthoxylated polyethers.

AMITRIPTYLINE

Aminophylline

Proprietary Name—Elavil*.

Chemical Class—Tricyclic dibenzocycloheptene derivative.

Pharmacological Class—Tricyclic antidepressant.

Source—Synthetic.

Solubility, Stability and Storage—Amitriptyline is readily soluble in water and alcohol. Its formulations may be stored at room temperature and protect from light.

Pharmacological Actions—Amitriptyline increases the levels of amine transmitters particularly serotonin and norepinephrine. Its action on serotonin level is responsible for its anti-anxiety and psychoactive properties. Amitriptyline has strong antihistaminic and anticholinergic actions.

Mechanism of Action—Amitriptyline blocks amine pump leading to increased levels of amine neurotransmitters particularly serotonin and norepinephrine. It has affinity for muscarinic and histamine H_1 receptors.

Indications—Amitriptyline is useful in pet animals for control of separation anxiety, inappropriate urination in cats, and for obsessive grooming behaviors in both dogs and cats.

Dosages—

Dog.   1-2 mg/kg every 12 hours or 2-4 mg/kg once a day.

Cat.   5-10 mg/kg once or twice a day.

Route(s) of Administration—Per os.

Absorption—Amitriptyline is rapidly absorbed from the GIT. Peak plasma concentration is attained within 2-12 hours.

Bioavailability (oral)—48 ± 11

Onset of Action—Delayed; 7-21 days (humans).

Distribution—Vd = 15 ± 3 litres/kg (humans). Amitriptyline crosses the blood-brain—barrier. It is secreted in milk at levels higher or equal to that in plasma.

Plasma Protein Binding—Amitriptyline is highly protein bound (94.8 ± 0.08).

Metabolism—Metabolized in the liver to both active (nortriptyline) and inactive products.

Plasma Half-life—6-8 hours (dog); 9-25 hours (human).

Clearance (ml/min/kg)—11.5 ± 3.4 (human).

Route(s) of Excretion—Amitriptyline is eliminated mainly in urine with 18% of the dose as unchanged drug). Small amount of the drug is eliminated in bile.

Toxicity and Adverse Effects—The most common side effect associated with amitriptyline is drowsiness/sedation. Its anticholinergic action results in dry mouth (characterized by frequently licking of the lips), urinary retention, constipation, and dried respiratory secretions. A potentially dangerous side effect that happens with a realistic frequency is the exacerbation of a cardiac rhythm disturbance. In humans, side effects involving virtually every organ system have been reported. This means that potentially any side effect (hematologic, gastrointestinal, endocrine etc.) could be attributed to the use of this medication. Overdose may cause arrhythmias, and cardiorespiratory collapse.

Management of Overdose/Toxicity—Treat symptomatically; control anticholinergic effects with physostigmine and seizure with diazepam, phenytoin or phenobarbitone.

Contraindications—Concurrent use with monoamine oxidase inhibitors; hypersensitivity to amitriptyline; diabetes mellitus; pregnancy; seizure disorders; lactation; cardiac rhythm disturbances.

Precautions—Use amitriptyline cautiously in patients with impaired liver function.

Drug Interactions—Amitriptyline and other tricyclic antidepressants cannot be safely used with monoamine oxidase inhibitors such as Deprenyl. Concurrent use of amitriptyline and methimazole may result in dangerously low white blood cell count. Cimetidine can interfere with the metabolism of amitriptyline and increase the risk of toxicity. Use of amitriptyline in conjunction with anticholinergic drugs, sympathomimetic and psychoactive drugs may cause additive effects.

Pharmaceutical Formulations—Available in 10 mg, 25 mg, 50 mg, 75 mg, 100 mg and 150 mg tablets. It is also available in 10 mg/ml injectable solution. No specific veterinary formulations are available.

AMMONIUM CHLORIDE

Synonyms—Muriate of ammonia; Sal ammoniac.

Proprietary Names—Ammonium chloride˙; MEq-AC ˙ (in combination with methionine); Uroeze˙ (in combination with methionine).

Pharmacological Class—Systemic and urinary acidifier; Diuretic.

Source—Synthetic.

Solubility, Stability and Storage—Ammonium chloride is soluble in water. Parenteral preparation of ammonium chloride is stored at room temperature; do not freeze.

Pharmacological Actions—Ammonium chloride decreases serum bicarbonate levels as well as blood and urine pH. It causes diuresis.

Mechanism of Action—Ammonium chloride dissociates into chloride and ammonium ions *in vivo*. The ammonium cation is converted by the liver to urea with the release of a hydrogen ion which combines with bicarbonate to form water and carbon dioxide. The chloride ion component combines with fixed bases in the ECF and decreases alkaline reserves in the body.

Indications—To prevent and dissolve certain types of uroliths (e.g., struvite); induce rapid renal excretion of certain toxins (e.g., strontium) or basic drugs (e.g. quinidine, amphetamine etc.); Ammonium chloride is used to enhance the efficacy of certain antimicrobials (e.g. chlortetracycline, methenamine mandelate, oxytetracycline, penicillin G or tetracycline) when treating urinary tract infections; It is also used to correct metabolic alkalosis.

Dosages—4-15 g orally in horses.

Route(s) of Administration—Ammonium chloride is administered orally or intravenously.

Absorption—The drug is rapidly and completely absorbed from the GIT. Absorption is complete within 3-6 hours in humans.

Metabolism—Metabolized in the liver.

Route(s) of Excretion—Urine.

Toxicity and Adverse Effects—Ammonium chloride may cause metabolic acidosis. Gastric irritation, nausea, and vomiting may be observed following oral administration. It causes pain at the site of IV injection unless administered slowly. Overdose of ammonium chloride causes acidosis, hyperventilation, hypokalemia, nausea, vomiting, excessive thirst, bradycardia or other arrhythmias, and progressive CNS depression.

Management of Overdose/Toxicity—Administer sodium bicarbonate or sodium lactate intravenously to control acidosis; give potassium as supplement to control hypokalemia.

Contraindications—Severe hepatic and/or renal impairment; uremia; urate calculi; respiratory acidosis.

Precautions—Ammonium chloride should not be administered subcutaneously, rectally or intraperitoneally. Use cautiously in patients with impaired pulmonary function or cardiac edema.

Drug Interactions—Ammonium chloride enhances the actions of urinary antiseptics (e.g. Methenamine mandelate). It reduces the effectiveness of aminoglycosides (e.g. gentamicin) and erythromycin when these drugs are used to treat urinary tract infection since they are more effective in alkaline media. Ammonium chloride may increase the renal excretion of quinidine due to urine acidification.

Pharmaceutical Formulations—Available in tablets (357 mg and 200 mg) and granules (535 mg and 200 mg) for veterinary use. A 26.75% parenteral preparation is available.

AMOXICILLIN (AMOXYCILLIN)

Amoxicillin

Proprietary Names—Amoxil*, Larotid*, Polymox*, Trimox*, Ultimox*, A—Cillin*, Wymox*, Imox*, Izoltil Piramox*, Suprapen* (amoxicillin and flucoxacillin), Augumentin* (amoxicillin and clavulanic acid.)

Chemical Class—6-Aminopenicillanic acid derivative.

Pharmacological Class—Aminopenicillin. Broad spectrum penicillin; Beta-Lactam antibiotic; Semi-synthetic penicillin.

Source—Semisynthetic.

Solubility, Stability and Storage—Once mixed, the oral suspension should be refrigerated. Unused portion should be discarded after 2 weeks.

Pharmacological Actions—Amoxicillin is bactericidal to Gram-negative and Gram-positive bacteria. It is less effective than ampicillin in human shigellosis. Amoxicillin is inactivated by penicillinase.

Mechanism of Action—Amoxicillin inhibits transpeptidase enzymes thus blocking the synthesis of peptidoglycan (a component of the bacteria cell wall) during active bacterial multiplication resulting in the formation of spheroblasts and ultimately, lysis of the bacteria cells.

Indications—Treatment of gastrointestinal, urinary and respiratory tract infections. It is also effective in mastitis, metritis, polynephritis and other infections caused by susceptible organisms. Amoxicillin is especially helpful in anaerobic infections.

Dosage—11 mg/kg orally two times daily.

Route(s) of Administration—Per os.

Absorption—Amoxicillin is very well absorbed from the GIT. Food does not retard its absorption. Peak plasma concentration is reached within 1-2 hours.

Bioavailability—93 ± 10% depending on the dose.

Distribution—Vd = 0.21 ± 0.03 L/kg. Amoxicillin is excluded from the CSF except when meninges are inflamed. It will cross the placenta but it is safe for use during pregnancy.

Plasma Protein Binding—18%

Plasma Half-Life—17 hours in animals; 1.7 ± 0.3 hours in humans. Half-life is increased in humans with uremia and in the aged.

Clearance (ml/min/kg). 2.6

Withdrawal Period—Two days.

Route(s) of Excretion—Urine with 86 ± 8% excreted as unchanged drug.

Dialysis Status—Amoxicillin can be removed from the blood by hemodialysis.

Toxicity and Adverse Effects—Seizures, skin rash (especially in humans with mononucleosis), diarrhea (usually less severe than that observed with ampicillin), and superinfection are common adverse reactions at therapeutic doses. Overdose may cause neuromuscular hypersensitivity, electrolyte imbalance, and renal failure.

Contraindications—Hypersensitivity to amoxicillin, the penicillins, their products or components.

Precautions—Reduce the dose in renal impairment. Use cautiously in animals hypersensitive to cephalosporin.

Drug Interactions—Disufiram and probenecid delay amoxicillin excretion.

Pharmaceutical Formulations—Available as amoxicillin trihydrate in 250 mg, 500 mg capsules; 125 mg and 250 mg chewable tablets; 125 mg/5 ml and 250 mg/5 ml oral suspension. Also available in combination with clavulanic acid (a beta-lactamase inhibitor) and flucoxacillin. Amoxicillin trihydrate is available in oral powder for addition to drinking water.

AMPHOTERICIN B

Proprietary Names—Fungizone*, Fungilin*, Mysteclin*

Chemical Class—Polyene macrolide.

Pharmacological Class—Antifungal; antimycotic; antimicrobial drug; Macrolide antibiotic.

Source—*Streptomyces nodosus*.

Solubility, Stability and Storage—Amphotericin B is practically insoluble in water, ethanol, chloroform and ether. It is soluble in propylene glycol and 1 in 20 of dimethylsulfoxide.

Pharmacological Actions—Amphotericin B has antifungal activities against organisms which produce systemic mycotic diseases such as *Cryptococcus neoformans*, *Blastomyces dermatitidis*, *Histoplasma capsulatum*, *Torulopis glabrata*, *Coccidiodes immitis*, *Paracoccidiodes braziliensis*, *Aspergillus* species and *Candida* species. It has limited activity against *Leishmania braziliensis* and *Naegleria fowleri*.

Amphotericin B

Mechanism of Action—Amphotericin B interferes with the membrane ergosterol of susceptible fungi to form pores or channels with a resultant increase in membrane permeability and the leakage of cell components which causes cell death.

Indications—Treatment of systemic mycoses such as histoplasmosis, blastomycosis, and coccidiomycosis.

Dosage—Dog, 1.8 mg/kg IV daily for seven days followed by a 7-day interval and a further seven days' administration.

Route(s) of Administration—Intravenous; intrathecal; topical.

Absorption—Absorption from the GIT is negligible.

Distribution—Vd = 0.76 ± 0.52 L/kg (volume of central compartment). Amphotericin B binds extensively to tissues with the highest concentrations in liver and spleen, and lesser amounts in kidney and lung. It penetrates minimally into the CSF, vitreous humor and normal amniotic fluid.

Plasma Protein Binding—Protein binding is higher than 90%. It binds largely to β-lipoprotein.

Metabolism—Metabolized in the liver. Biliary occlusion interferes with its metabolism in the dog.

Plasma Half-Life—Biphasic; 18 ± 7 hours initially and a terminal half-life of 15 ± 2 days due to extensive tissue binding.

Clearance—0.46 ± 0.2 (ml/min/kg).

Route of Excretion—Urine with 2-5% excreted as unchanged drug).

Dialysis Status—Poorly dialyzable.

Toxicity and Adverse Effects—Fever, chills and azotemia are the most common amongst the large number of adverse effects. Intravenous LD_{50} is 5 mg/kg in the rat. Renal toxicity is dose-dependent and occurs in 80% of cases. Other effects include hypochromic, normocytic anemia, vomiting, malaise, weight loss and phlebitis at intravenous site.

Management of Toxicity—Supportive measures.

Contraindications—Hypersensitivity to amphotericin B or any component.

Precautions—Avoid concomitant therapy with other nephrotoxic agents such as corticosteroids or cyclosporine. Monitor blood urea nitrogen and serum creatinine levels frequently during treatment. Supplemental potassium may be required during prolonged therapy.

Drug Interactions—Cyclosporine and aminoglycosides may increase the risk of amphotericin B causing nephrotoxicity. Corticosteroids may increase the risk of hypokalemia. Amphotericin B may precipitate in solutions of some electrolytes, in acid solutions and solutions with preservatives.

Pharmaceutical Formulations—Available in complex with sodium deoxycholate and sodium phosphate buffer in 50 mg sterile lyophilized powder for reconstitution in 5% dextrose in water. Also, available in 3% cream, 3% lotion and 3% ointment.

AMPICILLIN

Ampicillin sodium

Synonyms—Aminobenzylpenicillin.

Proprietary Names—Ampilag˙, Binota'l, Copharcillin˙, Extrapen˙, Lacilin˙, Penbrintin˙, Pentrexy'l Rivocillin˙, Semicillin˙, Standacillin˙, Amcill˙, Amplin˙; Omnipen˙, Penam®; Polycillin˙. Principen˙. Ampliclox˙ (ampicillin and cloxacilin) Ampen˙, Pentracrine˙, Unasyn˙ (ampicillin sodium and sulbatam sodium).

Chemical Classification—A 6-aminopenicillanic acid derivative.

Pharmacological Class—Aminopenicillin; Broad spectrum penicillin, Beta-lactam antibiotic; Semi synthetic penicillin.

Source. Semi synthetic.

Solubility, Stability and Storage—Anhydrous ampicillin and ampicillin trihydrate are soluble 1 in 170 of water but practically insoluble in organic solvents. Ampicillin sodium is soluble 1 in 2 of water and 1 in 50 of acetone; slightly soluble in chloroform but practically insoluble in ether. It is recommended that ampicillin capsules and powder for oral suspension be stored in tight containers at 15-30°C. Following reconstitution, oral suspension of ampicillin trihydrate is stable for 7 days at room temperature or 14 days at 2-8°C. Following reconstitution, ampicillin sodium solutions for IM or direct IV injection should be used within 1 hour and should not be frozen.

Pharmacological Actions—Ampicillin is bactericidal to Gram-positive and Gram-negative bacteria. It is ineffective against penicillinase-producing *Staphylococci* since it is inactivated by penicillinase.

Mechanism of Action—Ampicillin inhibits transpeptidase enzyme action thus blocking the synthesis of peptidoglycan, a component of bacteria cell walls. This action may be followed by the production of filamentous forms of the susceptible bacteria which ultimately die. This is what is observed in *E. coli*.

Indications—Treatment of gastrointestinal, urinary and respiratory tract infections; also effective in mastitis; pyonephritis and other infections caused by susceptible organisms.

Dosage—4-10 mg /kg orally or 2-7 mg/kg parenterally.

Route(s) of Administration—Per os, parenteral, intra mammary (in animals).

Absorption—Ampicillin is well absorbed from the GIT. Peak plasma concentration is attained within two hours. Food reduces the extent of absorption.

Bioavailability—62 ± 17% (human).

Distribution—Vd = 0.28 ± 0.07 L/kg (in human and dog); 0.167 L/kg (in cat). Ampicillin is distributed throughout the body tissues; concentrated in the liver and kidneys; excluded from the CSF with normal meninges; 5-10% enters the CSF when meninges are inflamed.

Plasma Protein Binding—15-20%. The level of binding is reduced in neonates.

Metabolism—Small portion is metabolized by hydrolysis to inactive penicilloic acid.

Plasma Half-Life—1.3 ± 0.2 hours in human beings. Half-life is higher in uremia, hepatic cirrhosis, and neonates. Half-life in animals is 12 hours. It undergoes enterohepatic circulation.

Residue Limit—0.01 ppm.

Withholding Period—Cattle, 6 days; milk, 48 hours; pig, 1 day.

Route(s) of Excretion—Mainly urine with high proportion as unchanged drug.

Dialysis Status—Dialyzable.

Toxicity and Adverse Effects—Skin rash, diarrhea, and vomiting may be observed in 10% of cases. Severe abdominal or stomach cramp, encephalopathy, seizure, and lymphocytic leukemia may be observed in few cases at therapeutic doses. Ampicillin may cause superinfection following oral administration. Overdose may cause neuromuscular hypersensitivity, electrolyte imbalance, and renal failure.

Contraindications—Hypersensitivity to ampicillin, the penicillins, their products, or components.

Precautions—Adjust the dose downwards in renal dysfunction.

Drug Interactions—Disulfiram and probenecid increase the plasma level of ampicillin.

Pharmaceutical Formulations—Available in the anhydrous form in 250 mg and 500 mg capsules; as the trihydrate salt in 250 mg and 500 mg capsules and oral suspension of 100 mg-500 mg/ml. It is also available as ampicillin sodium for parenteral injection and in combinations with cloxacilin (125 mg of each), and sulbatam sodium. Ampicillin is available in tablets, creams, and intra mammary preparations for livestock.

AMPROLIUM

Amprolium

Proprietary Names—Amprol*; Amprolium*; Ancoban*; Ancoxin* (in combination with sulfaquinoxalin); Coccisan* (in combination with sulfaquinoxalin and vitamin K); Coccimed* (in combination with sulfaquinoxalin and vitamin K); Biccocin* (in combination with sulfaquinoxalin); Amprolin®; Amprosulvit * (in combination with sulfaquinoxalin and vitamin K); Keprococ* (in combination with sulfaquinoxalin and vitamin K); Amprolmix* (in combination with ethopabate.

Chemical Class—Pyrimidine derivative; Thiamine analog.

Pharmacological Class—Thiamine antagonist; Anticooccidial drug.

Source. Synthetic.

Solubility, Stability and Storage—Amprolium is water soluble but slightly soluble in alcohol. Its products can be stored at room temperature.

Pharmacological Actions—Amprolium has anticoccidial activity chiefly against the first generation schizonts of *Eimeria tenella* and *E. acervulina*. It prevents the development of schizonts to merozoites.

Mechanism of Action—Amprolium competitively inhibits the active transport of thiamine.

Indications—Treatment and prevention of coccidiosis in poultry and other animal species—Amprolium is used singly or in combination with other anticoccidial drugs, e.g. sulfaquinoxalin.

Dosages—Birds, 36-113 g/ton of feed or 0.012% in drinking water.

Route(s) of Administration—Per os.

Residue Limit—Chickens and turkeys; 0.5 ppm (muscle), 1.0 ppm (liver and kidney), 7.0 ppm (egg).

Withdrawal Period—24 hours before slaughter of cattle.

Toxicity and Adverse Effects—Amprolium is well tolerated. However, depression, anorexia, and diarrhea have been reported. Overdose has caused thiamine deficiency in the host and also polioencephalomalacia in sheep.

Drug Interactions—Excess dietary thiamine may reduce the efficacy of amprolium.

Pharmaceutical Formulations—Available as amprolium hydrochloride in form of water soluble powder for addition to feed or water. Formulations with other anticoccidial agents and vitamins are available.

APOMORPHINE

Apomorphine

Chemical Class—Aporphine; Morphine derivative.

Pharmacological Class—Dopamine receptor agonist; Central emetic.

Source—Semi-synthetic; derived from morphine.

Stability and Storage—Apomorphine is stored at room temperature away from light. Do not use discolored or precipitated products.

Pharmacological Actions—Apomorphine stimulates the chemoreceptor trigger zone to induce emesis. Emesis occurs in dogs within 2-10 minutes following administration by subcutaneous or conjunctiva routes. Subsequent doses may not cause vomiting if the first failed because apomorphine can depress the vomiting center directly. It can stimulate and depress the CNS, although it causes more stimulation. Apomorphine depresses the medulla, thus causing respiratory depression. It induces penile erection in humans without causing sexual excitement.

Mechanism of Action—Apomorphine activates both D_1 and D_2 dopamine receptors.

Indications—To induce vomition in dogs and cats. It is used to relieve difficulty in emptying the urinary bladder in cases of Parkinson's disease in humans

Dosages—0.04 mg/kg IV or 0.07 mg/kg IM or 0.25 mg/kg in the conjunctiva sac.

Route(s) of Administration—Apomorphine may be administered orally parenterally (intravenous, intramuscular and subcutaneous). It may also be administered into the conjunctiva sac. Parenteral routes are preferred.

Absorption—Apomorphine is poorly absorbed from the GIT. Its effect is unpredictable if given by this route.

Bioavailability—Poor bioavailability following oral administration.

Onset of Action—2-10 minutes.

Metabolism—Apomorphine is conjugated in the liver.

Route(s) of excretion. Urine.

Toxicity and Adverse Effects—Emesis may be protracted at therapeutic doses. Higher doses may produce excitement, restlessness, cardiac and respiratory depression.

Management of Overdose—Wash conjunctiva with sterile saline. Naloxone can reverse the respiratory and CNS effects. Atropine may reverse the bradycardia.

Contraindications—Emesis should not be induced in the following conditions: hypoxia, dyspnea, shock, severe CNS depression, coma, absence of pharyngeal reflex, seizure, extreme physical weakness, repeated vomition, ingestion of corrosive agents such as strong acids, alkalis and other caustic agents, ingestion of petroleum products if the risk of toxicity is not as high as the risk of aspiration. Apomorphine is contraindicated in cases receiving other CNS depressants and those hypersensitive to apomorphine or morphine.

Precautions—Do not repeat a dose if the first did not cause emesis. Apomorphine should be used under the supervision of an experienced professional.

Drug Interactions—Emetic action may be antagonized by anti-dopaminergic drugs e.g. phenothiazines. Additive effects may be produced by concurrent administration of CNS or respiratory depressants (e.g. opioids and barbiturates).

Pharmaceutical Formulations—None is commercially available.

ASPARAGINASE

Synonyms—l-asparaginase, l-asparagine amidohydrolase, Coloaspase, A-as, ASN-ase.

Proprietary Names—Elspar®, Erwiniar®.

Chemical Class. Protein (Enzyme).

Pharmacological Class—Antineoplastic drug; Anticancer drug; Cytotoxic drug.

Source—Natural; derived from *Escherichia coli* and *Erwinia chrysanthemi.*

Solubility, Stability and Storage—Store lyophilized powder below 8⁰C. Reconstitute with normal saline or sterile water for injection. Refrigerate reconstituted product and use within 8 hours. Do not shake solution vigorously to avoid foaming. Use only clear solutions.

Pharmacological Actions—Asparagine has cytotoxic action against tumor cells that depend on preformed l-asparagine for protein synthesis.

Mechanism of Action—Normal cells synthesize l-asparagine, which they utilize for protein synthesis. Certain cancer cells have low levels of l-asparagine synthase and are thus unable to synthesize l-asparagine. These tumor cells depend on preformed l-asparagine. L-asparaginase converts l-asparagine to aspartic acid and ammonia, thus depriving the susceptible cells of an essential material.

Indications—Adjunctive treatment of lymphosarcoma. It is used in combination with other drugs to induce remission of the condition.

Dosages. Dogs, 20,000 IU weekly. Cats, 10,000 IU every 1-3 weeks.

Route(s) of Administration—Parenteral.

Absorption—Not absorbed from the oral route.

Bioavailability (IM)—50%.

Distribution—Vd = 4-5 liters/kg. Poorly distributed; asparaginase stays predominantly within the blood vessels due to high molecular weight. It does not cross the blood-brain-barrier.

Plasma Protein Binding—30%.

Metabolism—Asparaginase is almost completed degraded.

Plasma Half-life—8 to 30 hours following intravenous administration and up to 49 hours with intramuscular administration.

Clearance—0.035 (ml/min/kg).

Route(s) of Excretion—Trace amounts are found in urine.

Dialysis Status—Nondialyzable.

Toxicity and Adverse Effects—Hypersensitivity reaction characterized by vomition, diarrhea, urticaria, pruritis, dyspnea, restlessness, hypotension and collapse is common. The reaction is related to antigenicity of the enzyme. Hemorrhagic pancreatitis, hyperglycemia due to insulin deficiency, hepatotoxicity and coagulation defects due to deficient clotting factors are associated with its action on protein synthesis.

Contraindications—Hypersensitivity to asparaginase; pancreatitis.

Precautions—Administration of repeated doses of asparaginase should be with caution. It is advisable to change to a preparation from another source if allergic reaction is noticed. Preparations from two sources do not cross-react immunologically.

Drug Interactions—Asparaginase terminates methotrexate action if its administration precedes that of methotrexate since asparaginase prevents cell entry into the S-phase due to inhibition of protein synthesis. Methotrexate causes synergistic cytotoxicity with asparaginase if methotrexate's administration precedes that of the enzyme. Vincristine and prednisolone enhance asparaginase induced cytotoxicity.

Pharmaceutical Formulations—Three preparations of the enzyme are available. These are the native preparation from *Escherichia coli*, the *Escherichia coli* enzyme conjugated to polyethylene glycol (PEG-asparaginase) and the *Erwinia chrysanthemi* derived enzyme. Preparations contain 10,000 IU lyophilized powder in 10 ml vials.

ASTEMIZOLE

Proprietary Names—Hismanal'.

Chemical Class—Piperidine.

Pharmacological Class—Antihistamine, H_1 receptor antagonist.

Source—Synthetic.

Solubility, Stability and Storage—Astemizole is practically insoluble in water but soluble in ethanol and other organic solvents.

Pharmacological Actions—Astemizole inhibits the peripheral actions of histamine thereby causing reductions in capillary permeability, bronchoconstriction, intestinal contraction and other peripheral effects of histamine. It has little or no CNS sedative effect.

Mechanism of Action—Astemizole competes with histamine for H_1 receptor sites. It binds more avidly with histamine receptors at the lungs, gastrointestinal tract and blood vessels than at the cerebellum apparently due to poor transport across the blood—brain—barrier, hence the reduced CNS sedative effect.

Astemizole

Indications—Control of urticaria; facial-conjunctival edema of allergic origin; allergic rhinitis.

Dosage—10 mg daily (maximum).

Route(s) of Administration—Per os.

Absorption—Astemizole is well absorbed; peak plasma concentration is attained within 2-4 hours.

Bioavailability—Astemizole undergoes extensive first-pass metabolism.

Distribution—Vd = 250 L/kg. The drug is poorly distributed because of low lipid solubility. Transport across the blood-brain-barrier is also poor. Astemizole and its metabolites are passed into maternal milk in dogs.

Plasma Protein Binding—97%.

Metabolism—Astemizole is metabolized in the liver to active desmethylastemizole and other inactive metabolites.

Plasma Half-Life—24 hours for parent compound; t½ of desmethylastemizole is 12 days. The half-life of the drug and active metabolites may increase to 18-20 days following prolonged administration.

Plasma Protein Binding—96%.

Clearance—Plasma, 11 mL/min/kg.

Route(s) of Excretion—Astemizole is eliminated in urine and feces (it is excreted into bile).

Dialysis Status—Non dialyzable.

Toxicity and Adverse Effects—Increased appetite, weight gain, drowsiness, fatigue, dry mouth and palpitations may be observed in 10% of cases. Overdose causes sedation, apnea, and ventricular arrhythmias.

Management of Overdose—Undertake gastric lavage or induce emesis followed by administration of activated charcoal. Administer cholinesterase inhibitors such as neostigmine and physostigmine to overcome its anticholinergic effects. Give other symptomatic treatment.

Contraindications—Hypersensitivity to astemizole.

Precautions—Withdraw astemizole well ahead of skin allergic test. Use cautiously in cases of hepatic dysfunction; in patients under heart medication or with QT-prolongation; and in combination with erythromycin, ketoconazole, itraconazole, and quinine.

Drug Interactions—CNS depressants may enhance its sedative potentials. Erythromycin, ketoconazole, itraconazole and quinine decrease the metabolism of astemizole.

Pharmaceutical Formulations—Available in 10 mg tablets; 1 mg/ml and 2 mg/ml oral suspension.

ATENOLOL

Atenolol

Proprietary Names—Tenormin®.

Pharmacological Class—Beta$_1$-adrenergic receptor antagonist, Cardioselective beta-adrenergic blocker, Beta adrenergic blocking agent.

Source—Synthetic.

Solubility, Stability and Storage—Atenolol is slightly soluble in water. Atenolol products store well at room temperature but must be protected from light and moisture. The drug is compatible with normal saline.

Pharmacological Actions—Atenolol has negative inotropic and chronotropic actions resulting in reduction in sinus heart rate, blood pressure, cardiac oxygen demand, cardiac output, tachycardia and slowed AV conduction. It has no intrinsic sympathomimetic actions of its own. It has little or no membrane stabilizing action, unlike propranolol. Atenolol has little effect on the beta-receptor mediated peripheral vasodilator action of adrenaline being mainly a beta$_1$-adrenergic receptor antagonist.

Mechanism of Action—Atenolol competitively antagonizes the actions of beta-adrenergic agonists principally at beta$_1$ receptor sites. The beta$_2$ sites are antagonized only at high doses.

Indications—Treatment of systemic hypertension, supraventricular tachycardia, premature ventricular contractions in dogs and cats. Also used to treat hypertrophic cardiomyopathy in cats.

Dosages—2 mg/kg once a day in dogs and cats.

Route(s) of Administration—Per os.

Absorption—Rapidly but incompletely absorbed after oral administration. Peak plasma concentration is attained within 1-3 hours.

Bioavailability (Oral)—50%.

Effective Concentration—500-4,000 ng/ml.

Peak Effect—2-4 hours.

Distribution—Vd = 0.5 to 1.5 L/kg. Small amounts reach the CNS. It crosses the placenta and attains high levels in milk.

Plasma Protein Binding—5-15%.

Metabolism—Partly metabolized in the liver to 2-hydroxyatenolol and atenolol glucuronide.

Plasma Half-Life—6-9 hours (higher in renal impairment and in neonates).

Plasma Clearance—0.3-2 ml/min/kg.

Route(s) of Excretion—Eliminated as 40% and 50% unchanged drug in urine and feces respectively.

Dialysis Status—Dialyzable.

Toxicity and Adverse Effects—Atenolol is well tolerated at therapeutic doses. Bradycardia, lethargy and depression have been reported. Vomition and increased salivation have also been observed at therapeutic doses. High doses cause incoordination, ataxia, mydriasis, hyperemia and tremor in dogs.

Management of Toxicity/Overdose—Give general antidotal therapy.

Contraindications—Heart failure; sinus bradycardia; hypersensitivity to atenolol.

Precautions—Atenolol or other adrenergic blockers either of the cardioselective or nonselective groups should be used cautiously in patients with preexisting heart disease since compensatory dominance of sympathetic activity may be in place to maintain hemodynamics in such cases. A sudden blockade of sympathetic input to the cardiac beta$_1$-adrenoceptors in a compensated heart may precipitate heart failure.

Drug Interactions—Sympathomimetic drugs selective for beta-adrenergic receptors (especially beta$_1$ subtype) may have their actions reduced by atenolol. These agents may also reduce the action of atenolol. Myocardial depression will be enhanced with concurrent use of atenolol and cardiac depressants like anesthetic agents. Phenothiazines, furosemide, and hydralazine may enhance the hypotensive action of atenolol. Atenolol may prolong the hypoglycemic action of insulin.

Pharmaceutical Formulations—Atenolol is available in 25 mg, 50 mg and 100 mg tablets and as 0.5 mg/ml solution for injection. No specific veterinary formulation is available.

ATRACURIUM

Atracurium

Proprietary Names—Tracrium˙.

Chemical Class—Benzylisoquinoline.

Pharmacological Class—Competitive neuro-muscular blocker, Nondepolarizing neuromuscular blocker, Intermediate acting competitive neuromuscular blocker.

Source—Synthetic.

Solubility, Stability and Storage—Solubility in solvent is in the order normal saline < water < alcohol. Refrigerate atracurium solution for injection. Atracurium is compatible with intravenous fluids but incompatible with alkaline drugs e.g. barbiturates and sodium bicarbonate.

Pharmacological Actions—Atracurium causes skeletal muscle paralysis. Unlike tubocurarine, atracurium has no ganglion blocking effects and it is less potent than tubocurarine in releasing histamine.

Mechanism of Action. The drug competes with acetylcholine for the nicotinic receptors at the motor endplate. It does not activate the receptors but prevent access of Ach molecules to the receptors. Thus, Ach-induced end plate potential are reduced to sub threshold levels or abolished. Consequently, impulse transmission is blocked and the muscle becomes paralysed without preceding stimulation.

Indications—As adjunct to general anesthesia to induce muscle relaxation especially in patients with renal/or hepatic failure; to facilitate endotracheal intubation; to relax skeletal muscle during mechanical ventilation. Intramuscular injection of neuromuscular blocking agents is occasionally used to immobilize non domestic animals.

Dosages—0.5 mg/kg followed by increments of 0.2 mg/kg. Horses are sensitive; hence the recommended dose in this species is 0.055 mg/kg.

Route(s) of Administration—Intravenous.

Absorption—Poorly absorbed orally.

Onset of Action—2 minutes.

Peak Action—3-5 minutes

Duration of Action—15-35 minutes.

Distribution—Vd = 0.16-0.18 L/kg (human).

Plasma Protein Binding—80%.

Metabolism—Rapidly metabolized by plasma esterases; also significantly undergo spontaneous nonenzymatic degradation to laudanosine which may have some stimulatory action on the CNS. Atracurium does not have cumulative tendency because of nonenzymatic degradation.

Plasma Half-life—30 minutes.

Clearance (ml/min/kg)—5.3-6.1 (human).

Route(s) of Excretion—Excreted in urine and bile, mostly as metabolites.

Dialysis Status—Nondialyzable.

Toxicity and Adverse Effects—Atracurium is well tolerated. The few adverse effects reported are due to histamine release and these include hypotension, bronchospasm, and increased bronchial secretions. However, these effects are mild. Overdose causes respiratory depression and circulatory collapse.

Management of Overdose/Toxicity—Conservative approach to the management of persistent n-m paralysis and/or inadvertent overdose is advised. Artificial respiration and withholding administration of the drug constitute the initial steps to be undertaken. Atracurium effects can be reversed by anticholinesterase agents e.g. neostigmine (0.022mg/kg). Atropine (0.04mg/kg) should be administered prior to or in conjunction with neostigmine to circumvent the muscarinic effect of neostigmine.

Contraindications—Myasthenia gravis; hypersensitivity to atracurium.

Precautions—Use atracurium cautiously in patients with cardiovascular and respiratory diseases. These patients may be highly susceptible to histamine action. Neuromuscular blockers generally have low therapeutic index. Hence, they should be used with caution and preferably under the supervision of qualified and experienced personnel. Also, avoid administration of precalculated doses. It is advisable to administer the drugs to effect. Care should be taken when neuromuscular blockers are used with general anaesthetics to insure that the patient has not recovered from the anaesthesia but is unable to move because of paralysis caused by the n-m blocker.

Drug Interactions—The concurrent use of more than one competitive neuromuscular blocker results in additive effect. Some general anaesthetic agents (e.g. halothane, methoxyflurane, enflurane and isoflurane) synergize with the neuromuscular blocking action of atracurium. Verapamil, quinidine, furosemide, local anaesthetics, and immunodepressants enhance the blocking action of atracurium. Aminoglycoside antibiotics are potential neuromuscular blockers. Hence, their actions are synergistic with those of other neuromuscular blockers.

Pharmaceutical Formulations—Available as atracurium besylate in 10 mg/ml solution for injection. No specific veterinary formulation is available.

ATROPINE

Synonyms—dl-Hyoscyamine.

Proprietary Names—Isopto˚ Atropine; Atropisol˚; l-Tropine˚.

Chemical Class—Belladonna alkaloid.

Pharmacological Class—Parasympatholytic, antimuscarinic, cholinolytic, anticholinergic, mydriatic, spasmolytic, or antispasmodic agent.

Source. Natural; obtained from Belladonna plants such as *Atropa belladonna* (deadly nightshade), and *Datura stramonium* (Jimson weed; stinkweed; thorn-apple; evil-apple).

Solubility, Stability and Storage—Atropine is water soluble and 10 times less soluble in alcohol than water. Formulations may be safely stored at room temperature. Tablets are stored in tight containers. Atropine is compatible with most drugs except pentobarbital, methohexital, norepinephrine, metaraminol and sodium bicarbonate.

Pharmacological Actions—Atropine causes tachycardia and increased cardiac output. It relaxes the gastrointestinal smooth muscle in all species. It also reduces exocrine secretions especially from salivary glands. Gastric secretions are reduced at high doses. Atropine dilates the bronchioles and reduces bronchial secretions. It relaxes the urinary smooth muscle, dilates the pupil, and causes loss of accommodation (cyclopegia).

Mechanism of Action—Atropine competitively inhibits the actions of acetylcholine and other cholinomimetic agents at muscarinic receptor sites. Muscarinic receptors of salivary and sweat glands are most sensitive while those of GI, urinary bladder and gastric glands are most resistant to atropine blockade.

Indications—Treatment of intestinal spasm and hypermotility; treatment of anticholinesterase and cholinomimetic agent poisoning; used in conjunction with a cholinesterase reactivator (e.g. pralidoxime) in the treatment of organophosphate poisoning; treatment of hypertonicity of smooth muscles; adjunct in general anesthesia to reduce salivary and bronchial secretions; to facilitate ophthalmic examination.

Dosages—0.045 mg/kg. A higher dose is required in cholinergic agent toxicity e.g. 0.2-2.0 mg/kg with ¼ of the dose given IV and the remainder by IM or SC.

Route(s) of Administration—Per os, intravenous, intramuscular, subcutaneous, intraocular, endotracheal and inhalation (in human beings).

Absorption—Atropine is readily absorbed from the GIT.

Bioavailability (oral)—50% (human).

Onset of Action—15-20 minutes (intraocular).

Peak Action—3-4 minutes (IV); 2 hours (intraocular).

Duration of Action—Days (intraocular).

Distribution—Vd = 2.0 ± 1.1 (human). Atropine is widely distributed. It crosses the blood-brain-barrier and placenta and is detectable in milk.

Plasma Protein Binding—14-22 % (human).

Metabolism—Metabolized in the liver.

Plasma Half-life—3.5 ± 1.5 hours (human.

Clearance—8 ± 4 ml/min/kg in human).

Route(s) of Excretion—Eliminated in urine with 57 ± 8% as unchanged drug.

Toxicity and Adverse Effects—Qualitatively, the intensity of adverse effects is species and route dependent. Atropine causes dilated and fixed pupil, dry mouth, dry skin, transient bradycardia followed by tachycardia with palpitations and arrhythmias. It also causes reduction in tone and motility of the gastrointestinal smooth muscle resulting in constipation. Atropine causes CNS stimulation characterized by mania, excitement, extensive motor activity in animals at high doses. CNS effects in human beings are characterized by hallucination and disorientation. Herbivores are more resistant than carnivores to atropine effects. Rabbits are tolerant because they possess high levels of esterase enzymes. Parenteral administration produces more intense toxic effects than oral administration. Poisoning is characterized by dry mouth, mydiriasis, tachycardia, hyperpnoea, restlessness, hyperpyrexia and respiratory failure.

Management of Toxicity/Overdose—Give general antidotal therapy. Anticholinesterase agents (e.g. physostigmine) are antidotes.

Contraindications—Acute angle glaucoma; tachycardia; obstruction of the GIT and/or urinary tract; cardiac ischemia; acute hemorrhage; paralytic ileus; myasthenia gravis; hypersensitivity to atropine.

Precautions—Use cautiously in hepatic, renal, and cardiac diseases; hyperthyroidism, and in old animals.

Drug Interactions—Procainamide, amantadine, quinidine, butryophenones, phenothiazines, tricyclic antidepressants, pethidine, benzodiazepines, and antihistamines may enhance the effect of atropine since they possess some anticholinergic actions. Primidone, disopyramide, prolonged use of corticosteroids may enhance the toxic potential of atropine. Atropine may enhance the actions of nitrofurantoin, thiazide diuretics and sympathomimetic agents. Large doses of muscarinic receptor agonists or agents that prevent the hydrolysis of acetylcholine (e.g. anticholinesterases) can overcome the actions of atropine and other antimuscarinic drugs.

Pharmaceutical Formulations—Available as atropine sulfate in 0.4 mg and 0.6 mg tablets, solutions of various strength for injection, 0.5% ophthalmic solution and 0.5 % ophthalmic ointment.

AURANOFIN

Auranofin

Proprietary Names—Ridaura˙.

Chemical Class—Metallic gold preparation.

Pharmacological Class—Antiarthritic drug.

Source—Synthetic.

Solubility, Stability and Storage—Store auranofin capsules at room temperature; protect from light and moisture.

Pharmacological Action—Auranofin suppresses or prevents degenerative lesions associated with arthritis. It decreases complement activation and inhibits prostaglandin synthesis. It has minimal anti-inflammatory action in other inflammatory conditions.

Mechanism of Action—This is not certain but may be due to its ability to inhibit the maturation and function of mononuclear phagocytes, inhibit lysosomal enzyme release, decrease the level of rheumatoid factor and immunoglobulins, and suppress cellular immunity.

Indications—Treatment of rheumatoid arthritis and gold-responsive dermatoses.

Dosage—Dog, 0.1-0.2 mg/kg every 12 hours.

Route(s) of Administration—Per os.

Absorption—Absorption rate is 25%.

Bioavailability (oral)—15-25 %.

Distribution—Vd = 0.045 litres /kg.

Plasma Protein Binding—60%.

Plasma Half-Life—17-25 days; t½ for whole body may be as high as 80 days.

Clearance (ml/min/kg)—0.025 ± 0.016.

Route(s) of Excretion—Feces (major), urine (15%).

Toxicity and Adverse Effects—Skin rash and gastrointestinal disorders are common. Other toxic effects of parenteral gold preparations (aurothioglucose and gold sodium thiomalate) are produced but to a lesser degree.

Contraindications—Renal disease; congestive heart failure; hepatic dysfunction or a history of infectious hepatitis; history of hematological disorder; pregnancy; lactation; recent radiation therapy; concomitant use with antimalarial drugs, immunosuppressants and pyrazolone derivatives.

Precautions—NSAIDs and corticosteroids may be discontinued following gold therapy. Monitor blood parameters during therapy.

Drug Interactions—Sulfhydryl agents increase the excretion of auranofin.

Pharmaceutical Formulations—Available in 3 mg capsules containing 29% gold.

AUROTHIOGLUCOSE

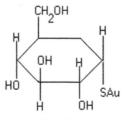

Aurothioglucose

Proprietary Names—Solganal`.

Chemical Class—Metallic gold preparation.

Pharmacological Class—Antiarthritic drug; Disease-modifying antirheumatic drug.

Source—Synthetic.

Solubility, Stability and Storage—Aurothioglucose is soluble in water but insoluble in alcohol and vegetable oil. Store product at 15-30°C in light resistant containers.

Pharmacological Actions—Aurothioglucose suppresses or prevents the degenerative lesions associated with arthritis. It has minimal anti-inflammatory actions in other circumstances.

Mechanism of Action—Like auranofin, another metallic gold preparation, the mechanism of action of aurothioglucose is not certain. Its action may be due to its ability to inhibit the maturation and function of mononuclear phagocytes as well as inhibit lysosomal enzyme release, decrease the level of rheumatoid factor and immunoglobulins, and suppress cellular immunity.

Indications—Treatment of rheumatoid arthritis.

Dosage—5 mg or 10 mg (test dose), then 1.0 mg/kg weekly in dogs and cats.

Route(s) of Administration—Intramuscular.

Absorption—Absorption is slow and erratic. Peak plasma concentration is attained within 4-6 hours.

Distribution—Aurothioglucose crosses the placental membrane and distributes into milk.

Plasma Protein Binding—95%

Plasma Half-Life—This is dependent on dose and length of therapy. It is usually 7 days for a 50 mg dose. Half-life increases with continued treatment and may be as long as 27 days.

Route(s) of Excretion—60% to 90% of administered aurothioglucose is excreted in urine while 10% to 40% are eliminated in feces.

Toxicity and Adverse Effects—Cutaneous reactions vary from simple erythema to exfoliative dermatitis. Grey-to-blue pigmentation (chrysiasis) on the skin and mucous membranes has also been reported. Metallic taste may be observed in 10% of human cases. Inflammations of cutaneous membranes such as stomatitis, pharyngitis, vaginitis, tracheitis, gastritis, colitis and glossitis have been reported. Other signs include proteinuria, blood dyscrasia and allergic reactions, which may be severe.

Management of Toxicity/Overdose—Administer dimercaprol or other chelating agent.

Contraindication—Renal disease; hepatic dysfunction; history of infectious hepatitis; history of hematological disorder; pregnancy; lactation; recent radiation therapy; concomitant use with antimalarial, immunosuppressant, and any pyrazolone derivative; history of hypersensitivity.

Precautions—Monitor blood parameters during use. Discontinue therapy if platelet, granulocyte and WBC counts fall below 100,000/mm^3, 1500/mm^3 and 4000/mm^3 respectively. Do not mix aurothioglucose with other medications during administration.

Drug Interactions—Sulfhydryl agents enhance the excretion of aurothioglucose.

Pharmaceutical Formulations—The drug is available as sterile suspension in fixed oil at 50 mg/ml.

AZAPERONE

Azaperone

Proprietary Names—Stresnil®; Suicalm®.

Chemical Class—Butyrophenone.

Pharmacological Class—Sedative-hypnotic; Tranquilizer.

Source—Synthetic.

Solubility, Stability and Storage—Azaperone is practically insoluble in water but soluble in dilute organic acids. Store azaperone products at 15-30°C.

Pharmacological Actions—Azaperone depresses the central nervous system, lowers blood pressure, stimulates respiration and cutaneous vasodilatation, and reduces aggression in pigs.

Mechanism of Action—Azaperone suppresses adrenergic reflexes. Butyrophenones block the actions of catecholamines by preventing their access to receptors.

Indications—To sedate pigs and prevent the rejection of piglets by nervous sows; also used to prevent fighting among groups of weaner pigs.

Dosage—1-4 mg/kg body weight depending on the level of sedation required.

Route(s) of Administration—Intramuscular.

Onset of Action—15 minutes.

Duration of Action—2-3 hours.

Metabolism—Azaperone is extensively metabolized in the liver to azaperol.

Route(s) of Excretion—13% of the dose is eliminated in feces. Azaperone is completely eliminated within 16 hours.

Toxicity and Adverse Effects—Azaperone may cause transient salivation. Shivering has been reported. Animals may be excited if disturbed before the peak effect of azaperone is established.

Contraindication—Hypersensitivity to azaperone.

Precaution—Do not administer azaperone intravenously.

Drug Interactions. The action of azaperone may be inhibited by 4-aminopyrine. Its action is potentiated by other CNS depressants.

Pharmaceutical Formulations—Available in 20 mg/ml solution for injection.

AZATHIOPRINE

Proprietary Names—Imuran®.
Chemical Class—Purine analog.
Pharmacological Class—Immunosuppressant.
Source—Synthetic. It is an imidazolyl derivative of 6-mercaptopurine.

Azathioprine

Stability and Storage—Azathioprine products are stored at room temperature away from light. Reconstituted solution for injection must be use within 24 hours if without refrigeration. Parenteral solution may be stable for up to two weeks if refrigerated. Parenteral preparations are compatible with dextrose or saline fluids. Azathioprine is hydrolyzed to mercaptopurine in alkaline media especially when the medium is heated or contains sulfhydryl group.

Pharmacological Actions—Azathioprine has immunosuppressive action, which is greater with cell-mediated than antibody-mediated responses.

Mechanism of Action—Azathioprine is converted to 6-mercaptopurine which in turn is converted to the active nucleotide form (6-thioinosine-5' phosphate) by hypoxanthine-guanine phosphoribosyl-transferase. The 6-thioinosine-5' phosphate inhibits several vital metabolic reactions as well as DNA and RNA synthases.

Indications—Adjunctive treatment of immune-mediated diseases in dogs.

Dosages—2 mg/kg orally.

Route(s) of Administration—Azathioprine may be administered orally or by intravenous route.

Absorption—The drug is absorbed considerably from the GIT. Peak plasma concentration is attained within 1-2 hours.

Bioavailability (oral)—60 ± 31 % (humans).

Distribution—Vd = 0.81 ± 0.65 L/kg (humans). Azathioprine crosses the placenta.

Plasma Protein Binding—30%.

Metabolism—Azathioprine is metabolized by xanthine oxidase to 6-mercaptopurine.

Plasma Half-life—Half-life is 12 minutes for parent drug and 0.7-3 hours for active product.

Clearance—57 ± 31 ml/min/kg in humans.

Route(s) of Excretion—Azathioprine is excreted in urine with < 2% as unchanged drug.

Dialysis Status—Poor.

Toxicity and Adverse Effects—Bone marrow depression characterized by anemia, leukopenia, and less severe thrombocytopenia is common. Nausea, vomiting, anorexia, reversible cholestatic jaundice and acute pancreatitis have all been reported. The risk for infection is heightened. Azathioprine is mutagenic and possibly teratogenic. Rapid withdrawal in the dog has resulted in rebound hyperimmune response.

Management of Overdose—Give symptomatic and supportive therapy.

Contraindications—Hypersensitivity to azathioprine; pregnancy.

Precautions—Feed kittens and pups with milk replacers if azathioprine is administered to nursing bitches and queens. Reduce the dose in patients with renal impairment. Use cautiously in animals with history of urolithiasis. Pregnant women must avoid handling antineoplastic agents. Concomitant use with other drugs that can cause hepatotoxicity or alteration in liver metabolic function must be with caution.

Drug Interactions—Allopurinol inhibits the metabolism of mercaptopurine, the active metabolite of azathioprine, thus causing increased toxicity of the latter. Hence, the dose of azathioprine must be reduced by as much as 75% if both drugs are administered concurrently. Azathioprine may produce additive bone marrow depression with antineoplastic agents and bone marrow depressants such as chloramphenicol, flucytosine, amphotericin B, and colchicine. Other immunodepressants may increase the risk of infection when used concurrently with azathioprine.

Pharmaceutical Formulations—Available as azathioprine sodium in 20 ml vial containing 100 mg and in 50 mg tablets.

BACITRACIN

Proprietary Names—AK-Tracin˙; Baciguent˙; Baci-IM˙; Polysporin˙; Medi—Quick˙; Mycitracin˙; Neomixin˙. Neosporin˙ Ocutricin˙; Septa˙; Triple Antibiotic˙; Cortisporin˙.

Chemical Class—Polypeptide.

Pharmacological Class—Narrow spectrum antibiotic, Polypeptide antibiotic.

Source—Tracy-I strain of *Bacillus subtilis* originally isolated from the damaged tissue and street dirt debrided from a compound fracture of one Margaret Tracy.

Pharmacological Actions—Bacitracin is bactericidal to most Gram-positive aerobic and anaerobic cocci, Gram-positive rods and some spirochaetes.

Mechanism of Action—The drug inhibits cell wall synthesis by interfering with the phospholipid carrier that transfers mucopeptides to the growing cell wall.

Indications—Treatment of open wounds and as a feed additive.

Route(s) of Administration—Bacitracin is administered orally and topically.

Absorption—Bacitracin is poorly absorbed from the GIT, intact skin, wound, mucous membranes, pleura or synovia. It is rapidly absorbed from muscular site. Peak plasma concentration is attained within 1-2 hours following intramuscular injection.

Distribution—The drug is widely distributed but it is excluded from the cerebrospinal fluid.

Plasma Protein Binding—Binding to plasma protein is minimal.

Duration of Action—6-8 hours.

Route(s) of Excretion—Urine.

Toxicity and Adverse Effects—Following parenteral administration, bacitracin causes severe nephrotoxicity characterized by proteinuria, hematuria and nitrogen retention. Topical application may cause hypersensitivity reactions such as skin rash. Oral administration may cause nausea and vomiting.

Contraindications—Hypersensitivity to bacitracin or any component; renal impairment.

Precautions—Do not administer bacitracin intravenously. Prolonged use may cause super infection.

Drug Interactions—Nephrotoxic drugs, neuromuscular blocking drugs and anaesthetics may increase the toxic potential of bacitracin.

Pharmaceutical Formulations—Bacitracin is available in solution for injection (50,000 units); topical and ophthalmic ointments (each containing 500 units/g); as zinc bacitracin for topical use and as feed additive for animals. Bacitracin is also available in ointment with neomycin, polymyxin B and hydrocortisone.

BENZATHINE PENICILLIN G

Synonyms—Benzathine Benzylpenicillin; Benzylpenicillin Benzathine; Penicillin G benzathine.

Proprietary Names—Penadur*; Penilente*; Retarpen*; Bicillin* L-A; Permapen*; Penidure-LA*; Longacillin*; Pencom*; Diapen*.

Chemical Class—6-aminopenicillanic acid derivative.

Pharmacological Class—Beta-lactam antibiotic, narrow spectrum antibiotic.

Source—Natural; 2 molecules of benzyl penicillin G, produced by the mold, *Penicillium* is complexed to 1 molecule of an ammonium base.

Solubility, Stability and Storage—Benzathine penicillin G is 0.02% soluble in water. Benzathine penicillin G suspension should be stored in a refrigerator.

Pharmacological Actions—Benzathine penicillin G is bactericidal to most Gram-positive organisms. Some Gram-negative organisms like *Neisseria gonorrhoeae*, some anaerobes, and spirochaetes are susceptible.

Mechanism of Action—The drug inhibits transpeptidase enzyme thus blocking the synthesis of peptidoglycan, a component of bacterial cell wall. This may be followed by activation of autolytic enzymes in the cell wall which causes lysis of the bacteria.

Uses—Treatment of streptococci bovine mastitis, anthrax, erysipelas, strangles, joint-ill, some clostridial diseases such as tetanus and blackleg.

Dosage—

Horse:	50,000 IU/kg every 48 hours
Cattle:	10,000-66,000 IU/Kg every 48 hours
Dog and Cat:	40,000-50,000 IU/Kg every 3 days

Route(s) of Administration—Intramuscular.

Absorption—The preparation releases the active benzyl penicillin G extremely slowly from muscular depot. Peak plasma concentration is attained within 12-24 hours. Plasma concentrations are generally low. Increased dosage only results in more sustained plasma level but not higher plasma concentration.

Duration of Action—antimicrobial activity has been detected for average of 26 days in humans.

Distribution—Vd = 0.35 L/ kg (humans); 0.65 L/kg (horses); 0.23 L/kg (sheep); 0.15 L/kg (camels).

Plasma Protein Binding—About 65%

Metabolism—30% of administered drug is metabolized in the liver to penicilloic acid.

Plasma Half-Life—Adequate blood levels are detectable for up to 4 weeks depending on the dose. Hence, benzathine penicillin G is useful for prophylaxis.

Route(s) of Excretion—Benzathine penicillin G is excreted in urine mainly by tubular secretion.

Dialysis Status—Benzathine penicillin G can be removed from blood by hemodialysis.

Toxicity and Adverse Effects—Hypersensitivity reactions ranging from mild transitory skin reactions to anaphylactic shock are the major adverse effects of benzathine penicillin G. Direct toxic effects are low. The drug causes local pain and thrombophlebitis at injection sites. Central nervous system related effects such as convulsion, confusion, and drowsiness may manifest following high doses especially in patients with renal insufficiency. Granulocytopenia, bone marrow depression, and hepatitis have also been reported.

Management of Overdose/Toxicity—Undertake hemodialysis. Give supportive and symptomatic treatment—

Contraindications—Hypersensitivity to penicillin, its breakdown products, or cephalosporin.

Precautions—Do not administer benzathine penicillin G orally. Patients with acute and severe infections should initially be given a loading dose with a soluble form of penicillin. This should be followed with maintenance doses of penicillin G benzathine.

Drug Interactions—Probenecid increases the half-life of penicillins. In uremia, other organic acids compete with penicillin for transport from the cerebrospinal fluid. Tetracyclines and other bacteriostatic antibiotics decrease the effectiveness of benzathine penicillin G. Aminoglycoside antibiotics have synergistic effect with penicillin.

Pharmaceutical Formulations—Benzathine penicillin G is available as dry powder in vials for reconstitution. Each ml contains 300,000 or 600,000 units when reconstituted. The drug is also available in suspension with other antibiotics.

BETAMETHASONE

Synonyms—Flubenisolone.

Proprietary Names—Betasone®, Betatrex®, Celestone®, Diprolene®, Urticort®, Valisone®.

Chemical Class—Corticosteroid.

Pharmacological Class—Glucocorticoid, anti-inflammatory drug.

Source—Synthetic.

Solubility, Stability and Storage—Betamethasone is insoluble in water and alcohol. Its products are unstable when exposed to light. Store products at room temperature or refrigerator.

Betamethasone

Pharmacological Actions—Betamethasone, like all glucocorticoids has effects on virtually every cell type and system in mammals. The drugs reduce capillary permeability and enhance vasoconstriction; inhibits fibroblast proliferation, platelet aggregation, macrophage and monocyte migration. They also inhibit lymphokines, sensitization of lymphocytes and the cellular response to mediators of inflammation. Glucocorticoids increase the numbers of circulating platelets, T-lymphocytes, neutrophils and red blood cells. They also stabilize lysosomal membranes; increase the secretion of gastric acid, pepsin, and trypsin; stimulate gluconeogenesis and enhances lipogenesis in certain areas of the body. Betamethasone has 25 times the anti-inflammatory potency of hydrocortisone. It is devoid of mineralocorticoid activity.

Mechanism of Action—Betamethasone activates glucocorticoid receptors to regulate protein synthesis.

Uses—Treatment of inflammatory dermatoses.

Dosages—

Guinea pig	0.1-0.2 ml IM, SC
Dog	0.25-0.5 ml aqueous suspension per 9 kg dog IM

Route(s) of Administration—Per os; Intramuscular; subcutaneous.

Absorption—Betamethasone is absorbed to a significant extent from the GIT.

Bioavailability (oral)—72% (humans).

Duration of Action—>48 hours.

Distribution—Vd = 1.4 ± 0.3 (humans).

Plasma Protein Binding—64% (humans).

Metabolism—Betamethasone undergoes extensive hepatic metabolism.

Plasma Half-life—5 hours (humans).

Clearance—2.9 ± 0.9 ml/min/kg.

Route(s) of Excretion—Urine with < 5% as unchanged drug.

Toxicity and Adverse Effects—Adverse effects are generally associated with long-term administration of high dosages. It retards growth of young animals. In dogs, it causes polydipsia, polyphagia, polyuria, dull and dry hair coat, weight gain, panting, vomiting, diarrhea, elevated liver enzymes, pancreatitis, GI ulceration, and lipidemias. It also causes activation or worsening of diabetes mellitus, muscle wasting and behavioral changes characterized by depression, lethargy, and viciousness. Cats tend to develop fewer adverse effects. Occasionally, polydipsia, polyuria, polyphagia with weight gain, diarrhea, or depression can be seen. Administration of betamethasone may play a role in the development of laminitis in horses.

Management of Overdose/Toxicity—Give supportive treatment.

Contraindications—Acute and chronic bacterial infections; systemic fungal infections (unless used for replacement therapy); diabetes mellitus; pregnancy; hypersensitivity to betamethasone.

Precautions—Corticosteroid therapy may induce parturition in large animal species during the latter stages of pregnancy. Patients taking corticosteroids should generally not receive live attenuated-virus vaccines. Do not give more than 4 injections in dogs during the treatment period. Discontinue anticholinesterase medication at least 24 hours prior to corticosteroid administration in patients with myasthenia gravis.

Drug Interactions—Concurrent use with NSAIDs could lead to gastric bleeding and ulceration. Amphotericin B and potassium-depleting diuretics (furosemide, thiazides) may cause hypokalemia when administered concomitantly with glucocorticoids. Glucocorticoid therapy may enhance insulin requirements in diabetics. Phenytoin, phenobarbital, rifampin may increase the metabolism of glucocorticoids while cyclosporine may inhibit their metabolism. Concomitant administration of glucocorticoid and anticholinesterase agent (*e.g.* pyridostigmine, neostigmine, etc.) may cause severe muscle weakness in cases with myasthenia gravis.

Pharmaceutical Formulations—Betamethasone is available as betamethasone base in tablets; betamethasone dipropionate in topical preparations; betamethasone sodium phosphate and betamethasone sodium acetate in solutions for injection

BETHANECHOL

Bethanechol

Synonyms—β-methyl carbaminoylcholine.

Proprietary Names—Duvoid˚; Myotonachol˚; Urabeth˚; Urecholine˚; PMS-Bethanechol Chloride˚.

Chemical Class—Choline ester.

Pharmacological Class—Parasympathomimetic agent; Cholinomimetic agent.

Source—Synthetic.

Solubility, Stability and Storage—Bethanechol is water soluble and heat resistant. Its products may be stored at room temperature.

Pharmacological Actions—Bethanechol acts mainly at muscarinic sites and selectively on the gastrointestinal and urinary tract smooth muscles. It acts also on the bronchus to cause dyspnea. Bethanechol stimulates the gastrointestinal tract causing increased peristaltic movement in addition to gastric and pancreatic secretions. Its actions on the bladder cause frequent urination respectively. The actions of bethanicol are restricted mostly to the gastrointestinal and urinary tract smooth muscles if administered orally or subcutaneously. Its effect on urinary smooth muscle is intense following subcutaneous administration.

Mechanism of Action—Bethanechol directly activates muscarinic cholinergic receptors.

Indications—Control of nonobstructive urinary retention which may be due to neurogenic factors in small animals.

Dosages—The recommended dose of bethanechol is 2.5-10 mg subcutaneously or 5-25 mg orally every 8-12 hours. The drug may be given at 5 mg orally every 8 hours if used with phenoxybenzamine.

Route(s) of Administration—Per os, subcutaneous.

Absorption—Absorption from the GIT is poor and variable.

Bioavailability (oral)—Bioavailability of bethanechol is low due to poor absorption.

Onset of Action—30-90 minutes (oral route in humans); 5-15 minutes (subcutaneous route in humans).

Duration of Action—6 hours following oral route in human beings but 2 hours following subcutaneous administration.

Distribution—Bethanechol is poorly distributed. It does not enter the CNS.

Plasma Protein Binding—Unknown.

Metabolism—Bethanechol is resistant to hydrolysis by either acetylcholinesterase or pseudo cholinesterase.

Plasma Half-life—It has a long half-life.

Dialysis Status—Nondialyzable.

Toxicity and Adverse Effects—Nausea, emesis, salivation, and anorexia are the most common signs at therapeutic doses. Overdose causes hypotension, bronchospasm, and urination in addition to enhancement of the common signs. Severe cholinergic activity may result if bethanechol is given intravenously or intramuscularly.

Management of Overdose—Atropine sulfate is the antidote for bethanechol toxicity.

Contraindications—Urinary or gastrointestinal retention caused by obstruction; following recent bladder or gastrointestinal surgery; hyperthyroidism; peptic ulcer; seizures; obstructive pulmonary disease; hypotension; bradycardia; hypersensitivity to bethanechol.

Precautions—Do not administer by intravenous or intramuscular routes as these routes may cause severe and more diffuse cholinergic reactions. Atropine should be readily available especially if administered parenteral.

Drug Interactions—Concomitant use of bethanechol with other cholinergic and anticholinesterase agents may cause additive effects and enhance its toxicity. Procainamide, quinidine, sympathomimetic amines may reduce the effect of bethanechol.

Pharmaceutical Formulations—Available as bethanechol chloride in 5, 10, 25, and 50 mg oral tablets and in 5 mg/ml solution for injection.

BISACODYL

Bisacodyl

Proprietary Names—Bisacolax˚; Dulcolax˚.

Chemical Class—Diphenylmethane derivative.

Pharmacological Class—Stimulant laxative.

Source—Synthetic.

Solubility, Stability and Storage—Bisacodyl is practically insoluble in water and in alkaline solutions. Store bisacodyl formulations at room temperature in a well-closed container.

Pharmacological Actions—Bisacodyl helps to evacuate the bowel and prevent chronic constipation by promoting soft, formed feces (stool). Bisacodyl exert its action on the colon. It therefore does not act promptly. It acts as from 6 hours after oral administration.

Mechanism of Action—The precise mechanism of action is unknown. Stimulant laxatives are thought to increase peristalsis by a direct action on the intestinal smooth muscle through stimulation of intramural nerve plexus. It has also been shown to promote fluid and ion accumulation in the colon to increase the laxative effect.

Indications—Short-term relief of constipation and evacuation of the rectum in small animals.

Dosages—5 mg once daily.

Route(s) of Administration—Per os.

Absorption—Bisacodyl is minimally absorbed from oral and rectal routes.

Bioavailability (oral)—Low

Onset of Action—¼ to 1 hour (rectal administration in humans); 6-8 hours (oral); onset is faster if taken on empty stomach.

Distribution—Bisacodyl may be distributed into breast milk and produce loose stools in nursing animals.

Metabolism—Bisacodyl is metabolized by deacetylation to the active metabolite, bisacodyl diphenol.

Route(s) of Excretion—30% of the dose is excreted in urine in 48 hours as bisacodyl diphenol glucuronide while 50% is eliminated in faeces as unconjugated bisacodyl diphenol.

Toxicity and Adverse Effects—Gastric irritation may occur if the enteric coating is destroyed by chewing. Weakness, incoordination, and orthostatic hypotension may be exacerbated in elderly human patients as a result of significant electrolyte loss when stimulant laxatives are used repeatedly to evacuate the colon. Electrolyte imbalance characterized by confusion, irregular heartbeat, muscle cramps, unusual tiredness or weakness may result from acute overdose or chronic misuse. Cramping, diarrhea and nausea have been less frequently reported.

Management of Overdose/Toxicity—Give symptomatic treatment.

Contraindications—Hypersensitivity to bisacodyl.

Precautions—To aid stool softening and to protect the patient against dehydration give drinking water or liquids when using any laxative. Do not administer with milk or antacids. Bowel function may become dependence on bisacodyl if overused. Do not administer within 2 hours of other medicine.

Drug Interactions—Chronic use or overuse of laxatives may reduce serum potassium concentrations by promoting excessive potassium loss from the intestinal tract. This may also interfere with potassium-retaining effects of potassium-sparing diuretics. Administration of antacids or histamine H_2-receptor antagonists, such as cimetidine, famotidine, nizatidine, and ranitidine or milk within one hour of bisacodyl tablets may cause the enteric coating to dissolve too rapidly, resulting in gastric or duodenal irritation.

Pharmaceutical Formulations—Bisacodyl is available as 5 mg enteric coated tablets and 10 mg suppositories. No specific veterinary preparations are available.

BITHIONOL

Proprietary Names—Bithin®; Douvivet® (Bithionol sulfoxide).

Chemical Class—Phenolic compound; Diphenylsulfide.

Pharmacological Class—Antifungal; anthelmintic; bacteriostat.

Source—Synthetic.

Solubility, Stability and Storage—Bithionol is insoluble in water but soluble in alcohol, ether and acetone. It is sensitive to light.

Pharmacological Actions—Bithionol has bacteriostatic, anthelmintic and antifungal actions. It is effective against *Taenia* species in dogs and cats; *Rallietina* species in chickens; most tapeworms of geese; *Monieza* and *Thysanosoma* species in ruminants; *Paramphistomum* in ruminants and skin flukes of fish. *Dipylidium caninum* is less susceptible than *Taenia* species in dogs and cats. Bithionol causes increased intestinal motility.

Bithionol

Mechanism of Action—Increased intestinal motility is due to cholinomimetic action.

Indications—Treatment of tapeworm infection in dogs, cats, poultry, and ruminants. Also used to treat rumen flukes of ruminants, and skin flukes of fish.

Dosages—

Bithionol

Dog, cat.	200 mg/kg
Sheep, goat	200 mg/kg
Goose	600 mg/kg as single treatment
Chicken	200mg/kg twice within 4 days

The dose of bithionol sulfoxide is 60 mg/kg.

Route(s) of Administration—Per os.

Absorption—Bithionol undergoes limited absorption.

Distribution—The drug attains higher concentration in bile than in blood.

Route(s) of Excretion—Bile.

Toxicity and Adverse Effects—Bithionol is well tolerated. It causes occasional emesis and transient diarrhea (arising from its cholinomimetic action).

Management of Overdose/Toxicity—Adverse effects may not warrant any action. However, give antidiarrheal drug if diarrhea becomes excessive.

Contraindications—Hypersensitivity to bithionol.

Drug Interactions—Cholinomimetic agents may enhance its action on the intestinal smooth muscle.

Pharmaceutical Formulations—Available as bithionol and bithionol sulfoxide in capsules, tablets and boluses.

BLEOMYCIN

Synonyms—BLM; NIM

Proprietary Name—Blenoxane®.

Chemical Class—Glycopeptide.

Pharmacological Class—Antineoplastic drug; anticancer drug; cytotoxic drug; anticancer antibiotic.

Source—Natural; obtained from *Streptomyces verticillus*.

Stability and Storage—Bleomycin sterile powder for injection should be refrigerated and reconstituted preferably with normal saline. Reconstituted product is stable for 14 days at room temperature and 28 days if refrigerated. Bleomycin is less stable in dextrose solution and it loses potency in a solution of 5% dextrose in water (D_5W) if kept in PVC or glass containers. Bleomycin is incompatible with amino acid solutions, antibacterials such as penicillin G, nafcillin, cefazolin and other drugs such as mitotane, furosemide, vitamin C, hydrocortisone and aminophylline.

Pharmacological Actions—Bleomycin has antibacterial activity against both Gram-positive and Gram-negative organisms. It is also active against some fungi and tumors. Its action on tumors is more pronounced at the G_2 phase. It has minimal myelosuppressive and immunosuppressive activities.

Mechanism of Action—Bleomycin binds to iron and copper to generate superoxide or hydroxyl radicals which attack DNA causing strand scission. The amino terminal tripeptide intercalates between guanine–cytosine base pair and cause fragmentation of DNA.

Indications—Adjunctive treatment of lymphomas, squamous cell carcinomas, and thyroid tumors in dogs and cats. Bleomycin has been used in combination with dl-alpha—difluoromethylornithine (DFMO) in the treatment of human African trypanosomosis (HAT).

Dosages—10 U/m² every day for 3-4 days followed by 10 U/m² every 7 days up to a maximum of 200 U/m².

Route(s) of Administration—Intravenous and subcutaneous.

Absorption—Bleomycin is poorly absorbed from the oral route. The extent of absorption from intramuscular route is low.

Bioavailability—The bioavailability of bleomycin following intramuscular administration is 30% with peak concentration attained within 30 minutes.

Distribution—Bleomycin is widely distributed with highest concentrations found in the skin and lungs where there is little metabolism. Concentrations in testes and GIT are low. Bleomycin does not cross the blood-bran-barrier. The apparent volume of distribution of bleomycin in human is 0.27±0.3 liters/kg.

Plasma Protein Binding—Bleomycin is poorly protein bound (about 1 % in human).

Metabolism—The drug is metabolized by bleomycin hydrolase, an aminopeptidase-like enzyme present in most tissues except skin and lungs.

Plasma Half-life—Estimated at 3.1 ± 1.7 hours in human; t½ is prolonged in renal impairment.

Clearance (ml/min/kg)—1.1 ± 0.3 (human).

Route(s) of Excretion—Bleomycin is excreted in urine with 68 ± 8% as unchanged drug in human.

Dialysis Status—Nondialyzable.

Toxicity and Adverse Effects—Effects such as fever, anorexia, emesis and allergic reactions may be noticed immediately following treatment. Delayed toxicity is related to skin and lungs. Bleomycin causes pulmonary fibrosis, desquamation, hyperpigmentation, and pruritic erythema. In the dog, pulmonary fibrosis may begin with interstitial pneumonia. Intramuscular or subcutaneous injection may cause pain.

Management of Overdose—Give general antidotal therapy.

Contraindications—Severe pulmonary disease; hypersensitivity to bleomycin.

Precautions—Reduce the dose of bleomycin in patients with renal impairment. Use with caution in patients with pulmonary disease. Use general anesthetics with caution in animals that had previously received bleomycin.

Drug Interactions—Toxicities caused by bleomycin may be enhanced by prior cancer chemotherapy or radiotherapy. Bleomycin may decrease the plasma levels of phenytoin and cardiac glycosides. Cisplatin causes delayed elimination of bleomycin.

Pharmaceutical Formulations—Available as bleomycin sulfate in powder of 15 and 30 units per vial.

BUMETANIDE

Bumetanide

Proprietary Names—Bumex˚; Burinex˚; Burinex-K˚ (0.5 mg bumetanide plus 573 mg potassium chloride in slow release wax core).

Chemical Class—Orthochlorosulfonamide.

Pharmacological Class—High-ceiling diuretic; loop diuretic; high efficacy diuretic.

Source—Synthetic.

Pharmacological Actions—Bumetanide causes increased urinary excretion of water and electrolytes particularly Na^+, Cl^-, Ca^{++}, Mg^{++}, and K^+. It also causes increased renal blood flow, albeit short—lived.

Mechanism of Action—Bumetanide inhibits the Na^+-K^+-$2Cl^-$ cotransport mechanism at the luminal face of the epithelial cells of the ascending limb of the loop of Henle. It also inhibits carbonic anhydrase, though weakly.

Indications—Mobilization of edema fluid of most types; reduction of excess tissue water in show animals; prophylaxis for epistaxis in horses.

Route(s) of Administration—Bumetanide may be administered orally or parenterally (intramuscular and intravenous routes).

Absorption Profile—The drug is readily absorbed from the gastrointestinal tract.

Bioavailability (oral)—81 ±18%.

Distribution—Vd = 0.13 ± 0.03 L/kg.

Plasma Protein Binding—Bumetanide is highly protein bound (99 ± 0.3%).

Metabolism—The drug is partially metabolized in the liver; 50% unmetabolized drug appear in urine.

Plasma Half-Life—0.8 ± 0.2 hours.

Clearance—2.6 ± 0.5 ml/min / kg.

Route(s) of Excretion—Urine (62 ± 20% of original dose).

Toxicity and Adverse Effects—Hypokalemic metabolic alkalosis, hyperuricemia, magnesium wasting, gastrointestinal disturbances, depression of formed elements of the blood, skin rashes paraesthesia, hepatic dysfunction, and transient deafness have all been reported. There may be cross-sensitivity with other sulfonamides.

Management of Overdose—Symptomatic and supportive.

Contraindications—Hepatic coma, anuria, pregnancy.

Precautions—Reduce the dose of bumetanide to the minimum in patients with hepatic failure. Use bumetanide with caution in gout and renal insufficiency. Bumetanide may precipitate digitalis toxicity. Therapy with bumetanide may require potassium supplement.

Drug Interactions—Bumetanide potentiates antihypertensive therapy. It competes for protein binding sites with warfarin. Renal clearance of lithium is decreased during long term therapy with bumetanide.

Pharmaceutical Formulations—Bumetanide is available as 0.5, 1.0 and 2.0 mg tablets. Solution of 0.25 mg/ml for injection is also available.

BUPRENORPHINE

Proprietary Names—Bupregesic*, Pentorel*, Norphin*, Tidigesic*, Buprenex* Temgesic*.

Chemical Class—Opioid phenanthrene alkaloid; thebaine congener;

Pharmacological Class—Narcotic (opioid) analgesic; semisynthetic opioid.

Source—Semisynthetic.

Pharmacological Action—Buprenorphine causes analgesia, sedation and respiratory depression. These effects are slower in onset and longer lasting than those produced by morphine. Buprenorphine antagonizes the respiratory depression produced by fentanyl.

Mechanism of Action—Buprenorphine is a partial μ (mu)-opioid agonist with a seemingly antagonistic action on κ (kappa)-opioid receptors.

Indications—Relief of post-operative pain. Also commonly used for analgesia in laboratory animals.

Dosage—

Bird	0.01-0.05 mg/kg IM.
Cat	0.005-0.01 mg/kg IV, SC, IM every 8-12 hours.

Dog	0.005-0.02 mg/kg SC every 6-12 hours.
Mouse	0.05-0.1 mg/kg SC every 12 hours or 2.5 mg/kg IP every 6-8 hours.
NHP	0.005-0.01 mg/kg IM, IV every 12 hours.
Rat	0.01-0.05 mg/kg IV, SC every 8-12 hours.
Sheep	0.005-0.01 mg/kg IM every 4-6 hours.
Pig	0.005-0.02 mg/kg IM, IV every 6-12 hours. Up to 0.1 mg/kg can be used for major surgical procedures.
Horse	0.01-0.02 mg/kg.
Rabbit	0.05mg/kg administered IM, IV or SC every 8-12 hours.
Guinea pig	0.05mg/kg administered IM, IV or SC every 8-12 hours.

Route(s) of Administration—Intramuscular, intravenous, subcutaneous and sublingual.

Absorption—Between 30 and 40% of buprenorphine dose is absorbed from muscular and cutaneous sites. The drug is well absorbed from the sublingual route in humans. Peak plasma concentration is attained within 5 minutes (IM) and 2 hours (sublingual).

Bioavailability—Buprenorphine undergoes extensive first pass metabolism following oral administration. Thus, oral bioavailability is poor.

Distribution—Vd = 97-187 L/kg in humans; 4.2 L/kg in rats. It is highly lipid soluble.

Plasma Protein Binding—96%.

Metabolism—Buprenorphine undergoes N-dealkylation and conjugation. It is primarily metabolized in the dog by glucuronidation to buprenorphine glucuronide.

Plasma Half-Life—3-5 hours in humans (increases with repeated use), 2.8 hours in rats.

Clearance (ml/min/kg)—23.2 in rats.

Onset of Action—10-30 minutes (parenteral routes).

Duration of Action—6-8 hours (increases to 24 hours with repeated use).

Route(s) of Excretion—Excreted mainly as unchanged drug; (70%) appear in feces via bile and (20%) appear in urine in humans. In the dog, 96% of its metabolite is eliminated through bile.

Toxicity and Adverse Effects—These have been documented in humans where buprenorphine causes sedation, dizziness, headache, sweating, nausea and vomiting. An overdose may cause CNS depression, pin point pupils, hypotension, and bradycardia.

Management of Overdose—Administer naloxone.

Contraindications—During labor; hypersensitivity to buprenorphine or any component.

Precautions—Buprenorphine may produce withdrawal syndrome in patients who have been on morphine-like drugs for several weeks. Use with caution in patients with hepatic dysfunction.

Drug Interactions—Prior administration of naloxone abolishes the respiratory depressant effects of buprenorphine. Benzodiazepines and barbiturates increase its CNS and respiratory depressant effects.

Pharmaceutical Formulations—Available as buprenorphine hydrochloride in 0.3 mg/ml solutions for injection and 0.2 mg sublingual tablets (for humans).

BUSULFAN

Busulfan

Proprietary Names—Myleran®.

Chemical Class—Alkylsulfonate.

Pharmacological Class—Antineoplastic drug.

Source—Synthetic.

Stability and Storage—Busulfan tablets should be stored at room temperature in well-closed containers.

Pharmacological Actions—Busulfan has bifunctional properties and its action is pronounced on cells of the granulocytic series. It is cytotoxic, mutagenic and carcinogenic (leukemogenic). It causes myelosuppression at low doses.

Mechanism of Action—Busulfan forms highly reactive carbonium ion intermediates which react with strongly neucleophilic substituents like phosphate, amino,—SH, OH, COOH and imidazole groups to form covalent bonds. The target molecule is thus alkylated. The N-7 position of guanine in DNA is highly susceptible. Alkylation of guanine in the DNA leads to cross linkage of DNA strands, linking of DNA to a closely associated protein, base pairing of guanine with thymine instead of cytosine, or breakage of the DNA strand.

Indications—Adjunctive therapy of chronic granulocytic leukemia in small animals.

Dosages—3 to 4 mg/m² daily.

Route(s) of Administration—Per os.

Absorption—Busulfan is rapidly and completely absorbed from the GIT. Peak plasma concentration is attained within 4 hours.

Distribution—Vd = 0.99 ± 0.23 (human).

Plasma Protein Binding—14% (human).

Metabolism—Busulfan is extensively metabolized in the liver to several metabolites that are excreted in urine.

Plasma Half-life—2.6 ± 0.5.

Clearance (ml/min/kg)—4.5 ± 0.9.

Route(s) of Excretion—Busulfan is excreted mostly as methanesulfonic acid in urine with 1% as unchanged drug.

Toxicity and Adverse Effects—Myelosuppression is the major adverse effect of busulfan. Pulmonary fibrosis has been reported in humans. Hyperuricemia and renal damage due to precipitation of urates as a result of rapid destruction of cells have been reported during initial phase of treatment of chronic granulocytic leukemia.

Management of Overdose—Give supportive therapy

Contraindications—Hypersensitivity to busulfan; preexisting severe bone marrow depression.

Precautions—The risk associated with its use in pregnancy must be weighed against desired benefit. Monitor leukocyte levels during therapy with busulfan. Handle the drug with extreme caution.

Drug Interactions—Additive bone marrow depression will result if busulfan is used with other bone marrow depressants. Hepatotoxicity may result if used with thioguanine.

Pharmaceutical Formulations—Busulfan is available in 2 mg tablets.

BUTORPHANOL

Proprietary Names—Stadol* (Human preparation), Torbugesic*, Torbutrol*.

Chemical Class—Morphinan derivative.

Pharmacological Class—Opioid partial agonist, opioid (narcotic) analgesic, semi synthetic opioid.

Source—Semi synthetic.

Stability and Storage—Store butorphanol formulations at room temperature and protected from light.

Pharmacological Actions—Butorphanol produces analgesia, sedation, respiratory depression, and cough suppression. Its analgesic potency is 4-7 times that of morphine; 15-30 times that of pentazocine and 30-50 times that of meperidine on a weight basis. Its antitussive potency is 100 times that of codeine, 4 times that of morphine. Butorphanol antagonizes the actions of true opioid agonists like morphine. Its antagonistic potency is 30 times that of pentazocine and 1/40th that of naloxone. It causes CNS stimulation in horses and dogs at high doses.

Butorphanol

Mechanism of Action—Butorphanol activates kappa and sigma opioid receptors to induce agonistic effects. It is a weak antagonist at μ (mu)-opioid receptors.

Indications—Suppression of chronic non-productive cough associated with infections and inflammation of respiratory tracts in dogs; control of visceral pain associated with colic in horses; preanaesthetic medication in small animals.

Dosage—

Horse: 0.2 mg/kg.

Small animal: 0.1-0.4 mg/kg IM, IV or SC (or 0.5-1.0 mg/kg orally 2-3 times a day).

Route(s) of Administration—Butorphanol may be administered parenterally (intramuscular, intravenous, subcutaneous) and orally (in small animals). Administration by nasal route is undertaken in humans.

Absorption—Butorphanol is rapidly and completely absorbed from the gastrointestinal tract but it undergoes extensive first pass effect. It is completely absorbed from muscular sites. Peak effect is attained within 0.5-1 hour following intramuscular injection.

Bioavailability—Oral bioavailability of butorphanol is poor because of extensive first pass metabolism.

Distribution—Butorphanol is widely distributed into body tissues and fluids. It crosses the placenta and is distributed into milk. Highest levels are found in the liver, kidney and intestines.

Plasma Protein Binding—Butorphanol is highly protein bound (80%) in humans.

Metabolism—The drug is hydroxylated in the liver. It is also dealkylated and conjugated to inactive metabolites.

Plasma Half-Life—3 hours.

Onset of Action—3 minutes (IV) in horses.

Peak Action—15-30 minutes (IV) in horses.

Duration of Action—4 hours in humans but 15-90 minutes in horses.

Route(s) of Excretion—Butorphanol is excreted mainly in urine with 5% as unchanged drug; 11-14% of the dose are excreted in bile.

Toxicity and Adverse Effects—Drowsiness, weakness, sweating, feelings of floating and nausea have been reported in humans. Restlessness, ataxia and shivering have been observed in horses. Overdose will depress respiratory, cardiac and CNS functions. Nystagmus, salivation, seizures and decreased gastrointestinal motility have been observed in horses given very high doses of butorphanol. The drug causes physical dependence in humans. This effect is minimal in animals.

Management of Overdose—Administer naloxone.

Contraindications—Congestive heart failure, myocardial infarction, hypersensitivity to butorphanol.

Precautions—Use butorphanol cautiously in patients with hypothyroidism, severe renal insufficiency, adrenocorticoid insufficiency, old and severely debilitated patients and dogs with heartworm disease. Use the drug with extreme caution in patients with head trauma, increased CSF pressure and CNS dysfunction. Do not use butorphanol in productive cough.

Drug Interactions—CNS depressants, skeletal muscle relaxants and monoamine oxidase (MAO) inhibitors may increase butorphanol toxicity. Butorphanol is incompatible with pentobarbital sodium. It is beneficial to combine butorphanol with xylazine (0.66 mg/kg) or detomidine (2.5-5 mcg/kg) in horses.

Pharmaceutical Formulations—Available as butorphanol tartrate in solutions of 0.5 mg/ml and 10 mg/ml for injection; also available in 1 mg and 5 mg tablets.

CALCITRIOL

Synonyms—1,25 dihydroxycholecalciferol; Vitamin D; 1,25-dihydroxyvitamin D_3.

Proprietary Name—Rocaltrol®.

Chemical Class—Steroid.

Pharmacological Class—Vitamin.

Source—Natural.

Solubility, Stability and Storage—Calcitriol is sensitive to light; store its formulations in tight light resistant containers.

Pharmacological Actions—Calcitriol increases the amount of calcium and phosphorus circulating in the bloodstream by enhancing the absorption of both calcium and phosphate from the gastrointestinal tract, promoting release of calcium and phosphate from the bones, and preventing renal excretion of calcium and phosphate. Calcitriol functions in concert with parathyroid hormone (PTH) and calcitonin to regulate serum calcium and phosphorous levels. It also regulates the immune system and aids haematopoiesis.

Mechanism of Action—In the intestinal epithelium, calcitriol induces the expression of calbindin D_{28K}, a protein involved in intestinal calcium absorption. It decreases excessive serum phosphatase levels, enhances lysyl oxidase activity and collagen cross-linking of matrix during mineralization of bone organic matrix.

Indications—Management of hypocalcaemia; reduction of elevated parathyroid hormone levels associated with kidney failure.

Dosages—No information; check package insert.

Route(s) of Administration—Per os.

Absorption—Calcitriol is rapidly absorbed from oral site.

Onset of Action—2-6 hours (human).

Duration of Action—3-5 days (human).

Metabolism—Calcitriol is ddegraded to 1, 24, 25-trihydroxycholecalciferol and 1, 24, 25-trihydroxyergocalciferol.

Plasma Half-life—3-8 hours (human).

Route(s) of Excretion—Calcitriol is eliminated principally in bile and feces. About 4-6% of the dose is excreted in urine.

Toxicity and Adverse Effects—Hypervitaminosis D causes excessive Ca mobilization which may lead to the formation of calcium phosphate crystals in soft tissues. Hypercalcaemia may also result in vasoconstriction. Polyuria, polydipsia, lethargy, vomition, cardiac arrhythmias, and neurologic signs may be observed.

Contraindication—Hyperphosphatemia (>6 mg/dl).

Precautions—Monitor blood calcium levels and discontinue calcitriol administration temporarily.

Drug Interactions—Concomitant use with magnesium-containing antacids gives additive effects.

Pharmaceutical Formulations—Calcitriol is available singly in 0.25 mcg and 0.5 mcg capsules; and in 1 mcg/ml solution for injection. It is also available as part of multivitamin preparations.

CALCIUM DISODIUM EDETATE

Synonyms—Edetate Calcium Disodium; Calcium disodium edathamil; Calcium EDTA (CaEDTA); Calcium edentate; Calcium disodium ethylenediaminetetra-acetate; Sodium calcium edentate.

Proprietary Names—Calcium disodium versenate®.

Pharmacological Class—Chelating agent; heavy metal antagonist.

Source—Synthetic.

Solubility, Stability and Storage—CaEDTA is freely soluble in water and slightly soluble in alcohol. Its formulations can be stored at room temperature. CaEDTA injection is compatible with normal saline or 5% dextrose.

Pharmacological Actions—CaEDTA chelates divalent and trivalent metals. This results in the mobilization and excretion of the metals.

Mechanism of Action—CaEDTA forms a stable water soluble complex with divalent and trivalent metals which displace the Ca in CaEDTA.

Indications—CaEDTA is used as an antidote in heavy metal poisoning especially lead poisoning. It also binds cadmium, copper, iron and manganese, but to a much lesser extent than either lead or zinc. CaEDTA is relatively ineffective for use in treating mercury, gold or arsenic poisoning.

Dosages—

Bird	35 mg/kg twice a day for 5 days; repeat in 3-4 days if necessary.
Dog, cat	100 mg/kg every 6 hours for 5 consecutive days. Dilute with 5% dextrose saline to obtain 10 mg/ml. A second course may be given if necessary after a five day break.
Bovine	110 mg/kg IP, IM in 1-2% solution in 5% glucose; skip 2 days and repeat for 2 days for up to 10-14 days.
Horse	75 mg/kg IV slowly in saline daily for 4-5 days (may divide daily dose into 2-3 administrations per day). Stop therapy for 2 days and repeat for another 4-5 days. Give adequate supportive and nutritional therapy.

Route(s) of Administration—CaEDTA may be administered parenterally (intramuscular, intravenous and subcutaneous). The subcutaneous route is preferred in small animals.

Absorption—CaEDTA is well absorbed from muscular or cutaneous sites.

Distribution—The drug is distributed primarily in the extracellular fluid. It does not penetrate erythrocytes or enter the CNS in appreciable amounts.

Metabolism—CaEDTA is not metabolized.

Plasma Half-life—This varies with the route of administration; t½ is 20-60 minutes following intravenous injection in humans but 1.5 hours with intramuscular injection.

Route(s) of Excretion—CaEDTA is rapidly excreted in urine, either as unchanged drug or chelated with metals.

Toxicity and Adverse Effects—CaEDTA causes renal tubular necrosis. This is the most serious adverse effect associated with its use. In dogs, CaEDTA also causes depression and gastrointestinal symptoms characterized by vomiting, and diarrhea. Chronic administration may cause zinc deficiency. Lethal dose in dogs is 12 g/kg. Intramuscular administration causes pain.

Management of Overdose/Toxicity—Adverse effects associated with the gastrointestinal function can be alleviated by zinc supplementation.

Contraindications—Severe renal failure; Anuria.

Precautions—Use cautiously in patients with reduced renal function. Ca EDTA may accumulate in patients with renal impairment. This can increase its nephrotoxic potential. Oral administration may increase the absorption of lead.

Drug Interactions—Concurrent administration of CaEDTA with zinc insulin preparations will decrease the sustained action of the insulin preparation. The renal toxicity of CaEDTA may be enhanced by the concomitant administration of glucocorticoids and nephrotoxic compounds such as aminoglycosides and amphotericin B.

Pharmaceutical Formulations—CaEDTA is available in 50 mg/ml and 200 mg/ml solution for injection. Formulations contain 5.3 mEq of sodium per gram of CaEDTA.

CAMBENDAZOLE

Cambendazole

Proprietary Names—Eqiben®, Noviben®, Bonlam®—

Chemical Class—Benzimidazole compound.

Pharmacological Class—Anthelmintic.

Source—synthetic.

Pharmacological Actions—Cambendazole can eliminate the major adult parasite including *Bunostomum, Chabertia, Cooperia, Haemonchus, Nematodirus, Oesophagostomum, Ostertagia, Strongyloides* and *Trichostrongylus* species in sheep and cattle. It is also effective against *Stronglyes, Oxyuris, Ascaris* species in horses. Cambendazole is also ovicidal and larvicidal.

Mechanism of Action—Uncertain; cambendazole is considered to inhibit microtubule polymerization in susceptible helminthes by binding to β-tubulin. This action results in progressive energy depletion, inhibition of waste products and degenerative alteration in the integument and intestinal cells. Binding to parasite tubulin takes place at a lower concentration than does the binding to mammalian tubulin.

Indications—Treatment of thread worm, pin worm, nodular worm and lung worm infection in horses, sheep, cattle, pigs as well as parasites of the gastrointestinal and respiratory tracts of birds.

Dosages—20mg/kg (sheep and horses); 25mg/kg (cattle); 20-40mg/kg (pig).

Route(s) of Administration—Per os.

Absorption—Cambendazole is poorly absorbed. Peak plasma concentration is attained within 2-4 hours.

Withdrawal Period—28days for cattle and 21days for sheep.

Route(s) of Excretion—Cambendazole is eliminated in feces (major) and urine.

Toxicity and Adverse Effects—Anorexia, and listlessness has been observed in cattle at three times the therapeutic dose and mild transient diarrhea in horses at doses above 300mg/kg. A dose of 600mg/kg is lethal to cattle. Cambendazole has teratogenic effect in ewe treated on 2nd-4TH week of pregnancy. It causes reduced lambing rate when used in early (10-14days) pregnancy.

Contraindications—First month of pregnancy in sheep.

Precautions—The slaughter clearance periods are 28 days for cattle and 21days for sheep.

Drug Interactions—Cambendazole is compatible with other drugs.

Pharmaceutical Formulations—Cambendazole is available as suspension for drenching and as powder for administering in feed; also available as paste for horses and cattle.

CARBENICILLIN

Carbenicillin

Synonyms—Carindacillin sodium; indanylcarbenicillin sodium.

Proprietary Names—Pyopen˙; Geocillin˙ (carbenicillin indanyl sodium)—

Chemical Class—6-aminopenicillanic acid derivative.

Pharmacological Class—Carboxypenicillin; Anti-pseudomonas penicillin.

Source—Semisynthetic.

Solubility, Stability and Storage—Carbenicillin is soluble in water and alcohol. Its formulations should be stored below 30°C and protected from light.

Pharmacological Actions—Carbenicillin is bactericidal to *Pseudomonas aeruginosa*, indole positive strains of Proteus and Enterobacter species.

Mechanism of Action—Carbenicillin binds to one or more of the penicillin binding proteins to inhibit transpeptidase enzyme action thus blocking the synthesis of peptidoglycan, a component of bacteria cell wall. This may be followed by activation of autolytic enzymes in the cell wall which causes lysis of the bacteria.

Indications—Treatment of infections caused by *Pseudomonas aeruginosa*, Proteus species and certain strains of *E. coli* in small animals usually in combination with aminoglycoside antibiotics; treatment of urinary tract and prostrate infections using the indanyl ester; treatment of infections caused by susceptible microbes in psittacine birds.

Dosages—

Dog, cat.   55-100 mg/kg orally every 8 hours

Psittacine bird 100-200mg/kg orally twice daily for 5-10 days.

Route(s) of Administration—Carbenicillin dosage forms may be administered orally and parenterally (intramuscular and). Carbenicillin indanyl sodium is administered orally.

Absorption—Between 30-40% of carbenicillin oral dose is absorbed in humans. Carbenicillin is unstable in stomach acid. Peak plasma concentration is attained within 0.5 hours but is inadequate for treatment of systemic infections.

Bioavailability—Oral bioavailability of carbenicillin is low.

Distribution—Vd (L/kg) = 0.18 in humans, 0.19 in dogs, and 0.4 in horses. Carbenicillin crosses the placenta but is almost excluded from the cerebrospinal fluid except when meninges are inflamed. It is secreted into milk and bile. Its concentration in milk rises in mastitis but is insufficient for treatment.

Plasma Protein Binding—50% in human beings.

Metabolism—Between 2-5% of the dose of carbenicillin is hydrolyzed to inactive products in humans. Carbenicillin can be inactivated by beta lactamase enzymes.

Plasma Half-Life (Hours)—Human, 1.0 ± 0.2 (higher in uremia, hepatitis, neonate and premature); dog, 0. 75-1.25; horse, 1.0-1.5.

Clearance (ml/min/kg) is 0.68 ± 0.15 in humans; 1.8 in dogs; 4.6 in horses.

Withdrawal Period—Two days before milking.

Route(s) of Excretion—Eliminated mainly in urine with 82 ± 9% as unchanged drug.

Dialysis Status—Dialyzable.

Toxicity and Adverse Effects—Skin rash, urticaria, hematologic disorders, nausea, vomition, diarrhea, hypokalemia and abnormal aggregation of platelets are observed at therapeutic doses. Overdose may cause neuromuscular hypersensitivity and convulsions.

Management of Overdose/Toxicity—Set up hemodialysis. Give supportive and symptomatic treatment—

Contraindications—Hypersensitivity to carbenicillin, the penicillins, their products, or components

Precautions—Avoid the use of carbenicillin in patients with severe renal failure or do not exceed 2g every 12 hours in such patients. Use carbenicillin cautiously in patients with history of hypersensitivity to cephalosporins. Do not use the milk of treated animals for human food within 2 days after treatment has stopped. Do not mix carbenicillin with aminoglycoside antibiotics in the same syringe.

Drug Interactions—Carbenicillin is synergistic with gentamicin against pseudomonas infections but do not mix both drugs physically. Probenecid increases the half-life of carbenicillin.

Pharmaceutical Formulations—Available as carbenicillin disodium in vials of 1g and 5g for injection. Also available as carbenicillin indanyl sodium in 382 mg film coated tablets. No specific veterinary formulations of carbenicillin are available.

CARBIMAZOLE

Proprietary Names—Neo-mercazole®; Thyrozole®; Carbazole®; Carbotiroid®; Neo-Morphazole®; Neo-Thyreostat®; Neo-Tireol®.

Chemical Class—Thioureylene compound.

Pharmacological Class—Antithyroid drug.

Source—Synthetic.

Solubility, Stability and Storage—Carbimazole is soluble 1 in 500 of water, and 1 in 50 of ethanol.

Pharmacological Actions—Carbimazole inhibits the synthesis of thyroid hormones. This results in hypothyroidism and reduction of basal metabolic rate—

Mechanism of Action—Carbimazole inhibits thyroid peroxidase enzyme thereby preventing the oxidation of iodine and iodination of tyrosine.

Indications—Treatment of feline hyperthyroidism.

Carbimazole

Dosages—The recommended doses are 2.5-5 mg orally every 8-12 hours initially, followed by a maintenance dose of 5-20 mg orally every 24 hours or divided every 12 hours.

Route(s) of Administration—Per os.

Absorption—Carbimazole is readily and almost completely absorbed.

Peak Action—This may take weeks; usually until existing hormone stores are exhausted.

Duration of Action—12-24 hours—

Distribution—Vd of active metabolite, thiamazole is 0.5 L/kg. Carbimazole is widely distributed. It enters milk and crosses the placenta. Carbimazole concentrates in the thyroid gland.

Plasma Protein Binding—Less bound than propylthiouracil.

Metabolism—Carbimazole is activated to thiamazole.

Plasma Half-Life—6-10 hours.

Route(s) of Excretion—Carbimazole is eliminated mainly in urine, mainly as 3-methyl-2-thiohydantoin, the major metabolite. About 3% of a dose is eliminated in faeces.

Toxicity and Adverse Effects—Agranulocytosis is the most serious adverse effect caused by carbimazole. However, this is rare. Minor side effects include nausea, paraesthesia, joint pain, rash and loss or depigmentation of hair. Goiter is produced following excessive doses.

Management of Overdose—Give supportive and symptomatic therapy.

Contraindications—Lactation, tracheal obstruction, and hypersensitivity to Carbimazole.

Precautions—Undertake frequent leukocyte count during therapy. Reduce the dose during pregnancy to avoid fetal goiter.

Drug Interactions—The use of carbimazole and other thionamides during the week before and after radioiodine therapy may hinder response to radiation.

Pharmaceutical Formulations—Carbimazole is available in 5 mg tablets.

CARBOPLATIN

Carboplatin

Synonyms—CBDCA, JM-8.

Proprietary Names—Paraplatin ®.

Chemical Class—Inorganic platinum-containing complex.

Pharmacological Class—Antineoplastic drug; Anticancer drug; Cytotoxic drug.

Source—Synthetic.

Stability and Storage—Carboplatin dosage forms should be stored at room temperature and protected from direct sunlight. Reconstitute in 5 ml normal saline immediately before use. Reconstituted solutions are stable for 8 hours at room temperature. Discard unclear solutions or those with precipitates. Do not administer with aluminum containing needles or intravenous sets.

Pharmacological Actions—The actions of carboplatin are similar to those of cisplatin. They include cytotoxic, mutagenic, carcinogenic, teratogenic, myelosuppressive and emetogenic properties. Carboplatin is less reactive than cisplatin.

Mechanism of Action—Similar to those of cisplatin. It binds covalently to DNA forming interstrand and intrastrand linkages with resultant inhibition of DNA replication and transcription as well as breaks and miscoding.

Indications—Adjunctive treatment of estrogenic sarcomas usually post amputation. Treatment should be started within 7 days of amputation. Carboplatin therapy does not require forced saline diuresis.

Dosages: 300 mg/m² intravenously over 15 minutes every 3 weeks.

Route(s) of Administration—Intravenous.

Distribution—Carboplatin distributes rapidly into tissues and attains high concentrations in kidneys, liver, skin and tumor tissue.

Plasma Protein Binding—Carboplatin is not bound to plasma protein.

Metabolism—The drug is degraded to aquated and hydroxylated products.

Plasma Half-life—2-6 hours for active drug in humans.

Clearance (ml/min/kg)—1.5 ± 0.3 in humans.

Route(s) of Excretion—The drug is eliminated in urine with $77 \pm 5\%$ as unchanged drug in humans.

Toxicity and Adverse Effects—Bone marrow depression with severe leukopenia and thrombocytopenia is the dose-limiting adverse effect of carboplatin therapy. Other adverse effects listed for cisplatin occur with less frequency.

Contraindications—Severe bone marrow depression; hypersensitivity to carboplatin.

Precautions—Use carboplatin with caution in patients with pre-existing myelosuppression, active infection, renal and/or hepatic impairment.

Drug Interactions—Aminoglycoside antibiotics and other nephrotoxic drugs may enhance the nephrotoxic potential of carboplatin. Previous treatment with cisplatin may also enhance carboplatin potential for neurotoxicity and ototoxicity. The myelosuppressive action of carboplatin may be enhanced by other myelosuppressants. Carboplatin may modify immune response to live or killed virus vaccines.

Pharmaceutical Formulations—Carboplatin is available as lyophilized powder for injection in 50 mg, 150 mg and 450 mg vials. Vials contain equal parts of mannitol.

CARPROFEN

Proprietary Names—Rimadyl®; Zenecarp®.

Chemical Class—Propionic acid derivative.

Pharmacological Class—Nonsteroidal Anti-inflammatory Drug (NSAID); Analgesic; Selective cyclo-oxygenase-2 inhibitor.

Source—Synthetic.

Solubility, Stability and Storage—Carprofen is practically insoluble in water but freely soluble in ethanol at room temperature. Store its dosage forms at room temperature.

Pharmacological Actions—Carprofen has analgesic, antipyretic and anti-inflammatory properties.

Mechanism of Action—Carprofen selectively inhibits cyclo-oxygenase-2. It only slightly inhibits cyclo-oxygenase-1.

Uses—Relief of joint or post-surgical pain in small animals.

Dosages—

Cat	4 mg/kg IV, SC.
Dog	4 mg/kg IV, SC once daily. 1-2 mg/kg PO twice daily for 7 days.
Rat	5 mg/kg SC.
Rabbit	1.5 mg/kg PO twice daily.
Pig	2-4 mg/kg IV, SC once daily.

Route(s) of Administration—Per os, intravenous and subcutaneous.

Absorption—Carprofen is readily absorbed from the gastrointestinal tract.

Bioavailability—Oral bioavailability is high (90% in dogs).

Peak Action—1-3 hours.

Distribution—Vd = 0.12-0.22 l/kg. Carprofen undergoes some enterohepatic cycling.

Plasma Protein Binding—Carprofen is highly (99%) bound to plasma protein.

Metabolism—Undergoes extensive hepatic degradation primarily via glucuronidation and oxidative processes.

Plasma Half-life—8-12 hours in the dog.

Route(s) of Excretion—About 70-80% of a dose is eliminated in feces while 10-20% is eliminated in urine.

Toxicity and Adverse Effects—There is a 1 in 1000 chances of a dog on carprofen developing nausea, appetite loss, vomiting, or diarrhea. Hepatopathy which usually occurs within the first 3 weeks of treatment and characterized by nausea, appetite loss, and/or diarrhea as well as marked elevations in liver enzymes has been reported in 1 in 5000 dogs treated with carprofen. Excess water consumption and urination may be evident in some patients developing renal failure due to action of carprofen on cyclooxygenase I. Other rare side effects (1 in 5000 or less) of carprofen include loss of balance, hyperactivity, depression, and aggression.

Management of Overdose/Toxicity—Discontinue treatment if signs of hepatopathy are suspected and then monitor the dog's liver enzyme and haematology. Dogs with hepatopathy syndrome show improvement 5-10 days after discontinuing carprofen.

Contraindications—Bleeding disorders; pre-existing hepatic and/or renal disease; hypersensitivity to carprofen or other propionic acid derivative; pregnant or nursing females.

Precautions—Hepatopathy may be a rare syndrome (1 in 5000), but it can become life-threatening if ignored. Appetite loss or other intestinal signs do not necessarily indicate a hepatopathy but since they might, it is important not to ignore these signs should they occur. Give a 2-3 day rest period when changing over to carprofen or to another NSAID from carprofen. For aspirin, give 10-14 days for a switch over. Allow at least one week between prednisone and carprofen.

Drug Interactions—Other NSAID may increase the potential for side effects if used concurrently with carprofen. Carprofen and phenobarbitone may antagonize the action of one another if used concurrently. Carprofen may reduce the actions of ACE inhibitors such as enalapril or captopril. Carprofen may reduce the saluretic and diuretic effects of furosemide and increase serum levels of digoxin.

Pharmaceutical Formulations—Carprofen is available in 25 mg, 75 mg & 100 mg scored caplets.

CEFADROXIL

Cefadroxil

Proprietary Names—Duricef°; Ultracef°; Droxyl°; Cefadrox°; Kefloxin°.

Chemical Class—Cephalosporin; 7-aminocephalosporinic acid derivative.

Pharmacological Class—First generation cephalosporin; beta-lactam antibiotic; antibacterial drug.

Source—Semisynthetic.

Solubility, Stability and Storage—Cefadroxil is soluble in water but slightly soluble in alcohol. Formulations are stable at room temperature and in moisture free environment. Reconstituted oral suspension should be stored in the refrigerator and used within 14 days.

Pharmacological Actions—Cefadroxil is bactericidal to most Gram-positive and Gram-negative bacteria.

Mechanism of Action—Cefadroxil disrupts cell wall synthesis in actively dividing organisms by inhibiting the action of transpeptidase enzymes thus blocking the synthesis of peptidoglycan, a component of bacteria cell wall. This is followed by activation of autolytic enzymes (autolysins and murein hydrolases) which eventually lyse the bacteria.

Indications—Treatment of susceptible infections of skin, soft tissues, and genitourinary tract in dogs and cats.

Dosages—

    Dog: 22 mg/kg orally two times a day for 3 days (in skin and soft tissue infections) or 7 days (in genitourinary tract infections).

    Cat: 10-20 mg/kg orally every 8-12 hours. Maximum therapy is for 30 days.

Route(s) of Administration—Per os.

Absorption—Cefadroxil is completely absorbed from the gastrointestinal tract. Absorption from equine GIT is poor and erratic. Peak plasma concentration is attained within 70-90 minutes in humans, but 1-2 hours in dogs. Absorption is not hindered by food.

Bioavailability—Oral bioavailability of Cefadroxil is 100%.

Distribution—Vd = 0.22 ± 0.05 L/kg. Cefadroxil is widely distributed. It penetrates body tissues and fluids including pericardium and synovial fluids. It crosses the placenta; gets into breast milk but it is almost excluded from the cerebrospinal fluid except when the meninges are inflamed.

Plasma Protein Binding—Cefadroxil is poorly (20%) protein bound in humans and dogs.

Metabolism—The drug is not metabolized.

Plasma Half-Life—1.1 ± 0.2 hours in humans; 2 hours in dogs and 3 hours in cats. In humans, plasma half-life of cefadroxil is 20-24 hours in renal failure.

Clearance (ml/min/kg)—2.6 ± 1.6 (lower in uremia).

Route(s) of Excretion—Urine (93 ± 4% as unchanged drug).

Dialysis Status—Dialyzable.

Toxicity and Adverse Effects—At therapeutic doses, cefadroxil may cause skin rash, diarrhea, nausea, vomition, gastritis, bloating, and bleeding which may be due to hypoprothrombinemia, thrombocytopenia, and/or platelet dysfunction. It also causes bone marrow depression characterized by granulocytopenia at therapeutic doses. An overdose may cause positive Coomb's reaction and acute renal tubular necrosis. Prolonged use may produce superinfection.

Management of Overdose/Toxicity—Set up hemodialysis; give symptomatic and supportive therapy.

Contraindications—Hypersensitivity to cefadroxil, other cephalosporins, the penicillins, their products or components.

Precautions—Reduce the dose of cefadroxil in patients with renal impairment.

Drug Interactions—Probenecid reduces excretion of cephalosporins. Furosemide and aminoglycoside antibiotics may increase the risk of nephrotoxicity.

Pharmaceutical Formulations—Available as cefadroxil monohydrate in oral tablets of 50 mg, 100 mg, 200 mg, and 1g and in oral suspension containing 50 mg/ml in 15 or 50 ml bottles for veterinary use. Available in 500 mg capsules; 1 g tablets; 125 mg/5 ml, 250 mg/5 ml and 500 mg/5 ml oral suspension for human use.

CEFAZOLIN

Proprietary Names—Ancef'; Kefzol'; Zolicef'.

Chemical Class—7-Aminocephalosporinic acid derivative.

Pharmacological Class—Cephalosporin; beta-lactam antibiotic; first generation cephalosporin.

Source—Semi-synthetic.

Solubility, Stability and Storage—Cefazolin is readily soluble in water but slightly soluble in alcohol. The products of cefazolin are photolabile. The powder for injection may be stored at room temperature not exceeding 40°C. The product deteriorates readily following reconstitution. Reconstituted product should be immediately frozen and used within 90 days; 96 hours if refrigerated, or 24 hours if kept at room temperature. The solution for injection is preferably stored frozen. Cefazolin products are compatible with normal saline and other parenteral fluids but are incompatible with some barbiturates, some antibacterial drugs such as tetracycline, erythromycin, polymyxin B and vitamin C.

Cefazolin

Pharmacological Actions—Cefazolin is bactericidal to Gram-positive bacilli, some Gram-positive cocci, and Gram-negative bacilli including *E coli*, *Proteus* and *Klebsiella*. It is more susceptible to cephlosporniase than cephalothin.

Mechanism of Action—Cefazolin disrupts cell wall synthesis by inhibiting the actions of transpeptidase enzymes thus blocking the synthesis of peptidoglycan, a component of bacteria cell wall. This is followed by inactivation of autolytic enzymes (autolysins and murein hydrolases) which eventually lyse the bacteria cell.

Indications—Treatment of susceptible infections in which short-acting first generation cephalosporin is indicated.

Dosages—

Bird	25-50 mg/kg IM, IV every 12 hours.
Cat	15-25 mg/kg IM, IV, SC every 4-8 hours.
Dog	15-25 mg/kg IM, IV, SC every 6-8 hours.
Guinea pig	100 mg/kg IM every 12 hours.
NHP	25 mg/kg IM, IV every 12 hours for 7-10 days.
Horse	11mg / kg every 12 hours; 20mg / kg every 8-12 hours in foals.

Route(s) of Administration—Cefazolin is administered parenterally (intramuscular, intravenous and subcutaneous).

Absorption—The drug is poorly absorbed from the gastrointestinal tract. Peak plasma concentration is attained within 0.5-2 hours after intramuscular injection in humans or 0.5 hours in dogs.

Distribution—Vd (L/kg) = 0.12 ± 0.03 in humans (higher in uremia and neonates); 0.7 in dogs; 0.19 in horses; 0.165 in calves. Cefazolin distributes into milk and crosses the placenta. Penetration into CSF is poor.

Plasma Protein Binding—Protein binding vary widely among species; 89 ± 2% in humans (lower in uremia, neonates, and children); 16-28% in dogs; 4-8 % in horses.

Plasma Half-Life—This may depend on species and route of administration. It is evaluated at 1.8 ± 0.4 hours in humans (higher in uremia and neonates, lower in pregnancy); 48 minutes in dogs; 49-99 minutes in calf (IM) or 38 minutes (IV); 84 minutes (IM) in horses.

Clearance (ml/min/kg)—Humans, 0.95 ± 0.17; Dogs, 10.4; Horses, 5.51.

Route(s) of Excretion—Urine is the main route with 80 ± 16 % of the dose eliminated as unchanged drug.

Dialysis Status—Cefazolin is dialyzable.

Toxicity and Adverse Effects—Cefazolin is relatively well tolerated. Diarrhea may be observed in 10% of cases. It may cause skin rash or urticaria, seizure, hematologic disorders (such as leukopenia, neutropenia, and thrombocytopenia), chlolestatic jaundice, and elevated hepatic enzymes at therapeutic doses. Overdose may cause neuromuscular hyper irritability, positive Coomb`s reaction and nephrotoxicity.

Management of Overdose/Toxicity—Set up hemodialysis. Give symptomatic and supportive therapy.

Contraindications—Hypersensitivity to penicillin or cephalosporin, or their components.

Precautions—The dose of cefazolin should be reduced in patients with renal insufficiency. Prolong use of the drug may produce superinfection. Do not use the products of treated animals for human food during the period of treatment.

Drug Interactions—Probenecid increases the half-life of cefazolin. Aminoglycoside antibiotics are synergistic with it but may increase the risk of nephrotoxicity.

Pharmaceutical Formulations—Available as cefazolin sodium in 500 mg and 1 gm solution for injection; and 250 mg, 1 g, 5 g, 10 g and 20 g powder for injection. One gram of formulation contains 2 mEq of sodium.

CEFOPERAZONE

Proprietary Names—Cefobid;˙; Magnamycin˙; Cefomycin˙.

Chemical Class—Cephalosporin; 7-aminocephalosporinic acid derivative.

Pharmacological Class—Third generation cephalosporin; beta-lactam antibiotic; antibacterial drug.

Source—Semisynthetic.

Solubility, Stability and Storage—Cefoperazone is readily soluble in water but slightly soluble in alcohol. The powder for injection is photolabile but can be stored at room temperature of 25⁰C and below. Reconstituted product is viable for varying periods (24 hours at room

Cefoperazone

temperature; 5 days with refrigeration and 3-5 weeks when frozen). Cefoperazone is compatible with most parenteral fluids. It is physically incompatible with aminoglycoside antibiotics.

Pharmacological Actions—Cefoperazone is bactericidal to many Gram-positive and Gram-negative bacteria. It is less active than cefotaxime and moxalactam but more active than both drugs against *Pseudomonas aeruginosa*. Cefoperazone is slightly susceptible to beta-lactamase.

Mechanism of Action—Cefoperazone disrupts cell wall synthesis in actively dividing organisms by inhibiting the action of transpeptidase enzymes thus blocking the synthesis of peptidoglycan, a component of bacteria cell wall. This is followed by activation of autolytic enzymes (autolysins and murein hydrolases] which eventually lyse the bacteria.

Indications—Treatment of serious infections caused by susceptible Enterobacteriaceae when aminoglycoside antibiotics are contraindicated.

Dosage—Horse, 30-50 mg/kg every 8-12 hours.

Route(s) of Administration—Intramuscular; intravenous.

Absorption—Cefoperazone attains peak plasma concentration within 1-2 hours following intramuscular injection. It is not absorbed from the gastrointestinal tract.

Distribution—Vd = 0.09 ± 0.01 L/kg (higher in cirrhosis). It is widely distributed to body fluids and tissues with high concentration in bile (the major route of excretion). It crosses the placenta, appears in breast milk, and attains low levels in the CSF.

Plasma Protein Binding—Cefoperazone is highly (89-93%) protein bound.

Plasma Half-Life—The value is determined by several factors such as species, disease conditions, age etc. It is evaluates at 2.1 ± 0.3 hours in humans. This value is higher in cirrhosis, hepatitis and in the aged.

Clearance—1.2 ± 0.1 ml/min/kg in humans (lower in hepatitis).

Route(s) of Excretion—Cefoperazone is eliminated in bile (70-75% of dose) and urine (29 ± 4% as unchanged drug).

Dialysis Status—Dialyzable.

Toxicity and Adverse Effects—Cefoperazone may cause cutaneous maculopapular and erythematous rash at therapeutic dose. It may also cause diarrhea, nausea, vomition, dyspepsia, colitis, and bleeding due to hypoprothrombinemia. The drug causes pain and induration at injection site. Overdose may cause positive Coomb's reaction and nephrotoxicity. Mild and transient increases in liver enzymes have been reported in some humans.

Management of Overdose/Toxicity—Give symptomatic and supportive therapy.

Contraindications—Hypersensitivity to cefoperazone, the cephalosporins, or their component.

Precautions—Lower the dose of cefoperazone in hepatic dysfunction or biliary obstruction. A low incidence of cross hypersensitivity to penicillins exists. Use cefoperazone cautiously in pre-existing bleeding disorder or in patients receiving anticoagulants. Cefoperazone should not be mixed with aminoglycoside antibiotics in the same syringe.

Drug Interactions—In humans, cefoperazone produces a disulfiram-like reaction in the presence of alcohol within 48-72 hours after treatment. It exhibits synergism with aminoglycosides and β-lactamase inhibitors (e.g. clavulanic acid).

Pharmaceutical Formulations—Available as cefoperazone sodium in 1 g, 2 g powder for injection after reconstitution. It is also available in 1 g and 2 g premixed infusion fluid. One gram of formulation contains 1.5 mEq of sodium. No specific veterinary formulations of cefoperazone are currently available.

CEFOTAXIME

Proprietary Names—Claforan˙; Oritazim˙; Omnatax˙.

Chemical Class—Cephalosporin; 7-aminocephalosporinic acid derivative.

Cefotaxime

Pharmacological Class—Third generation cephalosporin; beta-lactam antibiotic; antibacterial drug; aminothiazolyl cephalosporin; antimicrobial agent.

Source—Semisynthetic.

Solubility, Stability and Storage—Cefotaxime is sparingly soluble in water and alcohol. Its powder for injection is photolabile but can be stored at room temperature. The solution for injection is preferably stored frozen. Cefotaxime products are compatible with parenteral fluids. Products may turn dark in color with loss of potency. The normal color of the powder is white or off-white.

Pharmacological Actions—Cefotaxime is bactericidal to many Gram-positive and Gram-negative bacteria. It is highly resistant to bacterial β-lactamases. Many anaerobes such as *Bacteroides fragilis*, *Clostridium* species are susceptible.

Mechanism of Action—Cefotaxime disrupts cell wall synthesis in actively dividing organisms by inhibiting the action of transpeptidase enzymes thus blocking the synthesis of peptidoglycan, a component of bacteria cell wall. This is followed by activation of autolytic enzymes (autolysins and murein hydrolases) which eventually lyse the bacteria.

Indications—Treatment of infections caused by organisms susceptible to third generation cephalosporins in animal species. Treatment of meningitis caused by Gram-negative enteric bacteria and other infections such as pneumonia caused by *Pneumococcus*, and *H. influenzae* (including strains that produce β-lactamase), or *Staphylococci* in human beings.

Dosages—

Dog, cat:	25-50mg/kg every 8 hours.
Foal:	20-30mg/kg every 6 hour.
Bird:	50-100mg/kg three times daily.
Reptile:	20-40 mg/kg IM once daily for 7-14 days.

Route(s) of Administration—Intramuscular; intravenous.

Absorption—Cefotaxime is readily absorbed from IM site. Peak plasma concentration is attained within 0.5 hours. It is poorly absorbed from the gastrointestinal tract.

Bioavailability—Dog, 87% (IM); 100% (subcutaneous). Cat, 93-98% (IM).

Distribution—Vd = 0.23 ± 0.06 L/kg in humans (higher in cirrhosis); dog, 0.48L/kg. Cefotaxime is widely distributed. It appears in bone, aqueous humor and other body fluids like synovial, pericardial, ascitic, and prostatic fluids. Cefotaxime crosses the placenta. It enters the cerebrospinal fluid when meninges are inflamed. It attains low concentration in milk.

Plasma Protein Binding—36% in humans.

Metabolism—Cefotaxime is metabolized by acetylation to an active deacetylcefotaxime with a plasma half-life of 1.5-1.9 hours.

Plasma Half-Life—Humans, 1.1 ± 0.3 hours (higher in uremia and cirrhosis). Dogs, 0.75 hours (IV); 1.72 hours (subcutaneous). Cats, 1 hour.

Clearance (ml/min/kg)—Humans, 3.7 ± 0.6 (lower in uremia, cirrhosis and females); Dogs, 10.5 (IV); Cats, 3.0.

Route(s) of Excretion—Urine is the main route of elimination with 50 ± 5% as unchanged drug.

Dialysis Status—20-50% dialyzable.

Toxicity and Adverse Effects—At therapeutic doses, cefotaxime may cause skin rash, diarrhea, nausea, vomition and colitis. It may also cause bleeding (due to hypoprothrombinemia especially in malnourished subjects) and bone marrow depression (characterized by granulocytopenia and anemia). Cefotaxime causes phlebitis. An overdose may cause positive Coomb's reaction and nephrotoxicity.

Management of Toxicity/Toxicity—Set up hemodialysis; give symptomatic and supportive therapy.

Contraindications—Hypersensitivity to cefotaxime and other cephalosporins or their components.

Precautions—Reduce the dose of cefotaxime in patents with renal and hepatic impairment. Prolonged use may result in superinfection. A low incidence of cross hypersensitivity with the penicillins exists. In vitro sensitivity test should be performed before and during therapy.

Drug Interactions—Probenecid reduces cefotaxime clearance. Aminoglycoside antibiotics and furosemide may increase the risk of nephrotoxicity.

Pharmaceutical Formulations—Available as cefotaxime sodium in 500 mg, 1 g, 2 g and 10 g powder for injection after reconstitution. Cefotaxime is also available in 1 g (50 ml) and 2 g (50 ml) premixed infusion fluid. One gram contains 2.2 mEq of sodium. No specific veterinary formulations are available.

CEFOXITIN

Cefoxitin

Proprietary Names—Mefoxin˚—

Chemical Class—Cephalosporin; 7-aminocephalosporinic acid derivative.

Pharmacological Class—Cephamycin; beta-lactam antibiotic; antibacterial drug; 7-methoxycephen drug.

Source—Semisynthetic (obtained from cephamycin which is produced by *Streptomyces lactamdurans*).

Solubility, Stability and Storage—Cefoxitin is readily soluble in water but slightly soluble in alcohol. The powder for injection should be stored at room temperature not exceeding 40°C. The solution for injection is preferably stored frozen. The reconstituted powder deteriorates readily. Reconstituted product should be immediately frozen and used within 4 months; 48 hours to—1 week if refrigerated, or 24 hours if kept at room temperature. Cefoxitin products are compatible with normal saline and other parenteral fluids.

Pharmacological Actions—Compared with cephalosporins, cefoxitin has enhanced bactericidal activity against Gram-negative organisms but less active against Gram-positive microbes. It is more active against *Serratia*, and indole-positive *Proteus*. Cefoxitin is active against anaerobes especially *B. fragilis*. It is highly resistant to beta-lactamase enzymes produced by Gram-negative bacilli.

Mechanism of Action—Cefoxitin disrupts cell wall synthesis in actively dividing organisms by inhibiting the action of transpeptidase enzymes. This results in blocking peptidoglycan synthesis followed by activation of autolytic enzymes (autolysins and murein hydrolases) which eventually lyse the bacteria.

Indications—Treatment of infections caused by organisms susceptible to second generation cephalosporins in several animal species. It is used in humans for the treatment of gonorrhea caused by penicillinase-producing *Neisseria*. Cefoxitin is also used in treating infections caused by anaerobic and mixed aerobic/anaerobic organisms as in pelvic inflammatory disease and lung abscess as well as obstetric and surgical infections in humans. Used for prophylaxis before and after surgery.

Dosages—

Dog, cat.	10-20 mg/kg every 8 hours.
Foal.	20 mg/kg every 4-6 hours.
Bird.	50-100 mg/kg every 8-12 hours.

Route(s) of Administration—Intramuscular, intravenous.

Absorption—Cefoxitin is rapidly absorbed from muscular site. Peak plasma concentration is attained within 20-30 minutes following intramuscular injection.

Distribution—Vd = 0.31 ± 0.12 L/kg in humans (higher in neonates); 110 ml/kg (horses); 318 ml/kg (calves). Cefoxitin is widely distributed to body tissues and fluids including synovial, pleural, and bile. It crosses the placenta but not the blood-brain-barrier. It is distributed into milk.

Plasma Protein Binding—Human, 73%; calf .50%.

Metabolism—Small portion (2%) of the dose is metabolized to descarbamylcefoxitin in humans.

Plasma Half-Life—Humans, 0.65 ± 0.09 hours (higher in neonates and uremia; lower in children); Horse, 0.81 hours; Cat, 1.12 hours (IV), 1.35 hours (IM).

Clearance (ml/min/kg)—Human, 3.3; Horse, 4.32.

Route(s) of Excretion—Urine with 78% as unchanged drug.

Dialysis Status—Dialyzable.

Toxicity and Adverse Effects—At therapeutic doses, cefoxitin may cause skin rash, diarrhea, nausea, vomition and colitis. It may also cause bleeding due to hypoprothrombinemia thrombocytopenia and/or platelet dysfunction. Bone marrow depression characterized by granulocytopenia and anemia has also been reported. It causes phlebitis. An overdose may cause positive Coomb's reaction and nephrotoxicity. Prolonged use may produce superinfection.

Management of Overdose/Toxicity—Set up hemodialysis; give symptomatic and supportive therapy.

Contraindications—Hypersensitivity to cefoxitin, other cephalosporins, or their components.

Precautions—Low incidence of cross hypersensitivity to penicillins exists. Reduce cefoxitin dose in patients of renal impairment.

Drug Interactions—Probenecid increases the t½ of cefoxitin. Aminoglycoside antibiotics and furosemide may increase the risk of nephrotoxicity.

Pharmaceutical Formulations—Available as cefoxitin sodium in 1 g, 2 g and 10 g powder for injection following reconstitution; and 1 g and 2 g premixed infusion. One gram contains 2.3 mEq of sodium. No specific veterinary formulations are available yet.

CEFTRIAXONE

Chemical Class—Cephalosporin; 7-aminocephalosporinic acid derivative.

Proprietary Names—Recephin˚; Oframax˚; Monocef˚; Monotax˚.

Pharmacological Class—Antimicrobial agent; beta-lactam antibiotic; third generation cephalosporin.

Source—Semisynthetic.

Solubility, Stability and Storage—Ceftrixone is soluble in water; its powder is photolabile. Following reconstitution with normal saline, the rate of loss of potency depends on the strength of final solution. The period of potency is inversely proportional to concentration. Solutions of 100 mg/ml are viable for 3 days at room temperature or 10 days if refrigerated. Solutions of 250 mg/ml should be used within 24 hours if kept at room temperature or 3 days if refrigerated. Frozen products could remain potent for 26 weeks.

Ceftriaxone

Pharmacological Actions—Ceftrixone is bactericidal to many Gram-negative and some Gram-positive bacteria. It is particularly effective against *Enterobacteriaceae* and *Borrelia burgdorferi*. Ceftrixone is resistant to beta-lactamase.

Mechanism of Action—This is similar to other cephalosporins **Indications**—Treatment of serious infections especially those caused by susceptible Enterobacteriaceae when less expensive or aminoglycoside antibiotics are not indicated.

Dosage—

Dog, cat.   20 mg/kg IV or subcutaneous every 12 hours for 7-10 days.

Horse.   25-50 mg/kg every 12 hours IM or IV.

Route(s) of Administration—Intramuscular, intravenous, and subcutaneous.

Absorption. Ceftrixone is not absorbed from the gastrointestinal tract.

Distribution—Vd = 0.16 ± 0.03 L/kg in humans (higher in neonates and in cirrhosis). Ceftrixone is widely distributed into body organs and fluids. It crosses the placenta and the blood-brain-barrier substantially when the meninges are inflamed. It distributes into milk.

Plasma Protein Binding—Humans, 90-95% (lower in liver cirrhosis, neonates and children). Binding is saturable.

Plasma Half—Life—Humans, 7.3 ± 1.6 hours (higher in uremia, aged and neonates).

Clearance—Humans, 0.24 ± 0.06 ml/min/kg. This value is lower in uremia, neonates and aged and higher in cirrhosis and cystic fibrosis.

Route(s) of Excretion—Eliminated in urine and bile with 46 ± 7% appearing in urine as unchanged drug).

Dialysis Status—Ceftrixone is poorly (0-5%) dialyzable.

Toxicity and Adverse Effects—Like other cephalosporins, ceftriaxone may cause skin rash, nausea, vomiting, hypothrombinemia, and/or platelet dysfunction. It may also cause bone marrow depression (characterized by granulocytosis and anemia), hematologic disorders (such as eosinophilia, leukopenia, neutropenia), vaginitis, and elevation of hepatic enzymes (such as alkaline phosphatase) at therapeutic doses. It causes pain and phlebitis at local sites of injection. An overdose may cause positive Coomb's reaction and nephrotoxicity. Prolonged use may cause superinfection.

Contraindications—Hypersensitivity to ceftriaxone, cephalosporins, or their components; hyperbilirubinemia.

Precautions—Reduce the dose of ceftriaxone in severe renal and hepatic impairment. A low incidence of cross-sensitivity to penicillins exist. Use ceftriaxone cautiously in patients under vitamin K therapy.

Drug Interactions—Ceftriaxone displaces bilirubin from albumen binding sites. Probenecid increases its half-life. Aminoglycoside antibiotics may cause synergistic antibacterial activity and also increase its nephrotoxic potential.

Pharmaceutical Formulations—Available as ceftriaxone sodium in 250 mg, 500 mg, 1 g, 2 g, and 10 g powder for injection after reconstitution. It is also available as 1 g and 2 g in premixed infusion fluids. One gram contains 3.6 mEq of sodium. There are no specific veterinary formulations.

CEPHALEXIN

Cephalexin

Synonyms—Cefalexin.

Proprietary Names—Alcephin®; Biocef®; Cefanex®; C-lexin®; Cephacillin®; Cephaxin®; Ceporex®; Copharlexin®; Entacef®; Flucexin® (cephalexin and flucloxacillin); Keflex®; Keftab® (cefalexin hydrochloride); Kekrinal®; Ospexin®; Sporidex®.

Chemical Class—Cephalosporin; 7-aminocephalosporinic acid derivative.

Pharmacological Class—First generation cephalosporin; beta-lactam antibiotic; antibacterial drug.

Source—Semisynthetic.

Solubility, Stability and Storage—Cephalexin is sparingly soluble in water and insoluble in alcohol. Its products may be stored at room temperature. Reconstituted oral suspension may be stable for up to two weeks.

Pharmacological Actions—Cephalexin is bactericidal to most Gram-positive and Gram-negative bacteria. It is less active against penicillinase producing Staphylococci.

Mechanism of Action—Cephalexin acts by disrupting cell wall synthesis, like other cephalosporins.

Indications—Treatment of susceptible infections in horses, dogs, cats and birds when first generation cephalosporins are indicated.

Dosages—

Bird	35-50mg / kg every 6 hours.
Dog, cat	10-30mg / kg orally every 8 hours.
Guinea pigs	15 mg/kg SC once a day for 14 days.
Mouse	60 mg/kg PO every 12 hours or 15 mg/kg IM every 12 hours.
Horse	22-33mg/kg orally every 6 hours.
NHP	20 mg/kg PO every 12 hours
Rat	60 mg/kg PO every 12 hours or 15 mg/kg SC every 12 hours.
Rabbit	15-20 mg/kg PO every 12 hours or 15 mg/kg SC every 12 hours.
Sheep	10 mg/kg SC once daily.
Pig	10 mg/kg SC once daily.

Route(s) of Administration—Per os, subcutaneous and intramuscular.

Absorption—Cephalexin is rapidly and completely absorbed from adult gastrointestinal tract. Peak plasma concentration is attained within 1 hour in humans; 1.8 hours in dogs and 2.6 hours in cats. Absorption is delayed in children and neonates.

Bioavailability (Oral). Humans, 90 ± 9%; dogs and cats, 75%.

Distribution—Vd = 0.26 ± 0.03 L/kg. Cephalexin is widely distributed. It penetrates body tissues and fluids including pericardium and synovial fluids; crosses the placenta; gets into milk. Its distribution into the cerebrospinal fluid is poor.

Plasma Protein Binding—Extent of cephalexin binding is 14 ± 3%.

Metabolism—Cephalexin is not metabolized.

Plasma Half-Life—Humans, 0.90 ± 0.18 hours (higher in uremia); dogs and cats, 1-2 hours; calves, 1.5 hours.

Clearance (ml/min/kg). Humans 4.3 ± 1.1 (lower in uremia and higher in pregnancy).

Route(s) of Excretion—Eliminates in urine with 91 ± 18% as unchanged drug.

Dialysis Status—Cephalexin is dialyzable.

Toxicity and Adverse Effects—Cephalexin is relatively well tolerated. Diarrhea may be observed in 10% of patients. It may cause skin rash, seizures, confusion, hematologic disorders (such as anemia and transient neutropenia), and elevation of hepatic enzymes at therapeutic doses. An overdose may cause neuromuscular hyper irritability and acute renal tubular necrosis. Prolonged use may produce superinfection. Nephrotoxicity is rare. It causes salivation, tachypnea and excitability in dogs. Emesis and fever may be observed in cats.

Management of Overdose/Toxicity—Set up hemodialysis; give symptomatic and supportive therapy.

Contraindications—Hypersensitivity to cephalexin, other cephalosporin, the penicillins, their products, or components.

Precautions—Reduce cephalexin dose in patients with renal impairment.

Drug Interactions—Probenecid reduces cephalosporin excretion. Furosemide and aminoglycoside antibiotics may increase the risk of nephrotoxicity.

Pharmaceutical Formulations—Available as cephalexin monohydrate in 250 mg and 500 mg capsules; 250 mg, 500 mg and 1 g tablets; 125 mg/5 ml and 250 mg/ 5 ml oral suspension; and 100 mg/ml pediatric drops. It is also available as cephalexin hydrochloride in 250 mg and 500 mg tablets. A combination of cephalexin (500 mg) and flucloxacillin (250 mg) is available. No specific veterinary formulation is available.

CEPHALOTHIN

Cephalotin

Proprietary Names—Keflin®—

Chemical Class—Cephalosporin; 7-Aminocephalosporinic acid derivative.

Pharmacological Class—Cephalosporin; beta-lactam antibiotic; first generation cephalosporin.

Source—Semi-synthetic.

Solubility, Stability and Storage—Cephalothin is readily soluble in water but sparingly soluble in alcohol. Cephalothin powder for injection is stable at room temperature. Reconstituted product is stable for 12 hours at room temperature or 96 hours if refrigerated. The presence of precipitate in refrigerated product or discoloration of product kept at room temperature may not affect potency. Precipitates may redissolve if shaken. Cephalothin products are compatible with most parenteral fluids.

Pharmacological Actions—Cephalothin has bactericidal action against Gram-positive and Gram-negative organisms. It is resistant to hydrolysis by cephalosporinase produced by staphylococci.

Mechanism of Action—Cephalothin disrupts cell wall synthesis like other cephalosporins.

Indications—Treatment of susceptible infections in which a relatively short-acting first generation cephalosporin is indicated.

Dosages—

Dog, cat.	10-35mg/kg.
Horse.	10-18 mg/kg.
Cattle.	55 mg /kg daily in 4 divided doses.
Birds.	10 mg /kg every 6-8 hours.
Reptile.	20-40mg/kg every 12 hours.

Route(s) of Administration—Intramuscular, intravenous.

Absorption—Cephalothin is poorly absorbed from the gastrointestinal tract. Peak plasma concentration is attained within 30 minutes following intramuscular injection.

Distribution—Vd (L/kg) = 0.26±0.11 in humans; 0.435 in dogs; 0.145 in horses. Cephalothin is almost excluded from the cerebrospinal fluid except when meninges are inflamed. It crosses the placenta, distributes into milk, synovial and pericardial fluids.

Plasma Protein Binding—Human, 71 ± 3%; horse, 20%.

Metabolism—Cephalothin is partially metabolized in the liver to desacetylcephalothin with 25% antibacterial activity.

Plasma Half-Life—Human, 0.57 ± 0.32 hours (higher in uremia); horse, 15 minutes (IV) and 49 minutes (IM); dogs, 42-51 minutes.

Clearance (ml/min/kg)—Human, 6.7 ± 1.7; dog, 11.6 15; Horse, 13.

Route(s) of Excretion—Mainly urine with 52% of dose as unchanged drug and 27-54% as desacetyl metabolite.

Dialysis Status—Dialyzable.

Toxicity and Adverse Effects—Hypersensitivity reaction ranging from skin rash to anaphylaxis and gastrointestinal disorders including nausea, vomition, diarrhea, dyspepsia, and pseudomembranous colitis are common. Bleeding and thrombocytopenia may be observed. Cephalothin causes pain at the site of intramuscular injection. Overdose may cause neuromuscular hypersensitivity, convulsions, positive Coomb's reaction, and nephrotoxicity.

Management of Overdose/Toxicity—Set up hemodialysis. Give symptomatic and supportive therapy.

Contraindications—Hypersensitivity to the penicillins or other cephalosporins, or their components.

Precautions—Reduce the dose in patients with renal insufficiency. Prolong use may produce superinfection.

Drug Interactions—Probenecid increases the half-life of cephalothin. Aminoglycoside antibiotics such as gentamicin and tobramycin are synergistic but may increase the risk of nephrotoxicity.

Pharmaceutical Formulations—Available as cephalothin sodium in 1 g, 2 g, and 20 g powder for injection or as 1 g, and 2 g in 5% dextrose premixed bag of 50 ml D5W. Each gram contains 2.8 mEq of sodium. There are no specific veterinary formulations.

CEPHAPIRIN

Proprietary Names—Cefadyl ®, Cefa—Dri ®.

Chemical Class—A 7-Aminocephalosporinic acid derivative.

Pharmacological Class—Cephalosporin; beta-lactam antibiotic; First generation cephalosporin.

Source—Semi-synthetic.

Solubility, Stability and Storage—Cephapirin is readily soluble in water but sparingly soluble in alcohol. The powder for injection has a shelf life of two years. The stability of reconstituted products depends on the diluents, final concentration, and storage. Stability varies between 12-24 hours at room temperature and 10 days if refrigerated.

Pharmacological Actions—Cephapirin is bactericidal for Gram-positive and Gram-negative bacteria.

Mechanism of Action—Same as for other cephalosporins.

Cephapirin

Indications—Treatment of mastitis in lactating (with cephapirin sodium) and dry cows (with cephapirin benzathine); treatment of susceptible infections in animal species for which a relatively short-acting first generation cephalosporin is indicated.

Dosages—

Dog, cat.	10-30mg/kg IM or IV every 6-8 hours.
Cattle.	Inject entire syringe content into each quarter of the udder.
Horse.	20mg/kg IM every 8 hours (or 12 hours if administered with probenecid).
Foals.	20-30mg / kg IV every 6 hours.

Route(s) of Administration—Intramuscular, intravenous, intra mammary (in cattle).

Absorption—Cephapirin is poorly absorbed from the gastrointestinal tract. Peak plasma concentration is attained within 30 minutes following IM injection.

Bioavailability—Bioavailability after intramuscular injection in the horse is 95%.

Distribution—Vd (L/kg) = 0.21±0.06 (human); 0.32 (dog); 0.335-0.399 (cattle); 0.17-0.188 (horse). Cephapirin is widely distributed into body tissues and fluids. It crosses the placenta but poorly distributes into the cerebrospinal fluid.

Plasma Protein Binding—Binding is evaluated at 62 ± 4 %.

Metabolism—Half of the dose is metabolized into active product.

Plasma Half-Life (Hours)—Human, 0.72 ± 0.18 (higher in uremia); Dog, 0.42; Cattle, 1.07-1.17; Horse, 0.42-0.92.

Clearance (ml/min/kg)—Human, 6.9 ± 2.0 (lower in uremia); dog 8.9; cattle 12.66; horse 7.8-10.

Maximum Residue Limit (ppm)—0.02 in milk; 0.1 in edible tissues of cattle.

Withdrawal Period—Cephapirin sodium: milk (96 hours), slaughter (4 days). Cephapirin benzathine: milk (72 hours), slaughter, (42 days).

Route(s) of Excretion—Urine (48 ± 7 % as unchanged drug).

Dialysis Status—Dialyzable.

Toxicity and Adverse Effects—Hypersensitivity reactions ranging from skin rash to anaphylaxis. Diarrhea, seizure, leukopenia, thrombocytopenia and elevated liver enzymes may be observed at therapeutic doses. Overdose causes neuromuscular hypersensitivity, positive Coomb's reaction, and acute nephrotubular necrosis.

Management of Overdose/Toxicity—Give symptomatic and supportive therapy.

Contraindications—Penicillin or cephalosporin hypersensitivity.

Precautions. Reduce dose in cases of renal insufficiency. Prolong use may produce superinfection. Do not milk treated lactating cows within 12 hours. Treat dry cows not later than 30 days prior to calving.

Drug Interactions. Probenecid increases cephapirin half-life. The actions of cephapirin and aminoglycoside antibiotics are synergistic but concurrent use of both classes of drugs may increase the risk of nephrotoxicity.

Pharmaceutical Formulations—Available as cephapirin sodium in 500 mg, 1 g, 2 g, 4 g, 20 g powder for injection and 200 mg/10 ml mastitis tube. Each gram contains 2.36 mEq of sodium. It is also available as cephapirin benzathine in mastitis tube containing 300 mg/10 ml.

CHLORAL HYDRATE

Chloral hydrate

Synonyms—Chloral; Hydrated chloral; Trichloroacetyldehyde monohydrate.

Proprietary Names—Aquachloral®; Supprettes®; Noctec®; Somnos®.

Chemical Class—Chlorinated alcohol.

Pharmacological Class—CNS sedative; sedative/hypnotic.

Source—Synthetic.

Stability and Storage—Chloral hydrate is unstable. It volatilizes on exposure to air producing aromatic penetrating odor. Products, including crystals, should be stored in light resistant, and air tight containers.

Pharmacological Actions—Chloral hydrate depresses the cerebellum. Its action on the CNS at low doses results in hypnosis. High doses produce anesthesia with depression of the respiratory and vasomotor centres. Its effect on the vasomotor center causes fall of blood pressure. Chloral hydrate has low analgesic, and muscle relaxing effect. It causes local irritation to skin and mucous membranes.

Mechanism of Action—It is uncertain how chloral hydrate CNS depression but the active metabolite, trichloroethanol has been shown in vitro to exert barbiturate-like effects on $GABA_A$ receptor channels.

Indications—Used in preanaesthetic medication and as a hypnotic in large animals especially horses. Chloral hydrate may also be used as a basal narcotic in conjunction with local anesthetic. Two mixtures, one containing chloral hydrate and magnesium sulfate in the ratio of 2:1 and the second containing chloral hydrate (30 g), Magnesium sulfate (15 g) and pentobarbital (6.6 g) have been used satisfactorily for anesthesia in horses, cattle and camels.

Dosages—

Horse.	5 g/45 kg orally or 4.9 g/ 45 kg intravenously.
Cattle.	50-70 mg/kg IV or 30-60g orally.
Pig.	12 g/ 23 kg orally.

Route(s) of Administration—Per os, rectal and intravenous.

Absorption—Chloral hydrate is readily absorbed from the gastrointestinal tract. Peak plasma concentration of active metabolite, trichloroethanol, is attained within 1-2 hours in horses. It is attained more rapidly in humans.

Onset of Action—Horse, 10-20 minutes (oral administration).

Peak Action—Human, 0.5-1 hour.

Duration of Action—Human, 4-8 hours.

Distribution—Chloral hydrate crosses the placenta. Negligible amounts get into milk. It is secreted into saliva in horses.

Metabolism—Chloral hydrate is rapidly reduced to trichloroethanol, an active metabolite. Trichloroethanol is conjugated with glucuronic acid in the livers of rabbits, dogs and humans to form urochloralic acid. About 3%—4% of IV dose is oxidized to trichloroacetic acid in the dog.

Plasma Half-Life—8-11 hours (human).

Route(s) of Excretion—Elimination of chloral hydrate is mainly through urine. Small portion is excreted as unchanged drug but this portion increases when the liver is damaged. Small amount of chloral hydrate is excreted in feces via bile.

Dialysis Status—Chloral hydrate is 50-100% dialyzable.

Toxicity and Adverse Effects—Chloral hydrate has marrow margin of safety as an anesthetic. It irritates the skin and gastrointestinal mucous membranes causing epigastric distress, nausea, vomition and diarrhea especially when taken on an empty stomach or inadequately diluted before oral administration. CNS related adverse effects include malaise, ataxia, and hallucinations. Acute intoxication may cause icterus. Prolonged use in humans may produce psychic and physical dependence. Sudden withdrawal following habitual use may result in seizures and delirium. Overdose causes hypotension, respiratory depression, coma and cardiac arrhythmia. Perivascular injection or leakage in animals receiving the drug intravenously causes severe pain, necrosis and sloughing at the site.

Management of Overdose—Give supportive and symptomatic therapy. Administer activated charcoal to reduce intestinal absorption.

Contraindications—Hypersensitivity to chloral hydrate; renal or hepatic dysfunction; gastritis or gastric ulcer.

Precautions—Do not administer chloral hydrate for extended periods. Reduce the dose gradually following prolonged administration. Use the drug cautiously in neonates and patients with porphyria. Do not administer on an empty stomach. Avoid IV solutions in excess of 7% in animals.

Drug Interactions—Chloral hydrate potentiates the effects of CNS depressants. Flushing and blood pressure changes may occur when used concomitantly with intravenous furosemide.

Formulations—Chloral hydrate is available in capsules of 250 mg and 500 mg; rectal suppositories of 324 mg, 500 mg and 648 mg; syrup of 250 mg/5 ml, and 500 mg/5 ml. Intravenous solution is available for veterinary use. Chloral hydrate exists as translucent crystals which contain not less than 99.5% of chloral hydrate. Chloral hydrate solution may be made from crystals. One gram of crystal is soluble in 0.25 ml water.

CHLORAMBUCIL

Chlorambucil

Proprietary Names—Leukeran®.

Chemical Class—Nitrogen mustard; Alkylating agent.

Pharmacological Class—Antineoplastic drug; Immunosuppressive agent.

Source—Synthetic.

Stability and Storage—Chlorambucil dosage forms are preferably stored in tight, light resistant containers at room temperature. Its normal shelf life is one year.

Pharmacological Actions—Chlorambucil has cytotoxic actions due to disruption of nucleic acid function by interfering with DNA replication, RNA transcription and replication. It is cell cycle nonspecific. It also has immunosuppressive action.

Mechanism of Action—The drug alkylates target molecules by forming highly reactive carbonium ion intermediates that react with strongly neucleophilic substituents like phosphate, amino,—SH, OH, COOH and imidazole groups to form covalent bonds. The N-7 position of guanine in DNA is highly susceptible. Alkylation of guanine in the DNA leads to cross linkage of DNA strands, linking of DNA to a closely associated protein, base pairing of guanine with thymine instead of cytosine, or breakage of the DNA strand.

Indications—Treatment of chronic leukocytic leukemia in dogs and humans; multiple myeloma; polycythemia vera; adjunctive treatment of immune-mediated glomerolunephritis, and non-erosive arthritis.

Dosages—

Immunosuppression in immune-mediated glomerolonephritis:

0.1-0.2 mg/kg (dog), 0.25-0.5 mg/kg (cat) daily or every other day.

Chronic leukocytic leukemia:

20 mg/m² orally every 1-2 weeks or 6 mg/m² daily in dogs; 2 mg/m² every other day or 20 mg/m2 every other week in cats.

Other tumors.

2-6 mg/m² daily or every other day.

Route(s) of Administration—Per os.

Absorption—Chlorambucil is rapidly and almost completely absorbed from the gastrointestinal tract in human beings.

Bioavailability (oral)—Evaluated at 87 ± 20 but may be reduced by 10-20% in the presence of food.

Distribution—Vd = 0.29 ± 0.21 for parent drug and active metabolite. Chlorambucil crosses the placenta; may cross the blood-brain-barrier.

Plasma Protein Binding—Human, 99%. Chlorambucil binds extensively to tissues.

Metabolism—Chlorambucil is almost completely metabolized to active phenylacetic acid mustard.

Plasma Half-life—1.3 ± 0.9 hours for parent drug; 2.0 ± 1.1 hours for active metabolite.

Clearance—Human, 2.6 ± 0.9 ml/min/kg.

Route(s) of Excretion—Urine, with less than 1% as active parent drug and metabolite.

Dialysis Status—Nondialyzable.

Toxicity and Adverse Effects—Bone marrow depression characterized by anemia, leukopenia and thrombocytopenia is common. Pulmonary fibrosis, alopecia and cerebellar necrosis have been reported at high doses.

Contraindications—Hypersensitivity to chlorambucil; pre-existing bone marrow depression, infection and immunodepression.

Precautions—Use chlorambucil cautiously with drugs that have myelosuppressive or immunosuppressive actions and in cases most likely to get infected. Handle the drug with extreme caution.

Drug Interactions—Chlorambucil may produce additive bone marrow depression with other antineoplastic drugs and bone marrow depressants (e.g. chloramphenicol, flucytosine, amphotericin B and colchicine). Azathioprine, cyclophosphamide, corticosteroids and other immunodepressants may increase the risk of infection when used concurrently with chlorambucil.

Pharmaceutical Formulations—Chlorambucil is available in 2 mg oral tablets. There is no specific formulation for veterinary use.

CHLORAMPHENICOL

Chloramphenicol

Proprietary Names—Chloromycetin*, Chloroptic*, Ophthochlor*, Ak-chlor*, Biophenicol*, Detreomycine*, Tifomycine*, Synthomycetine*, Suismycetin* Ormanicol*, Kemi-cycline*, Kemicetine*, Comycetin*, Chlorocide*, Animycetin*, Bemacol*.

Chemical Class—Nitrobenzene derivative.

Pharmacological Class—Broad spectrum antibiotic.

Source—Originally isolated from *Streptomyces venezuelae* but now synthesized chemically.

Solubility, Stability and Storage—The solubility of chloramphenicol is approximately 2.5 mg/ml of water at 25°C. It is freely soluble in alcohol. Chloramphenicol sodium succinate sterile powder for injection is preferably stored at 15–25°C. Following reconstitution with sterile water for injection, chloramphenicol sodium succinate injection is stable for 30 days at room temperature but do not use if solution becomes cloudy.

Pharmacological Actions—Chloramphenicol is bacteriostatic to Gram-positive and Gram-negative aerobic and anaerobic bacteria as well as Rickettsia, Chlamydia and Mycoplasma. It may be bactericidal to some bacteria such as *Haemophilus influenzae*.

Mechanism of Action—Chloramphenicol inhibits protein synthesis by binding to the 50s ribosomal subunit which subsequently interferes with the interaction between peptidyl transferase and its amino acid substrate thus inhibiting peptide bond formation in bacteria and mitochondrial of mammalian cells.

Indications—Treatment of urinary tract infections, salmonellosis, staphylococci and coliform infections that have become resistant to other antibiotics. Chloramphenicol has also been used to treat dermatophilus infections.

Dosage—

Small animals, 33mg/kg/day IM, IV or 12-45mg/kg orally in 3-4 divided doses.

Large animals, 5-20mg/kg, IM, IV, 3 times daily. Actual doses vary with species and severity of infection.

Route of Administration—Oral, intramuscular, intravenous and topical routes may be used.

Absorption—Chloramphenicol palmitate is rapidly and almost completely absorbed from the gastrointestinal tract. Peak plasma concentration is attained within 2 hours. Chloramphenicol palmitate is well absorbed from muscular site but oral absorption is slow and erratic in the newborn and gastrointestinal disease.

Bioavailability—Oral bioavailability is 75-90%.

Distribution—Vd (L\kg) = 0.94 ± 0.06 in humans; 1.02 in ponies; 1.8 in dogs; 1.4 in horses or 2.36 in cats. Chloramphenicol is distributed to most body fluids and tissues with the highest concentration in the liver, kidney, and bile. It diffuses into the CSF and pleural fluids; crosses the placenta and appears in milk and egg.

Plasma Protein Binding—Human, 53 ± 5% (lower in cirrhosis, premature and neonates); Animals, 30-46%.

Metabolism—Chloramphenicol is metabolized extensively in the liver by glucuronidation to inactive metabolites. Chloramphenicol palmitate is hydrolyzed by lipases in the duodenum to the active base while the sodium succinate ester is hydrolyzed by esterases to active base.

Plasma Half-Life—Human, 4.0 ± 2.0 hours with higher values in liver cirrhosis, premature and neonates. Half-life values in other species are 0.9 hours in ponies, 5.1 hours in cats, 1.1-5 hours in dogs, 26 minutes in pigeon, 5 hours in bald eagle and pea fowl.

Clearance (ml/min/kg)—Evaluated at 2.4 ± 0.2 in human but values are lower in liver cirrhosis, premature and neonates.

Withdrawal Period—Allow 3 days for edible tissues of chicken and 4 days for eggs.

Route(s) of Excretion—Chloramphenicol is eliminated in urine with 5-10% of dose excreted as unchanged drug in humans and 6.3% in dogs. The drug also excreted in bile in dogs, rats, humans.

Dialysis Status—Poorly dialyzable.

Toxicity and Adverse Effects—Low rates of bone marrow toxicity resulting in pancytopenia with a high mortality rate have been reported. This is predominant in humans following prolong and repeated use. Depressed hematopoiesis has been described in cats. It causes the "grey syndrome" characterized by vomiting, flaccidity, hypothermia, gray color, shock and collapse at high doses in human infants. Nausea, vomiting, diarrhea may follow oral administration. Hypersensitivity reactions involving skin are rare.

Management of Overdose—Give supportive treatment.

Contraindication—Hypersensitivity to chloramphenicol or its components.

Precautions—Do not use chloramphenicol in undefined situations or in diseases which are readily, safely and effectively treatable with other antibiotics. Use the drug with caution in patients with impaired renal and hepatic functions; in neonates and cases of glucose-6 phosphate dehydrogenase deficiency. Avoid concomitant use with immunizing agents. Chloramphenicol therapy should be avoided, if possible, in anaemic patients who are receiving iron preparations, vitamin B_{12}, or folic acid. Concomitant administration of chloramphenicol with other drugs that have the potential for causing bone marrow depression should be avoided.

Drug Interactions—Chloramphenicol inhibits microsomal enzymes with consequent inhibition of the metabolism of phenytoin, tolbutamide, chlorpropamide and dicoumarol. Prolonged use of phenobarbital or acute use of rifampin reduces chloramphenicol half-life. Also, concurrent administration of phenobarbital and chloramphenicol may result in decreased plasma concentrations of the latter. Chloramphenicol can prolong the duration of phenobarbital anesthesia in dogs and cats. It delays the response to iron preparations, vitamin B_{12}, or folic acid, when administered concurrently with these drugs.

Pharmaceutical Formulations—The drug is available as chloramphenicol palmitate in 500 mg capsules, 150 mg base/5ml oral suspension, 5.5% soluble powder for oral use. It is also available as chloramphenicol sodium succinate in 1 g dry powder for parenteral use (as a 40% solution for IM or 10% IV for animals). Other available dosage forms include 1% cream, ophthalmic ointment, 0.5% ophthalmic and otic solutions. Chloramphenicol sodium succinate contains approximately 2.3 mEq of sodium per gram of chloramphenicol.

CHLORDIAZEPOXIDE

Chlordiazepoxide

Synonyms—Methaminodiazepoxide hydrochloride.

Proprietary Names—Librum®; libritabs®; Mitran®.

Chemical Class—Benzodiazepine.

Pharmacological Class—CNS depressant; sedative-hypnotic; anxiolytic.

Source—Synthetic.

Solubility, Stability and Storage—Chlordiazepoxide is practically insoluble in water but chlordiazepoxide hydrochloride is soluble in water and in alcohol and slightly soluble in propylene glycol. Chlordiazepoxide hydrochloride is unstable in water, normal saline, and the commercially available diluent. The injectable solution should not be mixed with Ringer's solution, normal saline, ascorbic acid, heparin, phenytoin, promethazine or secobarbital. The injection should be prepared immediately before use, and any unused portion should be discarded. Protect chlordiazepoxide tablets, capsules and powder for injection from light.

Pharmacological Actions—Chlordiazepoxide has actions similar to diazepam but is less potent. It selectively depresses the CNS and produces sedation and hypnosis without loss of consciousness. It causes amnesia in humans, decreases anxiety and makes rather hostile and aggressive animals become docile.

Mechanism of Action—Chlordiazepoxide binds to $GABA_A$ receptor/ion channel complex in the presence of GABA and allosterically modulates the action of GABA to produce increase in neuronal chloride conductance resulting in hyperpolarization and reduced neuronal excitability.

Indications—Chemical restraint and preanaesthetic medication in pigs and wildlife.

Dosages—

Pig:	5-10 mg/kg IM.
Baboon:	13 mg/kg orally.

Route(s) of Administration—Per os, intramuscular and intravenous are preferred routes.

Absorption—Chlordiazepoxide is readily and almost completely absorbed from oral route. Peak plasma concentration is attained within 2 hours. Intramuscular administration results in lower peak plasma levels than oral route.

Bioavailability—Almost 100%.

Effective Concentration = 0.4 to 4 mg/L in plasma—

Onset of Action = 1 hour (pig).

Distribution—Vd = 3.3 L/kg (human). Chlordiazepoxide readily passes into the cerebrospinal fluid and breast milk. It crosses the placenta.

Plasma Protein Binding—Human, 90-98%.

Metabolism—Extensively metabolized in the liver to active products, namely, desmethylchlordiazepoxide and demoxepam. Demoxepam is further metabolized to desmethyldiazepam (nordazepam) which is hydroxylated to oxazepam. Both desmethyldiazepam and oxazepam are also pharmacologically active.

Plasma Half-Life—There is considerable interspecies and intersubject variations. In humans, $t\frac{1}{2}$ is 6.6-25 hours for chlordiazepoxide. Higher values are obtained in renal insufficiency and liver cirrhosis (30-60 hours). Plasma half-life for demoxepam and desmethyldiazepam are 14 to 95 hours (mean 40) and about 40 to 100 hours respectively.

Clearance—Plasma clearance is about 0.5 mL/min/kg.

Route(s) of Excretion—In humans, about 60% of a dose is excreted in urine with less than 1% as unchanged drug. About 10 to 20% of dose is eliminated in faeces.

Dialysis Status—Not dialyzable.

Toxicity and Adverse Effects—Normal therapeutic doses may cause ataxia, and prolongation of reaction time. Chlordiazepoxide causes liver damage and icterus following prolonged treatment. It decreases bile flow. It has been associated with teratogenic effects if used within the first six weeks of pregnancy in humans. It has also been shown to cause cleft palate in rodents following high doses. Chlordiazepoxide hydrochloride may cause hypotension and/or respiratory depression if the drug is administered too rapidly by intravenous route.

Management of Overdose—Give general antidotal therapy in addition to adequate supportive measures. Flumazenil will specifically antagonize the CNS depressant effect of chlordiazepoxide.

Contraindications—Pregnancy; pre-existing CNS depression; severe uncontrolled pain; hypersensitivity to chlordiazepoxide or any component.

Precautions—Use chlordiazepoxide with caution in patients with liver dysfunction, CNS impairment or obstructive pulmonary condition. The drug should be administered slowly intravenously, preferably over a 1-minute period.

Drug Interactions—Increased CNS depression will result if used concurrently with other CNS depressants.

Pharmaceutical Formulations—Available as chlordiazepoxide hydrochloride in 5 mg, 10 mg and 15 mg tablets; 5 mg, 10 mg and 15 mg capsules; 100 mg powder for injection after reconstitution.

CHLOROTHIAZIDE

Chlorothiazide

Proprietary Names—Diuril*; Saluric* Diurigen*.

Chemical Class—Sulfonamide derivative.

Pharmacological Class—Thiazide (benzothiadiazide) diuretic; antihypertensive agent.

Source. Synthetic.

Solubility, Stability and Storage—Chlorothiazide is slightly soluble in water and alcohol. Chlorothiazide sodium is soluble in water and alcohol. Chlorothiazide oral suspension should be protected from freezing. Following reconstitution, the unused portion of chlorothiazide injection solution should be discarded.

Pharmacological Actions—Chlorothiazide causes increased urinary excretion of sodium and water by inhibiting the reabsorption of sodium in the early distal tubule. It may reduce glomerular filtration due to direct action on renal vasculature. It decreases renal excretion of calcium and urate while increasing the excretion of mg^{++}. Chlorothiazide causes elevated blood sugar and reduced blood pressure in hypertensive patients.

Mechanism of Action—Chlorothiazide blocks the electroneutral Na$^+$/Cl$-$ cotransport mechanism at the luminal membrane of the kidney tubules which consists of glycoprotein receptors with 12 membrane spanning domain. Its action on uric acid excretion is due to its interference with tubular secretion of the compound. Elevated blood sugar is as a result of decreased insulin release.

Indications—Mobilization of edema fluid of most types such as parturient edema, cardiac and nephrotic edema, bowel edema and salt poisoning in pigs.

Dosage—12-15 mg/kg orally two times daily or 10 mg/kg/day intravenously.

Route(s) of Administration—Chlorothiazide is administered orally but chlorothiazide sodium is given intravenously.

Absorption—Only 10-21% of chlorothiazide oral dose is absorbed from the gastrointestinal tract of monogastric animals. Peak plasma concentration is attained within 4 hours. The presence of food appears to increase the extent of absorption of the drug.

Bioavailability—This is dose-dependent; decreasing with increasing dose.

Onset of Action—2 hours with oral administration.

Duration of Action—6-12 hours (oral); 2 hours (IV)—

Distribution—Vd = 0.20 ± 0.08 L/kg.

Plasma Protein Binding—94.6 ± 1.3%

Metabolism—Not metabolized.

Plasma Half-Life—Human, 1.5 ± 0.2 hours (increases in uremia).

Clearance—Human, 4.5 ± 1.7 ml/min/kg (decreases in uremia).

Route(s) of Excretion—Chlorothiazide is eliminated almost completely in urine (92 ± 5% of original dose).

Toxicity and Adverse Effects—These are rare but weakness, paraesthesia, hypokalemia, metabolic alkalosis, impaired carbohydrate tolerance, hyperuricemia, hyperlipidemia, hyponatremia and allergic reactions have been reported following therapeutic doses. Overdose may cause hyper motility, confusion, muscle weakness and coma.

Management of Overdose—Give supportive therapy with intravenous fluids and electrolytes.

Contraindications—Anuria; hepatic cirrhosis; renal insufficiency; digitalis therapy; hypersensitivity to chlorothiazide.

Precautions—Potassium supplement may be required. Use chlorothiazide with caution in borderline renal and/or hepatic insufficiency. Concurrent administration with digitalis glycoside and thiazides requires electrolyte monitoring since loss of K^+ may enhance the therapeutic and toxic actions of digitalis. Do not administer chlorothiazide injection subcutaneously or intramuscularly. Avoid extravasation of the alkaline solution.

Drug Interactions—Chlorothiazide potentiates the actions of other antihypertensive drugs. It may be alternatively administered with K^+ sparing diuretics.

Pharmaceutical Formulations—Chlorothiazide is available in 250 mg and 500 mg tablets; and also as the sodium salt in 500 mg lyophilized powder for intravenous administration. Oral suspension containing 250 mg chlorothiazide/5 ml is also available. Chlorothiazide sodium for injection is a sterile, lyophilized mixture of the drug and mannitol. It contains approximately 2.5 mEq of sodium.

CHLORPHENIRAMINE

Chlorpheniramine

Proprietary Names—Chlorpheniramine®; Chlor-Trimeton®; Teldrin®; Phenetron®; Telachlor®; Chlorate®; Aller-chlor®.

Chemical Class—Alkylamine (Propylamine) compound.

Pharmacological Class—Antihistamine; Histamine H_1 antagonist; Anti allergic drug.

Source—Synthetic.

Solubility, Stability and Storage—Chlorpheniramine is soluble in water and alcohol. It is photosensitive; its solutions should be stored in light-resistant containers at room temperature. Tablets and capsules should be stored in tight containers.

Pharmacological Actions—Chlorpheniramine blocks the actions of histamine at the H_1 receptor sites. Hence, the histamine released during allergic conditions is unable to constrict smooth muscle, make exocrine glands secrete, or increase capillary permeability. Chlorpheniramine possesses some anticholinergic and sedative actions.

Mechanism of Action—Chlorpheniramine competitively excludes histamine from H_1 receptor sites.

Indications—Symptomatic control of allergic conditions—

Dosages—

Dog	2-8 mg/kg twice a day.
Guinea pig	5 mg/kg SC

Mouse	1 mg/kg IP
NHP	0.5 mg/kg /day PO in divided doses

Route(s) of Administration—Oral, intramuscular and intravenous routes are used.

Absorption—The drug is well absorbed from the gastrointestinal tract of monogastric animals.

Bioavailability (oral)—41 ± 16%.

Distribution—Vd = 3.2 ± 0.3 L/kg. Chlorpheniramine is widely distributed and attains high concentration in the lungs, heart, kidney, brain, small intestine, and spleen.

Plasma Protein Binding—70 ± 3%.

Metabolism—Orally administered drug undergoes metabolic degradation to a significant level in gastrointestinal mucosa and liver.

Plasma Half-life. 20 ± 0.5 hours (human).

Clearance—1.7 ± 0.1 ml/min/kg in human.

Route(s) of Excretion—Chlorpheniramine is eliminated through urine with 0.3-26% of total dose eliminated as unchanged drug. Urine excretion increases with the rate of flow and lower pH.

Toxicity and Adverse Effects—Effects related to the CNS (somnolence, lethargy) and gastrointestinal tract (diarrhea, vomiting and anorexia) may be observed. It may also cause dry mouth, urinary retention due to its anticholinergic actions. Overdose is characterized by more prominent anticholinergic effects, CNS depression, respiratory depression, and death. Overdose may also cause CNS stimulation.

Management of Overdose/Toxicity—Undertake general antidotal therapy procedures. Control CNS excitement with phenytoin. Anticholinergic effects may be controlled with physostigmine.

Contraindications—Angle closure glaucoma; hypersensitivity to chlorpheniramine or other antihistamines belonging to the alkylamine group; bladder neck obstruction; pyloroduodenal obstruction; asthma.

Precautions—Do not mix chlorpheniramine with calcium chloride, kanamycin sulfate, norepinephrine bitartrate and pentobarbital sodium in the same syringe.

Drug Interactions—Concurrent use of chlorpheniramine with other CNS depressants may cause additive effect. It may counteract the anticoagulant actions of heparin and warfarin.

Pharmaceutical Formulations—Available as chlorpheniramine maleate in 2, 4, 8, and 12 mg tablets; 2 mg/ml oral syrup; 10 mg/ml and 100 mg/ml solution for injection; 12 mg capsules; 8 mg and 12 mg time release tablets. Chlorpheniramine maleate is available in combination with different classes of drugs such as antibiotics, analgesics and antitussives.

CHLORPROMAZINE

Synonyms—CPZ.

Proprietary Names—Thorazine®; Ormazine®; Largactil®.

Chemical Class—Phenothiazine derivative.

Pharmacological Class—Tranquilizer; CNS sedative; Sedative-hypnotic.

Source—Synthetic.

Solubility, Stability and Storage—CPZ is practically insoluble in water but the hydrochloride salt is soluble 1 in 2.5 of water. CPZ is soluble 1 in 2 of ethanol. It decomposes and darkens upon prolonged exposure to light. Store CPZ at room temperature protected from light. Avoid using products with precipitates or that have become darkened. Solution with slight yellow color may still be potent. Solutions diluted with normal saline will remain stable for 30 days. CPZ may adsorb to plastic if stored in plastic syringes or other plastic containers for prolonged periods.

Chlorpromazine

Pharmacological Actions—CPZ causes sedation, inhibits spontaneous motor activity, and reduces aggressive behavior and hostility. It decreases spontaneous motor activity and causes catalepsy at high doses. CPZ prevents and reverses the peripheral actions of epinephrine. For instance, the ventricular fibrillation induced by epinephrine during use of halogenated inhalant anesthetics can be prevented by chlorpromazine. It increases the synthesis and metabolism of dopamine and causes hyperglycemia through release of epinephrine. CPZ possesses endocrine effects such as increased prolactin blood level, inhibition of antidiuretic hormone, melanocyte-stimulating hormone and release of oxytocin. It has hypothermic, anticonvulsive, skeletal muscle relaxant, weak anticholinergic, antihistaminic and antispasmodic actions. CPZ has little effect on respiration except at high doses when respiration may be depressed. It causes splenic sequestration of erythrocytes resulting in reduced packed cell volume.

Mechanism of Action—CPZ antagonizes dopamine and other agonists of the DAe (Dopamine excitatory) receptor. These other agonists are amphetamine and apomorphine.

Indications—To prevent apomorphine and morphine induced emesis in dogs and morphine induced hyper excitement in cats. CPZ is also used in anesthetic premedication, chemical restraint of intractable animals and to prevent motion sickness. It has been used in adjunctive treatment of agalactia in pigs as well as treatment of severe pruritus associated with skin diseases in small animals.

Dosages—

Dog, cat	0.55-4.4 mg/kg IV or 1.1-6.6 mg/kg IM or 3 mg/kg PO 1-4 times daily.
Goat	2-3.5 mg/kg IV.
Cattle	0.2 mg/kg IM.
Tiger	4 mg/kg.
Jackal	2.0 mg/kg.
Rhesus monkey	1.4-2.0 mg/kg.
Dromedary	1.5-2.5 mg/kg.
Reptile	10 mg/kg.

Route(s) of Administration—Per os, intravenous and intramuscular (contraindicated in rabbits).

Absorption—CPZ is rapidly absorbed following administration by oral route.

Bioavailability—Oral bioavailability is low (32 ± 19%) due to extensive first pass.

Distribution—Vd = 21 ± 9 liters/kg in human.

Plasma Protein Binding—Human, 95-98%; goat, 91-99%.

Metabolism—CPZ is slowly metabolized to both active and inactive products. It stimulates hepatic microsomal enzymes in rats.

Plasma Half-life—Dog, 6 hours; goat, 1.51 ± 0.48 hours. Half-life is biphasic in humans (initial = 2 hours, terminal = 30 ± 7 hours).

Clearance—Human, 8.6 ± 2.9 ml/min/kg.

Route(s) of Excretion—Urine with <1% as unchanged drug.

Dialysis Status—Not dialyzable.

Toxicity and Adverse Effects—CPZ may induce cardiac arrhythmia in dogs. High doses in the cat produce tremor, shivering, lethargy, relaxation of anal sphincter, diarrhea and loss of righting reflex. CPZ blocks ovulation and suppresses estrus cycle at high doses. Intramuscular injection causes severe myositis followed by lameness, muscular atrophy and paralysis in rabbits. Chlorpromazine may cause severe dermatitis in sensitized persons.

Management of Overdose—Empty the gut if overdose was given by oral administration. Control seizure with diazepam or barbiturates. Use doxapram to reverse CNS depression. Hypotension should be controlled with noradrenaline or phenylephrine, not epinephrine.

Contraindications—Epidural anesthetic procedures; pregnancy; history of seizure.

Precautions—Do not administer epinephrine when CPZ is used. Use cautiously in debilitated animals and those with cardiac diseases or hypovolemic shock. Do not mix glycopyrrolate and phenothiazines in the same syringe.

Drug Interactions—CPZ potentiates the actions of atropine, analgesics, hypnotics, local and general anesthetics. It blocks the emetic action of apomorphine. CPZ increases the toxicity of physostigmine, dichlorvos and paraquat. It is physically incompatible with diazepam and glycopyrrolate. Other CNS depressants may produce additive effects when used concurrently with CPZ. Quinidine may produce additive cardiac depression. Antidiarrheal mixture and antacids may reduce the level of oral absorption of CPZ. The blood levels of CPZ and propranolol may increase when both drugs are administered concomitantly. Phenothiazines may enhance procaine activity and depress phenytoin metabolism.

Pharmaceutical Formulations—The drug is available as chlorpromazine hydrochloride in 10 mg, 25 mg, 50 mg, 100 mg and 200 mg tablets; 30 mg, 75 mg, 150 mg 200 mg and 300 mg extended release capsule; 2 mg/ml, 30 mg/ml and 100 mg/ml oral solution; 10 mg/5 ml syrup; 25 mg and 100 mg rectal suppository; and 25 mg/ml solution for injection. No specific veterinary formulations are available.

CHLORTETRACYCLINE

Chlortetracycline

Synonyms—Aureomycin.

Proprietary Names—Aureomycin®; AS 250®; Pfichlor®; Clorotet Plus® (in combination with vitamins); Aurofac®; CTC 20® (in combination with vitamins).

Chemical Class—Polycyclic naphthacenecarboxamide derivative.

Pharmacological Class—Antibacterial drug; broad spectrum antibiotic.

Source—Natural; elaborated by *Streptomyces aureofaciens*, a soil mold.

Solubility, Stability and Storage—Chlortetracycline is slightly soluble in water. Protect chlortetracycline products from light and store in tight containers.

Pharmacological Actions—Chlortetracycline has bacteriostatic action against a wide range of microorganisms including Gram-positive and Gram—negative bacteria, Rickettsia, Chlamydia and many spirochaetes. It could be bactericidal at high doses. Some protozoa such as *Anaplasma* are also susceptible. It has limited activity against intestinal coccidial organisms in animals.

Mechanism of Action—Chlortetracycline inhibits protein synthesis by binding principally to the 30s subunit of ribosome to prevent access of aminoacyl tRNA to the acceptor site of the mRNA-ribosome complex thereby preventing the addition of amino acids to the growing peptide chain.

Indications—Treatment of acute anaplasmosis, mastitis, metritis, cutaneous and ocular infections caused by susceptible organisms; treatment of early *Babesia equi* infection in horses; feed additive in farm animals and poultry to prevent liver abscesses, anaplasmosis, coccidiosis, and improve production.

Dosage—

Small animals.	25-50 mg /kg orally.
Large animals.	10-20 mg/kg orally.
Early *B. equi* infection.	0.5-2.6 mg/kg IV daily for 6 days.
Intrauterine administration.	500 mg-1 g
Feed additive.	350 mg/animal/day.

Route(s) of Administration—Topical, per os, intrauterine, intra mammary.

Absorption—30% of oral dose is absorbed in a fasting state. Absorption can be decreased by ingestion of foods, dairy products, antacids containing polyvalent cations, and adsorbents.

Distribution—Chlortetracycline is widely distributed. Significant amounts accumulate in most tissues. It distributes poorly into CSF, vitreous humor and fat. Vd (L/kg) = 0.2284 (turkey); 1. 39 (pig); and 1.93 (calf). It crosses the placenta and is distributed into milk.

Metabolism—Not metabolized to any significant extent.

Plasma Half-Life—Turkey, 0.88 hours; calf, 8.25 hours.

Clearance (ml/min/kg)—Pig, 0.31; turkey, 3.77.

Route(s) of Excretion—Eliminated in urine and feces.

Residue Limit—Maximum residue limit of 0.1 ppm is set for kidney, liver, and muscles of cattle and sheep.

Toxicity and Adverse Effects—Chlortetracycline irritates the gastrointestinal tract causing nausea, vomiting, and sometimes diarrhea in pigs, cats and dogs, or gastrointestinal upset in ruminants. It may cause superinfection. Topical application may be followed by faint yellowing of the skin, redness, swelling, irritation, and photosensitivity.

Contraindications—Hypersensitivity to chlortetracycline, other tetracyclines, or their components; young animals; intra mammary injection in dry cow.

Precautions—Do not use topical formulations in the eyes. Do not administer chlortetracycline parenterally in humans.

Drug Interactions—Absorption is reduced if coadministered with milk, antacids, calcium, magnesium and iron salts.

Pharmaceutical Formulations—Available as chlortetracycline hydrochloride in 50 mg and 250 mg capsules, 500 mg tablets, powder, aerosol sprays and 426 mg intra mammary formulation for animal treatment. Also available in 1% ophthalmic ointment, 3% topical ointment and intrauterine oblets containing 1000 mg/oblet. Formulations containing other antimicrobial agents such as sulfonamides, penicillin G, amprolium, ethopabate, buquinolate, monensin, robenidine, decoquinate, and buquinolate as well as vitamins are available.

CHORIONIC GONADOTROPIN

Synonyms—Human chorionic gonadotropin, HCG, hCG, CG, Chorionic gonadotrophin, Pregnancy-urine hormone, PU.

Proprietary Names—APL*; Choragon*; Chorex*; Choron*; Gonadotraphon LH*; Gonasi HP*; Gonic*; Physex*; Predalon*; Pregnesin*; Pregnyl*; Primogonyl*; Profasi*.

Chemical Class Atenolol A glycoprotein hormone.

Pharmacological Class—Gonad-stimulating peptide.

Source—Natural; obtained from the urine of pregnant women. It is secreted by the syncytiotrophoblasts of the chorionic villa of the human placenta.

Solubility, Stability and Storage—HCG is soluble in water and practically insoluble in alcohol. HCG powder for injection can be stored at room temperature. It should be protect from light. The solution following reconstitution is stable for 30-90 days (depending on the product) when stored at 2-15°C.

Pharmacological Actions—HCG has luteinizing hormone-like action. It also has some FSH activity. In males, HCG stimulates the differentiation of testicular interstitial (Leydig) cells and the production of androgen. It also stimulates testicular descent. In females, HCG stimulates the corpus luteum to produce progesterone and also induces ovulation. In the bitch, HCG induces estrogen secretion.

Indications—HCG is used induce luteinization and ovulation in females and to treat cryptorchidism in males. It is also used in cows for the treatment of nymphomania (frequent or constant heat) due to cystic ovaries.

Dosages—

Horse and cattle	1000 Units injected twice weekly for 4-6 weeks in foals with cryptorchidism.
	2000-4000 IU IV to induce ovulation
	1500-3300 IU 5-6 days after the second prostaglandin treatment or on the first or second day of estrus for synchronization of estrus.
Rodent	100 IU IM, SC; may repeat in 2 weeks

Route(s) of Administration—Intramuscular, subcutaneous and intravenous are recommended.

Absorption—HCG is destroyed in the GIT being a polypeptide. It is absorbed readily from the intramuscular route and peak plasma concentration is attained within 6 hours.

Distribution—HCG is distributed primarily to the gonads in males and females but some may also be distributed to the proximal tubules in the renal cortex.

Metabolism—The β-subunit of chorionic gonadotrophin is metabolized in the liver to a smaller component of 12,000 to 17,500 molecular weight.

Plasma Half-life—HCG undergoes biphasic elimination; initial elimination half-life is about 11 hours while the terminal half-life is approximately 23 hours.

Clearance (ml/min/kg)—3.4 to 3.9 in humans.

Route(s) of Excretion—20 to 30% of intramuscular dose is excreted in urine within 5 to 6 days.

Withdrawal Period—There are no withdrawal times for either milk or meat.

Toxicity and Adverse Effects—Hypersensitivity reactions are possible with HCG. It may cause abortion in mares prior to the 35th day of pregnancy.

Management of Overdose/Toxicity. No overdose has been reported with HCG.

Contraindications—Androgen-dependent neoplasias; hypersensitivity to HCG.

Precautions—HCG may be antigenic and stimulate antibody production.

Drug Interactions—Antibody production and interaction resulting in diminished effect may be observed following repetitive use.

Pharmaceutical Formulations—Available in 5,000, 10,000, and 20,000 Units per vial.

CIMETIDINE

Cimetidine

Proprietary Names—Tagamet®; Cimetidine®.

Chemical Class—Imidazole.

Pharmacological Class—Histamine H_2-receptor antagonist; antiulcer agent; gastric antisecretory agent.

Source—Synthetic.

Solubility, Stability and Storage—Cimetidine is sparingly soluble in water and soluble in alcohol. Cimetidine formulations may be stored at room temperature but must be protect from light. Do not refrigerate cimetidine solutions as this may cause precipitation. Precipitates can re-dissolve by warming. Cimetidine hydrochloride injection can be mixed with most IV infusion fluids (e.g., normal saline, 5 or 10% dextrose, lactated Ringer's, 5% sodium bicarbonate).

Pharmacological Actions—Cimetidine inhibits gastric acid and pepsin secretions during basal conditions and when induced by histamine, food, pentagastrin, and insulin. It does not affect biliary or pancreatic secretions. Cimetidine inhibits cytochrome P_{450} and reduces the metabolic rate of drugs normally biotransformed by the enzyme system. It reduces hepatic blood flow and thus influences the clearance of certain drugs such as propranolol. Cimetidine has also been noted to have immunomodulating and weak anti-androgenic properties.

Mechanism of Action—Cimetidine competes reversibly with histamine for H_2 receptors on the parietal cells.

Indications—Treatment of uremic gastritis, active duodenal and benign gastric ulcers.

Dosages—

Bird	2.5-5 mg/kg IV every 6-12 hours by slow injection over 30-40 min.
Dog	5-10 mg/kg 3-4 times daily.
Cat	5-10 mg/kg 3-4 times daily.
Rabbit	5-10 mg/kg every 6-12 hours.
Cattle	8-16 mg/kg 3 times daily.
Horse	1000-1200 mg in three divided doses per day

Route(s) of Administration—Per os, intramuscular, intravenous and subcutaneous.

Absorption—Cimetidine is rapidly absorbed following oral administration. Absorption can be delayed by food.

Bioavailability—Oral bioavailability is 70-95% in the dog.

Distribution—Vd = 1.2 L/kg. Cimetidine is widely distributed throughout the body. It crosses the placenta and also appear in milk.

Plasma Protein Binding—Human, 15-20%.

Metabolism—Cimetidine is partly metabolized in the liver to sulfoxide and 5-hydroxymethyl derivatives.

Plasma Half-Life—Evaluated at 1-1.3 hours. The half-life is longer in hepatic and/or renal dysfunction.

Route(s) of Excretion—In humans, 80-90% of the drug is excreted in urine within 24 hours; 50-73% is excreted unchanged and the remainder as the two metabolites. About 10% of the drug is excreted in feces.

Dialysis Status—Cimetidine may be removed from the circulation after 5 hours of hemodialysis.

Toxicity and Adverse Effects—Cimetidine is well tolerated in animals. It may cause pain at the site of intramuscular injection. Rebound gastric acid hypersecretion has been observed following discontinuation of cimetidine and other H_2 receptor antagonists. This has been associated with relapse of gastroduodenal ulcers notably in humans.

Management of Overdose—Give symptomatic and supportive treatment.

Contraindication—Hypersensitivity to cimetidine.

Precautions—Use cautiously in old animals and in those patients with hepatic or renal impairment.

Drug Interactions—Cimetidine influences the plasma levels and half-lives of several drugs in three ways. First, by altering gastrointestinal pH and thus influence drug absorption. Secondly, by inhibiting microsomal enzyme thus reducing metabolism of affected drugs. Thirdly, by reducing hepatic blood flow and reducing the clearance of drugs. The disposition of beta-adrenergic blockers, calcium channel blockers, benzodiazepines, ethanol, metronidazole, phenytoin, quinidine, theophylline, triamterene, cyclosporine and warfarin may be affected. Concurrent administration of aluminum and magnesium antacids under fasting and nonfasting conditions may decrease cimetidine absorption. Cimetidine may potentiate the myelosuppressive effects (e.g. neutropenia, agranulocytosis) of myelosuppressive drugs like alkylating agents and antimetabolites.

Pharmaceutical Formulations—The drug is available as cimetidine hydrochloride in 100 mg, 200 mg, 300 mg, 400 mg and 800 mg tablets; 300 mg/5 ml oral liquid; 150 mg/ml solution for injection; and 300 mg in 50 ml normal saline.

CIPROFLOXACIN

Proprietary Names—Ciloxan˙, Cipro˙, Ciprotil˙.

Chemical Class—Fluorinated 4-quinolone (Fluoroquinolone).

Pharmacological Class—Antimicrobial agent.

Source—Synthetic.

Solubility, Stability and Storage—Ciprofloxacin is practically insoluble in water but ciprofloxacin hydrochloride is slightly soluble in water. Store ciprofloxacin tablets in tight containers at less than 30°C. Keep prepared bags for 14 days only, preferably refrigerated.

Ciprofloxacin

Pharmacological Actions—Ciprofloxacin is rapidly bactericidal to several bacteria including *E. coli*, various species of *Salmonella, Shigella, Enterobacter, Campylobacter, Neisseria, Chlamydia, Mycoplasma, Legionella, Brucella, Staphylococci, Klebsiella, Pseudomonas aeruginosa, Haemophilus, Proteus, Yesinia, Serratia, Vibrio, Salmonella, and Aeromonas*. Ciprofloxacin is active in stationary and growth phases of bacterial multiplication. It is weakly active against anaerobic organisms.

Mechanism of Action—Ciprofloxacin inhibits gyrase-mediated DNA negative super coiling leading to inability of the bacteria to maintain DNA super helical structure and effect DNA repair.

Indications—Ciprofloxacin is effective for the treatment of complicated and uncomplicated urinary tract infections caused by susceptible organisms in dogs and cats. It is also used to treat bacterial prostitis, respiratory tract and gastrointestinal tract infections, infections of skin and soft tissues, staphylococci endocarditis pseudomonal meningitis and otitis media.

Dosages—

Bird	Psittacines: 80 mg/kg total daily dose.
	Pigeons: 5-20 mg/kg PO every 12 hours for 5-7 days.
Dog, cat	5-15 mg/kg PO every 12 hours.
NHP	16-20 mg/kg PO every 12 hours in sterile water.
Rabbit	40-50 mg/kg every 8 hours.

Route(s) of Administration—Per os, intravenous and topical.

Absorption—Oral ciprofloxacin is rapidly absorbed in simple stomach animals with plasma concentration reaching its peak within 0.5-2 hours. Antacids containing aluminum, magnesium and/or calcium reduce absorption of ciprofloxacin. Absorption is poor in ponies.

Bioavailability—Human, 60 ± 12%; pony, 2-12%; calf, 50%; pig, 40%.

Distribution—Vd (L/kg) = 1.8 ± 0.4 in humans (value is lower in the aged); 1.47 in rabbits; 3.83 in pigs; 2.50 in calves. Ciprofloxacin is widely distributed in body tissues and fluids. It crosses the placenta, appears in milk and CSF. Concentrations in the CSF are usually less than 10% of peak plasma concentrations although higher concentrations are found if the meninges are inflamed.

Plasma Protein Binding—The values are 40% (human); 70% (calf); 23% (pig).

Metabolism—Ciprofloxacin is partially biotransformed in the liver to inactive products. Ciprofloxacin is itself a metabolite of enrofloxacin.

Plasma Half-Life (hours)—Human, 4.1 ± 0.9 (longer in uremia and shorter in cystic fibrosis); dog, 4.65-7.48; calf, 2.44; pig 2.57; rabbit, 2.21.

Clearance—The rate is 6.0 ± 1.2 ml/min/kg in humans (lower in uremia and higher in cystic fibrosis).

Route(s) of Excretion—As much as 65 ± 12% of dose is excreted as unchanged drug in urine; 20-40% of a dose appears in feces following biliary excretion.

Dialysis Status—Only small amounts are removed by haemodialysis or peritoneal dialysis.

Toxicity and Adverse Effects—Gastrointestinal effects such as vomiting and anorexia are most common. Ciprofloxacin causes bubble-like abnormalities in articular cartilage at high doses especially in growing animals. CNS effects characterized by dizziness, confusion, and seizures are common especially in humans. Crystalluria have been reported. Cutaneous rash may also occur. Ciprofloxacin may cause photosensitization in humans. In humans, flouroquinolones induce tendinopathy mainly at the Achilles tendons. They also induce arthralgia and myalgia.

Management of Toxicity—Reduce its gastrointestinal absorption and give supportive therapy.

Contraindications—Young (2-8 months) small and medium breeds of dogs; hypersensitivity to ciprofloxacin, any component or other quinolones; pregnancy.

Precautions—Reduce the dose in patients with severe renal impairment. Use cautiously in CNS disorders.

Drug Interactions—Ciprofloxacin inhibits the metabolism of theophylline, caffeine, cyclosporine, and warfarin. Azlocillin, cimetidine, and probenecid increase quinolone blood levels. The absorption of ciprofloxacin is reduced if co-administered with antacids containing magnesium, calcium, and aluminum. Probenecid blocks tubular secretion of ciprofloxacin and increases its half-life. Nitrofurantoin may antagonize its antimicrobial activity. Flouroquinolones may enhance the nephrotoxic effect of cyclosporine. Corticosteroid therapy predispose patients to flouroquinolone tendinopathy.

Pharmaceutical Formulations—The drug is available as ciprofloxacin hydrochloride in 100 mg, 250 mg, 500 mg and 750 mg tablets; 200 mg and 400 mg solution for injection; 3.5 mg/ml ophthalmic solution; 200 mg and 400 mg infusion fluids.

CISPLATIN

Cisplatin

Synonyms—CDDP; *cis*-Platinum II; *cis* DDP; Platinum diamminodichloride.

Proprietary Names—Platinol®.

Chemical Class—Inorganic platinum-containing complex.

Pharmacological Class—Antineoplastic drug; anticancer drug.

Source—Synthetic.

Solubility, Stability and Storage—Cisplatin is slightly soluble in water but practically insoluble in ethanol and most common organic solvents, except dimethylsulfoxide. Store cisplatin formulations at room temperature protected from direct sunlight. Reconstitute the powder in 10 ml normal saline immediately before use. Reconstituted solutions are stable for 20 hours at room temperature. Discard solutions with precipitates. Do not administer cisplatin solution with needles or IV sets containing aluminium. Cisplatin products are incompatible with sodium bicarbonate.

Pharmacological Actions—Cisplatin has cytotoxic, mutagenic, carcinogenic, teratogenic, myelosuppressive, and emetogenic properties.

Mechanism of Action—Cisplatin is activated by aquation of its chloride moieties. Activated drug reacts with N-7 of guanine residues and other DNA neuclophiles to form interstrand and intrastrand linkages with resultant inhibition of DNA replication and transcription as well as breaks and miscoding.

Indications—Treatment of transitional cell carcinoma, squamous cell carcinoma, osteosarcoma and adenocarcinoma in dogs.

Dosages—60 mg/m^2 IV over 20 minutes every 3 weeks following a 12 hour fast, and hydration with normal saline at 110 ml/kg before and after administration of cisplatin. Saline administration should last for 6 hours and cisplatin administered 4-5 hours after saline hydration was begun. Inject cisplatin at 1 mg/ml concentration.

Route(s) of Administration—Intravenous.

Effective Concentration—The peak plasma therapeutic concentration is 1 to 5 mg/L (free fraction).

Distribution—Vd = 0.28 ± 0.07 liters/kg (human). Cisplastin distributes rapidly into tissues and attains high concentrations in kidneys, liver, prostrate, intestine, ovaries, uterus and lungs.

Plasma Protein Binding—> 90% (human). The platinum from cisplatin, but not cisplatin itself, is rapidly and extensively bound to tissue and plasma proteins. Binding to tissue and plasma proteins appears to be essentially irreversible and increases with time. Less than 2–10% of platinum in blood remains unbound several hours after intravenous administration of cisplatin.

Metabolism—Cisplastin undergoes inactivation in blood and tissues.

Plasma Half-life—Cisplastin exhibits biphasic elimination half-life; initial phase is 22 minutes and terminal phase is 5 days in dogs; 20-30 minutes (initial) and 24 hours (terminal) in humans.

Clearance—Human, 6.3 ± 1.2 ml/min/kg.

Route(s) of Excretion—In humans 2.3 ± 9% of dose is excreted in urine as unchanged drug. In dogs, 80% is recovered in urine as free platinum.

Dialysis Status—Hemodialysis is of little effect in removing platinum from the body because of cisplatin's rapid and high degree of protein binding.

Toxicity and Adverse Effects—Nephrotoxicity, intractable nausea and emesis are prominent. Other major adverse effects are ototoxicity, anaphylactic-like reaction, neurotoxicity and mild myelosuppression. Skin reactions associated with accidental exposure to the drug may occur. Overdose may result in acute renal failure, severe myelosuppression, intractable nausea and vomiting, neuritis and ototoxicity leading to irreversible deafness.

Management of Overdose—Discontinue the drug and give general supportive therapy. Administer chlorpromazine to control vomition. Nucleophilic (reducing) sulfhydryl (thiol) compounds (e.g., glutathione, acetylcysteine, mesna) can inactivate cisplatin and act as chemoprotectants (e.g., protecting against nephrotoxicity) if these are administered early. Dithiocarbamates [e.g. dithiocarb (diethyldithiocarbamate, DDTC), amifostine (ethiofos)] can react with platinum even after protein binding has occurred and can stimulate substantial biliary excretion of the metal.

Contraindications—Cats; pre-existing severe renal impairment and myelosuppression; hypersensitivity to cisplatin.

Precautions—Give saline fluid before and after dosing with cisplatin to ensure good urinary output and minimize nephrotoxicity. Avoid contact with skin and mucous membranes. Avoid the use of aminoglycoside antibiotics and amphotericin B within 2 weeks of cisplatin therapy to reduce incidence of nephrotoxicity. Protective gloves should be used during handling of commercially available cisplatin injection and during preparation of cisplatin solutions. If cisplatin solution comes in contact with the skin or mucosa, the affected area should be washed with soap and water (skin) or flushed with water (mucosa) immediately and thoroughly.

Drug Interactions—Cisplatin is inactivated by sodium thiosulfate. It binds covalently to glutathione. Cisplatin reduces the serum levels of phenytoin.

Pharmaceutical Formulations—Cisplatin is available as powder for injection containing 10 mg and 50 mg per vial. It is also available in 1 mg/ml solution for injection.

CLEMASTINE

Clemastine

Synonyms—Meclastine, mecloprodin.

Proprietary Names—Tavegyl˚; Tavist˚.

Chemical Class—Ethanolamine derivative.

Pharmacological Class—Histamine H_1-receptor antagonist; Antihistamine; First generation antihistamine.

Source—Synthetic.

Solubility, Stability and Storage—Clemastine fumarate is slightly soluble in water and sparingly soluble in alcohol. The oral solution and tablets should be stored in tight, light-resistant containers at a temperature not exceeding 25°C.

Pharmacological Actions—Clemastine reduces capillary permeability, bronchoconstriction, intestinal contraction and other effects of histamine. It has antipruritic and mild sedative and anticholinergic actions.

Mechanism of Action—Clemastine competes with histamine for H_1 receptors. It has higher affinity than histamine for the receptors but it does not activate the receptors thus blocking the receptors and prevent histamine from combining and activating them.

Indications—Clemastine is useful in the management of allergic conditions such as urticaria, pruritus, insect stings and bites. It is used also as adjunct to the treatment of acute and chronic eczema, contact dermatitis, drug eruptions, anaphylactic shock and angioneurotic edema.

Dosage—0.05 mg/kg PO every 12 hours.

Route(s) of Administration—Per os.

Absorption—Clemastine is readily and almost completely absorbed following oral administration and peak plasma concentration is attained within 2-4 hours.

Distribution—Clemastine is widely distributed. It appears in breast milk.

Plasma Protein Binding—95%

Metabolism—The drug is extensively metabolized in the liver.

Plasma Half-Life—It exhibits biphasic half-lives evaluated at 3.6 ± 0.9 hours and 37 ± 16 hours.

Duration of Action—10-12 hours.

Peak Action—5-7 hours.

Route(s) of Excretion—Clemastine is eliminated in urine.

Toxicity and Adverse Effects—CNS related effects such as fatigue, sedation and occasional CNS stimulation have been reported. Other effects are associated with its anticholinergic effects. These may be observed as dry mucous membranes. Increased appetite, weight gain, diarrhea, and skin rash may be observed at normal doses. Overdose may cause tachycardia, urinary retention, hyperthermia and hypotension. Intravenous administration may cause hypersensitivity reaction in rare cases.

Management of Overdose—Set up general antidotal therapy. Cholinesterase inhibitor (e.g. physostigmine) may help in reducing the anticholinergic affects.

Contraindications—Hypersensitivity to clemastine or members of the ethanolamine group of antihistamines; narrow-angle glaucoma; asthmatic attack.

Precautions—Use clemastine cautiously in patients with stenosing peptic ulcer, pyloroduodenal obstruction, prostatic hypertrophy with urinary retention, and bladder neck obstruction. Antihistamines should be used with caution in patients with increased intraocular pressure, hyperthyroidism, cardiovascular disease, or in patients who have a breathing problem (e.g. emphysema, chronic bronchitis).

Drug Interactions—Clemastine potentiates the sedative effects of sedative-hypnotics, MAO inhibitors, tricyclic antidepressants and alcohol.

Pharmaceutical Formulations—The drug is available as clemastine hydrogen fumarate in 1 mg tablets, 0.1 mg/ml and 1 mg/ml solution for injection. Suspension of 0.5 mg/5 ml is also available.

CLENBUTEROL

Clenbuterol

Proprietary Names—Ventipulmin®.

Pharmacological Class—Sympathomimetic agent; beta$_2$-adrenergic agonist.

Source—Synthetic.

Solubility, Stability and Storage—Clenbuterol hydrochloride is very soluble in water, methanol and ethanol. Clenbuterol syrup can be stored at room temperature.

Pharmacological Actions—Clenbuterol selectively inhibits smooth muscle contraction thereby causing smooth muscle relaxation or dilatation. It causes bronchodilatation and vasodilatation.

Mechanism of Action—It activates beta$_2$-adrenergic receptors followed by activation of adenylyl cyclase and increased level of cAMP.

Indications—Clenbuterol is used as a bronchodilator in the treatment of chronic obstructive pulmonary disease in horses.

Dosages: 0.8 mcg/kg twice daily for 3 days. Increase the dose progressively to 1.6 mcg/kg, 2.4 mcg/kg, 3.2 mcg/kg if there is no improvement with smaller doses. Follow the regimen for 30 days.

Route(s) of Administration—Per os.

Absorption—Clenbuterol is rapidly and almost completely absorbed after oral administration. Peak plasma level is attained within 2 hours.

Duration of Action—6-8 hours.

Plasma Protein Binding—89 to 98%.

Metabolism—Clembuterol is extensively metabolized by first-pass sulfation.

Plasma Half-Life—10 hours.

Route(s) of Excretion—Urine.

Toxicity and Adverse Effects—CNS excitement, tachycardia, muscle tremors, sweating and dizziness have been reported. Ataxia may occur.

Management of Overdose—Institute symptomatic and supportive therapy. Beta-adrenergic blockers may be used to control heart rate and rhythm.

Contraindications—Food producing animals; cardiovascular impairment; pregnancy nearing full term; hypersensitivity to clenbuterol.

Drug Interactions—Clenbuterol antagonizes dinoprost (prostaglandin F$_2\alpha$) and oxytocin. Concomitant use with other sympathomimetic agents may increase the likelihood of cardiovascular adverse effects. Beta-adrenergic blockers may inhibit the action of clenbuterol. Monoamine oxidase inhibitors and tricyclic antidepressants may enhance the pressor effects of clenbuterol. Administration of clenbuterol in animals under halogenated hydrocarbon induced anesthesia may enhance its potential to cause cardiac arrhythmias. Concurrent use with digitalis may induce cardiac arrhythmia. Bronchodilation may be enhanced by concomitant administration of methylxanthine (e.g. aminophylline) in cases that have experienced receptor down regulation as a result of prolonged administration of clenbuterol.

Pharmaceutical Formulations—Available as clenbuterol hydrochloride in oral syrup containing 72.5 mcg/ml.

CLONAZEPAM

Proprietary Names—Klonopin®; Clonazepam®.

Chemical Class—Benzodiazepine.

Pharmacological Class—CNS depressant; sedative-hypnotic; anxiolytic.

Source—Synthetic.

Solubility, Stability and Storage—Solubilities of clonazepam in mg/mL at 25° in different solvents are: acetone 31, chloroform 15, methanol 8.6, ether 0.7, benzene 0.5, water <0.1. Clonazepam is stable, with a shelf-life of five years. Store clonazepam tablets at room temperature in air-tight and light resistant containers.

Pharmacological Actions—Clonazepam selectively depresses the CNS and produces sedation and hypnosis without loss of consciousness. It exhibits anticonvulsant properties by depressing nerve transmission in the motor cortex and suppressing spike and wave discharge.

Clonazepam

Mechanism of Action—Clonazepam binds to $GABA_A$ receptor/ion channel complex in the presence of GABA and allosterically modulates the action of GABA to produce increase in neuronal chloride conductance resulting in hyperpolarization and reduced neuronal excitability.

Indications—Clonazepam is used as an adjunct in the treatment of seizures in dogs. It is also used to control status epilepticus.

Dosages: 0.5 mg/kg orally every 8-12 hours. Adjust dosage slowly according to individual requirements and response.

Route of Administration—Per os.

Absorption—Clonazepam is well absorbed after oral administration. Peak plasma concentration is attained within 1-2 hours.

Bioavailability—Oral bioavailability is high (98%).

Effective Concentration: 0.015-0.07 mcg/ml.

Onset of Action—Human, 20-60 minutes.

Distribution—Vd = 3.2 ± 1.1. Clonazepam crosses the blood-brain-barrier and placenta. It is not known if clonazepam is secreted in milk.

Plasma Protein Binding: 86 ± 0.5.

Metabolism—Extensively metabolized in the liver to several glucuronide and sulfate conjugates.

Plasma Half-Life—23 ± 5 hours.

Clearance (ml/min/kg)—1.55 ± 0.28.

Route(s) of Excretion—Urine, with 1% as unchanged drug.

Dialysis Status—The drug can be removed from the body by dialysis.

Toxicity and Adverse Effects—The most frequent adverse effects of clonazepam are sedation or drowsiness and ataxia. Increased salivation, hypersecretion in upper respiratory passages, chest congestion, rhinorrhea, and shortness of breath have also been reported. Adverse gastrointestinal effects of clonazepam include constipation, diarrhea, increased or decreased appetite, weight gain or loss, dyspepsia, nausea, dry mouth, abnormal thirst, and sore gums. Clonazepam may also produce haematologic effects characterized by anemia, leukopenia, thrombocytopenia, and eosinophilia. Overdose of clonazepam may produce somnolence, confusion, ataxia, diminished reflexes, or coma. Tolerance has been reported in dogs usually after three months of therapy. Adverse effects have been reported in rabbits and rats when used during pregnancy.

Management of Overdose—Follow general antidotal therapy in addition to adequate supportive measures. Flumazenil will specifically antagonize the CNS depressant effects of clonazepam and may be used as adjunct to general antidotal therapy.

Contraindications—Hypersensitivity to clonazepam or other benzodiazepines; acute narrow-angle glaucoma; severe liver dysfunction.

Precautions—Use the drug cautiously during pregnancy. The dose of clonazepam should be tapered especially following prolonged high dose therapy to avoid precipitating seizures, status epilepticus, or withdrawal symptoms.

Drug Interactions—Concurrent administration with other CNS depressants will give additive effects. Phenytoin and barbiturates may increase the clearance of clonazepam. Enzyme inducers may increase its metabolism. Its metabolism may be decreased by cimetidine, erythromycin, isoniazid, ketoconazole, propranolol and valproic acid.

Pharmaceutical Formulations—Clonazepam is available in 0.5 mg, 1 mg and 2 mg tablets. No specific formulation for veterinary use is available.

CLOPIDOL

Clopidol

Proprietary Names—Coyden 25®; Lerbek® (in combination with methylbenzoquate).

Chemical Class—Pyridinol.

Pharmacological Class—Coccidiostat; anticoccidial agent.

Source. Synthetic.

Solubility, Stability and Storage—Clopidol is insoluble in water but slightly soluble in ethanol.

Pharmacological Actions—Clopidol is effective against all Eimeria spp. It arrests sporozoite and trophozoite development. Sporozoites can resume development following withdrawal of the drug.

Mechanism of Action—Disrupts electron transport in mitochondrial cytochrome of Eimeria thereby inhibiting the parasite respiration.

Indications—Prevention of coccidiosis caused by *E. tenella, E. necatrix, E. acervulina, E. maxima, E. brunetti,* and *E. mivati* in broiler chickens and rabbits. Clopidol is effective against ionophore-resistant coccidia. It is also used in the prevention of leucocytozoonosis in turkeys.

Dosages—113.5 g/ton of feed for chickens (broilers and layer replacements) and turkeys; 227 grams clopidol per ton of feed for chicken layers.

Route(s) of Administration—Per os.

Residue Limit—

Chickens and turkeys. 15 ppm in uncooked liver and kidney; 5 ppm in uncooked muscle.

Cattle, sheep, and goats. 3 ppm in uncooked kidney; 1.5 ppm in uncooked liver; 0.2 ppm in uncooked muscle.

Pig. 0.2 ppm in uncooked edible tissues.

Milk. 0.02 ppm (negligible residue).

Withdrawal Period—Chicken (broilers) and turkeys. Observe withdrawal period of 5 days before slaughter if given at the level of 0.025 percent in feed or reduce the level of intake to 0.0125 percent 5 days before slaughter.

Toxicity and Adverse Effects—Clopidol is very safe for chickens; also safe in mammals.

Contraindications—Hypersensitivity to clopidol.

Precautions—Withdrawal of the drug may lead to relapse of infection. Drug resistance problems limit its use to shuttle programs (e.g. last 1 ± 3 weeks of broiler growout).

Drug Interactions—Clopidol potentiates the action of 4-hydroxyquinolines. There is no cross resistance between the two groups of drugs.

Pharmaceutical Formulations—Clopidol is available as 25% premix for addition to feed.

CLOPROSTENOL

Proprietary Names—Estrumate˙.

Chemical Class—Prostaglandin $F_2\alpha$ analog.

Pharmacological Class—Arbortifacient; Ecbolic; Oxytocic agent.

Source—Synthetic.

Solubility, Stability and Storage—Cloprostenol is freely soluble in water and alcohol. Formulations of cloprostenol sodium should be stored at room temperature (15-30°C) and protected from light.

Pharmacological Actions—Cloprostenol causes rapid regression of the corpus luteum and arrest its secretory activity. It also contracts the uterine smooth muscle and relaxes the cervix. Cloprostenol could cause estrus within 2-5 days in cycling animals. It could also cause abortion within 2–3 days if used between 10-50 days of gestation in cattle.

Mechanism of Action. Cloprostenol activates Prostaglandin F (FP) receptors.

Indications—To induce luteolysis; treat pyometra or chronic endometritis; expel mummified fetus; induce safe and early abortions after mismating; synchronize estrus and ovulation for controlled breeding.

Dosages—100 micrograms in cattle and horses.

Route(s) of Administration—Intramuscular.

Absorption—Cloprostenol is readily absorbed from the skin.

Withdrawal Period—Neither pre-slaughter withdrawal nor milk withdrawal is required.

Toxicity and Adverse Effects—Cloprostenol may cause increased risk of dystocia if used after the month of gestation. It may induce abortion or acute bronchoconstriction. Cattle may become restless and let down milk following overdose. Overdose in small animals may result in shock and death.

Contraindications—Pregnancy.

Precautions—Efficiency of cloprostenol may decrease if used after 5 months of gestation. Veterinarians or animal attendants with asthma or other respiratory diseases should use extreme caution when handling cloprostenol as it may cause acute bronchoconstriction. Spills on the skin must be washed off rapidly with soap and water. Do not administer intravenously.

Drug Interactions—Other oxytocic agents may enhance the action of cloprostenol.

Pharmaceutical Formulations—Available as cloprostenol sodium in 250 mcg/ml solution for injection.

CLORSULON

Clorsulon

Proprietary Names—Curatrem˙; Ivomec Super˙ (1% ivermectin and 10% Clorsulon).

Chemical Class—Benzenesulfonamide.

Pharmacological Class—Anthelmintic; Flukicide.

Source—Synthetic.

Solubility, Stability and Storage—Store clorsulon formulations at room temperature (15-30°C).

Pharmacological Actions—Clorsulon is active against adult forms of *Fasciola hepatica* and *Fasciola gigantica* in cattle. Immature flukes above 8 weeks are susceptible. Clorsulon is ineffective against the rumen fluke (*Paramphistomum*).

Mechanism of Action—Clorsulon inhibits the glycolytic enzymes 3-phosphoglycerate kinase and phosphoglyceromutase, thereby blocking the Emden-Myerhof glycolytic pathway. The fluke is deprived of its main metabolic energy source and dies.

Therapeutic Uses—Treatment of fluke infection in cattle.

Dosages. 7 mg/kg PO by placing the clorsulon suspension at the back of the tongue.

Route(s) of Administration—Per os. Ivomec Super® is administered subcutaneously.

Absorption—Clorsulon is rapidly absorbed after oral administration. Peak blood levels are attained within 4 hours. Peak drug levels are attained in the flukes within 8-12 hours after administration.

Withdrawal Period—72 hours for milk; 8 days for edible tissues.

Toxicity and Adverse Effects—Clorsulon is very safe. No adverse effects have been reported at the therapeutic doses.

Contraindications—Female dairy cattle of breeding age; hypersensitivity to clorsulon.

Pharmaceutical Formulations—Available as 8.5% (85 mg/ml) oral drench. Also available in combination with ivermectin in injectionable solution.

CLOXACILLIN

Cloxacillin

Synonyms—Sodium cloxacillin; chlorphenylmethyl isoxazolyl penicillin sodium; methylchlorophenyl isoxazolyl penicillin sodium.

Proprietary Names—Cloxapen˚, Tegopen˚, Kloxyl˚, Orbenin˚, Dariclox˚, Dicloxin˚, Ampiclox˚ (125mg or 250mg each of cloxacillin and ampicillin).

Chemical Class—6-Amino penicillinic acid derivative.

Pharmacological Class—Isoxazolyl penicillin; penicillinase-resistant penicillin; beta-lactam antibiotic; anti-staphylococci penicillin.

Source—Semisynthetic.

Solubility, Stability, and Storage—Cloxacillin sodium is readily soluble in water and alcohol. Cloxacillin benzathine is only slightly soluble in water and alcohol. Store cloxacillin formulations at room temperature. Reconstituted oral suspension is stable for 7 days at room temperature and 14 days if refrigerated.

Pharmacological Actions—Cloxacillin is bactericidal to penicillinase-producing *Staphylococcus aureus* and penicillin G-sensitive staph. It is less active than penicillin G against other Gram-positive microorganisms except Staphylococcus. It has narrower spectrum than natural penicillins.

Mechanism of Action—Same as other penicillins.

Indications—Cloxacillin is effective in the treatment and prevention of mastitis during lactation and dry period. It is also used to treat skin and soft tissue infections, wounds, burns, and septicemia caused by gram positive microbes.

Dosages—

Small animals: 4-10mg\kg every 12 hours.

Large animals: 1-2mg\kg every 12 hours.

For treatment of mastitis: 200mg of cloxacillin sodium or 500mg of benzathine cloxacillin intramammary per quarter.

Route(s) of Administration—Per os; intramammary (in animals).

Absorption—Cloxacillin is rapidly but incompletely absolved after oral administration. Peak plasma concentration is attained within 1 hour following oral administration. Food reduces the rate and extent of absorption. Cloxacillin is acid-resistant.

Bioavailability (oral)—43 ± 16%.

Distribution—Vd = 0.094 ± 0.015 liters\kg. Cloxacillin is widely distributed to body fluids and bones. It appears in milk and crosses the placenta. Penetration into cells, eye, and CSF is poor.

Plasma Protein Binding—94.6 ± 0.6% in human.

Metabolism—Cloxacillin is partly metabolized to active and inactive products.

Plasma Half-Life—Human, 30-60 minutes; values are higher in uremia.

Clearance—2.2 ± 0.5ml/min\kg in humans (lower in uremia).

Route(s) of Excretion—Cloxacillin is eliminated via urine with 75% of dose as unchanged drug. About 10% of a dose is excreted in the bile.

Dialysis Status—Not dialyzable.

Toxicity and Adverse Effects—Hypersensitivity reactions ranging from skin rash to serum sickness-like conditions. Nausea, diarrhea, vomiting, hematologic disorders, hepatotoxicity and hematuria have been observed at therapeutic doses. Overdose may cause neuromuscular hypersensitivity, electrolyte imbalance and renal failure.

Management of Overdose/Toxicity—Give supportive and symptomatic treatment—

Contraindications—Hypersensitivity to cloxacillin, the penicillins or their products.

Precautions—Administer cloxacillin 1 hour prior to, or 2 hours after meals.

Drug Interactions—The effects of anticoagulants may be increased by cloxacillin. Probenecid or disulfiram increase its plasma concentration.

Pharmaceutical Formulations—Available as cloxacillin sodium in 250 mg or 500 mg capsules; 125mg/5 ml or 250 mg/5 ml oral solution and also in combination with ampicillin. Cloxacillin sodium in an oil base is available for parental administration in the treatment of mastitis during lactation. Cloxacillin benzathine, also in an oil base, is available for administration via the teat canal during the dry period.

COLCHICINE

Colchicine

Proprietary Names—Colchicine˙.

Chemical Class—Phenanthrene alkaloid.

Pharmacological Class—Antimitotic agent; Antigout agent; Uricosuric agent.

Source—Natural; obtained from the plant, *Colchicum autumnale* (Meadow Saffron) and other *Colchicum* species.

Solubility, Stability and Storage—Colchicine is soluble 1 in 20 of water but freely soluble in ethanol. Colchicine formulations store well in tight light resistant containers. Dilute injection solution with normal saline or water for injection but not with 5% dextrose solution. Do not use products that have become turbid.

Pharmacological Actions—Colchicine possesses anti-inflammatory action only in acute gout. It interferes with mitotic spindle formation in dividing cells. It also inhibits the release of histamine-containing granules from mast cells. Cochicine blocks the synthesis and secretion of serum amyloid A by hepatocytes thus preventing the formation of amyloid enhancing factor and amyloid disposition. It decreases the formation and increases the breakdown of collagen.

Mechanism of Action—Colchicine binds to microtubular proteins and interferes with the function of the mitotic spindles by causing depolymerization and disappearance of the fibrillar microtubular in agranulocytes and other mobile cells. This results in the inhibition of migration of granulocyte into inflamed areas and the failure of spindle formation during mitosis. Colchicine also interferes with sodium urate deposition by directly decreasing polymorphonulear leukocytes lactic acid production and indirectly reducing acid production by decreasing phagocytosis.

Indications—Treatment of amyloidosis in small animals and of chronic hepatic fibrosis; Colchicine is used as a multiplier of chromosomes in animal breeding for the production of multiple offspring.

Dosages—None was sighted; see product insert. For animal breeding, semen is exposed to a solution of colchicine prior to artificial insemination.

Route(s) of Administration—Per os; intravenous. Colchicine causes severe local irritation if given subcutaneously or intramuscularly.

Absorption—Colchicine is rapidly absorbed from oral sites. Peak plasma concentration is attained within 0.5-2 hours.

Distribution—Colchicine is distributed into several tissues and fluids including milk and leukocytes.

Plasma Protein Binding—10-31%.

Metabolism—The drug is partly inactivated in the liver by deacetylation. It undergoes enterohepatic circulation.

Plasma Half-Life—20 minutes-1 hour (higher in cases of severe renal disease.) Colchicine half-life in leukocytes is about 60 hours.

Duration of Action—12 hours.

Route(s) of Excretion—Feces (via bile) and urine.

Dialysis Status—Dialyzable.

Toxicity and Adverse Effects—Gastrointestinal side effects including nausea, vomiting, diarrhea, abdominal pain and hemorrhagic gastroenteritis are common. Vascular damage, nephrotoxicity, muscular depression, and ascending paralysis of the CNS have all been reported. Temporary leukemia which is soon replaced by leukocytosis and agranulocytosis following long term therapy has also been observed. Colchicine may decrease spermatogenesis. An overdose may cause nausea, vomiting, shock, abdominal pain, kidney damage, muscle weakness, delirium and convulsions.

Management of Overdose/Toxicity—Undertake measures that could reduce absorption and prevent shock. Give other supportive and symptomatic treatment including peritoneal dialysis.

Contraindications—Severe cardiac, renal and gastrointestinal diseases; hypersensitivity to colchicine or any component.

Precautions—Use cautiously in patients with early stages of cardiac, renal and GI diseases. Use with caution in debilitated animals. Discontinue therapy if early signs of toxicity consisting of abdominal pain, anorexia, vomiting and diarrhea are noticed.

Drug Interactions—Concurrent use of colchicine with NSAIDs especially phenylbutazone may increase the risk of bone marrow depression. Antineoplastic agents and other bone marrow depressants may have additive effect. Colchicine may reduce the absorption of vitamin B_{12} and enhance the actions of sympathomimetic agents and CNS depressants.

Pharmaceutical Formulations—Colchicine is available in 0.5 mg and 0.6 mg tablets, and in 0.5 mg/ml sterile solution for injection. A formulation consisting of 500 mg probenecid and 0.5 mg colchicine is also available.

COLISTIN

Synonyms—Polymyxin E.

Proprietary Names—Coly-mycin*; Colistin 4800*; Colivet*; Virgocilline*; Cofacoli*; Keproceryl*. Colistin is in fixed dose combination with other drugs in the following products: Neoceryl*, Coryl SP*, Doseryl*, Mirth-O-Ceryl*, Belcospiral*, Combisan*, Colidox*, Poultaid C*, Ticol*, Ladseryl*, Aseryl*.

Chemical Class—Polypeptide.

Pharmacological Class—Antibiotic; Antibacterial agent.

Source—Natural; elaborated by *Bacillus (Aerobacillus) colistinus*.

Solubility, Stability and Storage—The powder for making oral suspension is stable for two weeks when refrigerated. The solution for injection should be stored below 25⁰C and protected from light.

Pharmacological Actions—Colistin is primarily bactericidal to Gram-negative bacilli such as *E. coli*, *Enterobacter aerogenes*, *Salmonella*, *Shigella*, *Pasteurella* and *Pseudomonas aeruginosa*.

Mechanism of Action—Colistin interacts strongly with phospholipids. It penetrates into and disrupts the structure, osmotic properties, and transport mechanisms of bacteria cell membranes causing leakage of macromolecules and death of the bacteria.

Indications—Colistin is effective in enteric infections caused by susceptible organisms in young animals, fowl typhoid and pullorum disease in broilers. The drug is used in topical treatment of skin, eye, and ear infections and of wounds, eczema, dermal ulcers, eye and external ear infections usually in combination with bacitracin and neomycin.

Dosages—50,000 IU or 2.5 mg/kg twice daily for three days.

Route(s) of Administration—Per os; intramuscular.

Absorption—Colistin is poorly absorbed from the gastrointestinal tract but the level of absorption may be unpredictable in young animals.

Bioavailability (oral)—Low.

Distribution—Colistin reversibly binds to and persists in body tissues such as the liver, kidneys, lung, heart, and muscle. It crosses the placenta and is distributed into milk.

Plasma Protein Binding—Colistin is more than 50% bound to serum proteins.

Plasma Half-life—Human, 2.8-4.8 hours (48-72 hours in anuria).

Route(s) of Excretion—Colistin is excreted via urine with 65-75% of a dose eliminated as unchanged drug.

Toxicity and Adverse Effects—Colistin may cause severe neural and renal toxicity if administered systemically. It causes less irritation than polymyxin B when applied to the cornea or conjunctiva. Colistin causes nausea, and vomiting. Prolonged use may cause superinfection.

Contraindications—Anuria; hypersensitivity to colistin.

Precautions—Use Colistin with caution in renal impairment. Note that the possibility of renal and neural damage exist especially following systemic administration. Do not administer colistin systemically with aminoglycosides or other nephrotoxic drugs.

Drug Interactions—Aminoglycoside antibiotics may increase the risk of nephrotoxicity.

Pharmaceutical Formulations—Available as colistin sulfate in tablets, ointment and injectable solution containing 1,000,000 IU/ml. Colistin sulfate is available as water soluble powder in combination with several antibacterial drugs and vitamins for addition to animal feed or water. It is also available in powder for oral suspension of 25 mg/5 ml for use in children. Colistin sulphomethane sodium formulation which slowly releases the active principle is also available for parenteral administration.

CORSYNTROPIN

Synonyms—Synacthen; Tetracosactide.

Proprietary Names—Cortrosyn®

Chemical Class—Polypeptide.

Pharmacological Class—Hormone.

Source—Synthetic; identical to human ACTH 1-24. Ten mcg of corsynthropin is approximately equivalent to 1 unit of porcine ACTH.

Pharmacological Actions—Corsynthropin stimulates growth of adrenal cortex and steroidogenesis. It may also cause adipose tissue lipolysis and increased skin pigmentation.

Mechanism of Action—Corsynthropin increases cellular cAMP resulting in increased activity of cholesterol desmolase which converts cholesterol to pregnenolone, the rate-limiting step in steroid synthesis.

Indications—Diagnostic aid in distinguishing between adrenocortical hyperplasia and primary adrenocortical neoplasia in dogs, cats, cattle, and horses.

Dosage—250 mcg (dog); 125 mcg (cat, preferably by intravenous injection).

Route(s) of Administration—Intravenous, and intramuscular.

Absorption—Corsynthropin is readily absorbed from muscular sites.

Distribution—It crosses the placenta.

Metabolism—Unknown.

Peak Action—60-90 minutes (dog).

Toxicity and Adverse Effects—Corsynthropin has few side effects, which includes flushing, fever, pruritus, chronic pancreatitis and hypersensitivity reaction.

Contraindications—Hypersensitivity to corsynthropin.

Precautions—Use corsynthropin cautiously in patients known to be allergic to corticotropin or with pre-existing allergic disorder.

Pharmaceutical Formulations—The drug is available as 0.25 mg powder for injection (equivalent to 25 units of corticotropin)

CORTICOTROPIN

Synonyms—ACTH; Adrenocorticotropin.

Proprietary Names—ACTH®ᶦ Acthar®; HP Acthar® gel; Adrenomone®.

Chemical Class—Polypeptide.

Pharmacological Class—Hormone.

Source. ACTH is naturally secreted from the anterior pituitary gland. It is commercially obtained from porcine pituitaries; 1 unit of porcine ACTH is equivalent to 10 mcg of corsyntropin, a synthetic human ACTH.

Solubility, Stability and Storage—Aqueous corticotropin formulation for injection is stable at room temperature before reconstitution. It is better refrigerated and used within 24 hours once reconstituted. The reconstituted product may be stable for 8 hours at room temperature. Corticotropin gel is stable for less than 72 hours at room temperature, hence it should be refrigerated. Warm the vial prior to use for ease of filling a syringe with the product.

Pharmacological Actions—ACTH stimulates the secretion of glucocorticoid hormones (primarily cortisol in mammals and corticosterone in birds) from the adrenal cortex. It also stimulates adrenal hypertrophy and hyperplasia.

Mechanism of Action—See Corsynthropin.

Indications—Diagnosis of adrenal insufficiency; treatment of secondary adrenocortical insufficiency and non-endocrine disorders that would normally respond to glucocorticoids; treatment of primary bovine ketosis.

Dosages—

Horses and cattle	1 IU/kg for ACTH stimulation test.
Dogs and cats	2.2 IU/kg for ACTH stimulation test.

Route(s) of Administration—Intramuscular, intravenous (aqueous formulation) and subcutaneous routes are preferred.

Absorption—ACTH is largely absorbed from the IM site. Peak blood concentration of aqueous corticotropin is attained within 1 hour. Corticotropin gel may be absorbed over 8-16 hours.

Onset of Action—Human, 6 hours.

Peak Action—Aqueous corticotropin, 30-90 minutes; corticotropin gel, 2 hours in horses, dogs and 1 hour in cats.

Duration of Action—Aqueous corticotropin, 2-4 hours; 12-48 hours (corticotropin gel).

Plasma Half-life—Aqueous corticotropin, 10-20 minutes.

Route(s) of Excretion—Eliminated via urine.

Toxicity and Adverse Effects—Prolonged use of corticotropin may cause fluid and electrolyte disturbances.

Management of Overdose/Toxicity—Potassium supplement may be necessary with prolonged administration.

Contraindications—Hypersensitivity to porcine proteins; systemic fungal infection.

Precautions—Use ACTH cautiously during pregnancy. Corticotropin may mask signs of infection. Do not administer live vaccines concurrently with corticotropin.

Drug Interactions—Effects of corticotrophin may be reduced by spironolactone, hydrocortisone and cortisone. Corticotropin can antagonize the actions of anticholinesterases such as neostigmine.

Pharmaceutical Formulations—Available as corticotropin in 25 and 40 units per vial, for injection. Other formulations are repository corticotropin for injection (corticotropin gel containing 40 and 80 units/ml) and corticotropin zinc hydroxide suspension containing benzyl alcohol.

CYCLOPHOSPHAMIDE

Cyclophosphamide

Synonyms—CPM; CTX; CYT

Proprietary Names—Cytoxan®; Neosar®.

Chemical Class—Nitrogen mustard derivative.

Pharmacological Class—Antineoplastic drug; Immunosuppressive agent; Alkylating agent.

Source—Synthetic.

Solubility, Stability and Storage—Cyclophosphamide is soluble in water and in alcohol. Store all products below 30⁰C. Use reconstituted powder within 24 hours if stored at room temperature or 6 days if refrigerated.

Pharmacological Actions—Cyclophosphamide has cytotoxic actions due to disruption of nucleic acid function by interfering with DNA replication, RNA transcription and replication. It also has immunosuppressive action. Cells that divide rapidly (and thus replicate their DNA rapidly) such as rapidly dividing cancer cells, bone marrow cells, stimulated lymphocytes (those engaged in proliferation and antibody production), fetal cells, hair follicle cells, and intestinal cells are especially affected by cyclophosphamide.

Mechanism of Action—Cyclophosphamide acts by forming highly reactive carbonium ion intermediates which react with strongly neucleophilic substituents like phosphate, amino,—SH, OH, COOH and imidazole groups to form covalent bonds. The target molecule is thus alkylated. The N-7 position of guanine in DNA is highly susceptible. Alkylation of guanine in the DNA leads to cross linkage of DNA strands, linking of DNA to a closely associated protein, base pairing of guanine with thymine instead of cytosine, or breakage of the DNA strand.

Indications—Treatment of immune mediated diseases (especially those of life-threatening nature such as immune mediated hemolytic anemia); also used in cancer chemotherapy (especially for bone marrow or blood cell cancers such as lymphoma). Cyclophosphamide is used in combination with prednisolone in the treatment of canine transmissible venereal tumor.

Dosages—50 mg/m² orally or IV 4 days per week.

Route(s) of Administration—Per os; intravenous.

Absorption—Cyclophosphamide is well absorbed from the gastrointestinal tract. Peak plasma concentrations are attained within 1 hour.

Bioavailability—Oral bioavailability in human is 74 ± 22%.

Distribution—Vd = 0.78 ± 0.57 l/kg. Cyclophosphamide is widely distributed. It crosses the blood-brain-barrier and placenta; attains sub therapeutic concentration in CSF. It distributes into milk.

Plasma Protein Binding—The level of binding is evaluated at 13%.

Metabolism—Cyclophosphamide is activated by hepatic cytochrome P-450 mixed functional oxidase, first to 4-hydroxycyclophosphamide and then aldophosphamide, carboxyphosphamide and 4-ketocyclophosphamide. Aldophosphamide is active and is further converted to active phosphoramide mustard and acrolein.

Plasma Half-life—7.5 ± 4.0 hours (human)

Clearance (ml/min/kg)—1.3 ± 0.5 (human)

Route(s) of Excretion—Urine (6.5 ± 4.3% as unchanged drug).

Dialysis Status—20-50% dialyzable.

Toxicity and Adverse Effects—Marked alopecia in wavy coated dogs such as poodles has been observed. Cats undergoing chemotherapy commonly lose their whiskers. In general, hair texture tends to get softer. Its emetogenic potential in dogs and cats is low and can be readily controlled with antiemetics when it occurs. Bone marrow depression, leukopenia, thrombocytopenia appear approximately 1-2 weeks following a dose of cyclophosphamide. This time period makes the patient especially vulnerable to infection. Up to 30% of dogs receiving cyclophosphamide for over 2 months develop hemorrhagic cystitis characterized by bloody urine.

Management of Overdose—Discontinue or reduce the dose in patients with severe bone marrow depression. Give antiemetics to reduce the incidence of vomition.

Contraindications—Hypersensitivity to cyclophosphamide; pre-existing infection and immunodepression.

Precautions—Hydrate the animal to prevent hemorrhagic cystitis. Cyclophosphamide is preferably administered in the morning and possibly with mesma (sodium 2-mecaptoethanesulfonate) to bind acrolein and prevent hemorrhagic cystitis. Use cyclophosphamide cautiously in animals with impaired hepatic and renal functions. Avoid the drug in patients taking other bone marrow suppressing agents such as azathioprine or methimazole.

Drug Interactions—Prolonged administration of enzyme inducers (e.g. phenobarbital and phenytoin) may increase metabolism and enhance toxicity by cyclophosphamide active metabolites. Cimetidine reduces cyclophosphamide activation by inhibiting its metabolism. Pseudo cholinesterase concentration is decreased by cyclophosphamide thus affecting drugs that are usually metabolized by the enzyme system (e.g. succinylcholine). Allopurinol and thiazide diuretics may enhance myelosuppression caused by cyclophosphamide. Chloramphenicol increases cyclophosphamide half-life. Cyclophosphamide may potentiate the action of cardiotoxic drugs (e.g. doxorubicin).

Pharmaceutical Formulations—Available as cyclophosphamide hydrate in 25 mg and 50 mg tablets and as 100 mg, 200 mg, 500 mg, 1 g, and 2 g lyophilized, and non-lyophilized powder for injection.

CYCLOSPORINE

Synonyms—Cyclosporin A; Ciclosporin.

Proprietary Names—Atopica*; Neoral*; Sandimmune*; Cremophor* Optimmune*; Labrafil* (ophthalmic).

Chemical Class—Cyclic polypeptide.

Pharmacological Class—Disease-modifying antirheumatic drug; Immunosuppressive agent.

Source. Natural; produced by the soil fungus *Beauveria nivia*.

Solubility, Stability and Storage—Cyclosporine is relatively insoluble in water (aqueous solubility = 0.04 mg/ml at 25°C). It is generally soluble in lipids and organic solvents. Solubility in alcohol at 25°C is more than 80 mg/ml. Cyclosporine preparations should be stored at room temperature and protected from light. Do not refrigerate or freeze the preparations. Containers which have been opened should be used within 2 months.

Pharmacological Actions—Cyclosporine possesses immunosuppressive activity. It inhibits cell-mediated immune responses such as allograft rejection and delayed hypersensitivity. Cyclosporine also inhibits primary and secondary responses to T cell-dependent antigens. It may also inhibit humoral immune responses to some extent. Cyclosporine causes increased survival of allogeneic (homologous) transplants involving skin, heart, kidney, liver, pancreas, bone marrow, small intestine, and lung.

Mechanism of Action—Cyclosporine binds to and inhibits calcineurin, a calcium and calmodulin dependent phosphatase, which inhibits transcription and hence production of interleukin-2 by T-helper cells. Cyclosporin may also inhibit expression of receptors for interleukin-2. The inhibition of interleukin-2 expression by cyclosporine reduces the production of a wide range of other cytokines.

Indications—Cyclosporine relieves the symptoms and discomfort associated with "dry eye" (keratoconjunctivitis sicca), a condition caused by immune-mediated inflammation in the tear glands in dogs. The drug is used also to treat atopic dermatitis and immune-mediated hemolytic anemia as well as prevention of rejection of kidney, liver, or heart allografts.

Dosages—Cyclosporine is generally given once or twice daily depending on the disease being treated. Dogs with atopic dermatitis begin with once daily usage and then taper to a schedule more like every other day or less. Concurrent use of low dose of ketoconazole may allow the cyclosporine dose to be cut in half.

Route(s) of Administration—Per os and intravenous.

Absorption—Cyclosporine is variably and incompletely absorbed from the gastrointestinal tract. Cyclosporine is best given on an empty stomach (either 1 hour before a meal or 2 hours after a meal).

Bioavailability (oral)—The drug undergoes extensive first-pass metabolism following oral administration.

Distribution—Vd = 13 L/kg (human). Cyclosporine is widely distributed into body fluids and tissues. Most of the drug is distributed outside the blood volume. Cyclosporine crosses the placenta and is distributed into milk at a maximum concentration of 2% of the maternal dose.

Plasma Protein Binding—90–98%.

Metabolism—Extensively metabolized by the cytochrome p-450 hepatic enzyme system and less extensively in the gastrointestinal tract and the kidney to at least 30 metabolites found in bile, feces, blood, and urine.

Plasma Half-life—Biphasic: initial phase $(t_{1/2\alpha})$ = 1.2 hours and terminal elimination phase $(t_{1/2}\beta)$ = 8.4–27 hours. Values are higher in renal impairment.

Clearance (ml/min/kg)—5 to 7 (human).

Route(s) of Excretion—Excreted principally via bile almost entirely as metabolites; 6% of a dose is excreted in urine, with 0.1% of a dose being excreted unchanged.

Toxicity and Adverse Effects—The most common side effect seen in one of three treated dogs is upset stomach characterized by appetite loss, vomiting, and diarrhea. This generally resolves within one week even if the medication is continued. Other side effects include heavy callusing on the footpads, red/swollen ear flaps, and proliferation of the gums. Dogs infected with the papilloma virus may develop large numbers of papillomas (warts) while on cyclosporine.

Management of Overdose/Toxicity—Reduce the frequency of administration until the gastrointestinal upset resolve and then resume the usual dose.

Contraindications—Patients with malignancy, infection, primary or secondary immunodeficiency, severe chronic organ dysfunction and those hypersensitive to cyclosporine. Cyclosporine should not be used during pregnancy or lactation.

Precautions—Use cyclosporine cautiously in patients with liver disease. Vaccinations may not "take" when given to patients on cyclosporine. Modified live vaccines should not be given to patients on cyclosporine.

Drug Interactions—Drugs such as ketoconazole, itraconazole, diltiazem, erythromycin, fluconazole, high dose steroids, warfarin, cimetidine, and verapamil which are known to inhibit the cytochrome P-450 enzyme system, will inhibit the metabolism of cyclosporine and may necessitate dosage reduction. Lower levels of cyclosporine may occur when taken concomitantly with carbamazepine, phenytoin, phenobarbitone, and rifampicin. Increased nephrotoxicity is possible when cyclosporine is used with other nephrotoxic agents particularly aminoglycosides, amphotericin B, trimethoprim and NSAIDs. Cyclosporine can increase blood levels of digoxin. It may decrease blood levels of trimethoprim-sulfa, omeprazole or phenobarbitone.

Pharmaceutical Formulations—Cyclosporine is available in 0.2% ophthalmic ointment, 10 mg, 25 mg, 50 mg and 100 mg capsules and as oral liquid for veterinary use. Human dosage forms are available commercially in conventional (unmodified) oral solution containing the drug in an olive oil and peglicol 5 oleate vehicle with 12.5% (v/v) alcohol. Also available as 50 mg/ml solution for injection in polyoxyl 35 castor oil or polyethoxylated castor oil with 32.9% (v/v) alcohol. Modified liquid formulation of the drug that forms aqueous dispersion is available both as oral solution and oral 25 and 100 mg liquid-filled capsules.

CYTARABINE

Cytarabine

Synonyms—Cytosine arabinoside; ARA-C; l-beta-d-Arabinofuranosylcytosine; Arabinosylcytosine; Arabinosylcytosine; Cytosine Arabinoside.

Proprietary Names—Cytosar-U®; Tarabine®.

Chemical Class—Pyrimidine analog.

Pharmacological Class—Antineoplastic drug; Antimetabolite Antineoplastic agent.

Source—Synthetic.

Solubility, Stability and Storage—Cytarabine is Soluble 1 in 10 of water, 1 in 1000 of ethanol or chloroform. Cytarabine powder for injection is better stored in a refrigerator. Reconstituted solution is stable for 48 hours at room temperature.

Pharmacological Actions—Cytarabine is cytotoxic mainly at the S phase of cell cycle. It inhibits DNA synthesis and repair. It is a potent immunosuppressant which can suppress humoral and/or cellular immune responses; however, cytarabine does not decrease preexisting antibody titers and has no effect on established delayed hypersensitivity reactions.

Mechanism of Action—Primarily, cytarabine inhibits DNA polymerase enzyme through its activated product, Ara-cytidine triphosphate (Ara-CTP) which competes with deoxycytidine triphosphate for the enzyme. Ara CTP is also incorporated into DNA. Incorporation of Ara-CTP into the DNA chain inhibits chain growth and repair. This latter mechanism may be responsible for its cytotoxic action.

Indications—Treatment of lymphoreticular neoplasms such as feline and canine lymphosarcoma, myeloproliferative disease and CNS lymphoma in small animals.

Dosages—100 mg/m^2 daily for 2-4 days.

Route(s) of Administration—Intravenous, subcutaneous and intramuscular routes are used.

Absorption—Cytarabine is freely absorbed from muscular and cutaneous sites; attains peak plasma concentration within 20-60 minutes.

Bioavailability (oral)—Cytarabine attains low (20%) oral bioavailability due to rapid metabolism in the gastrointestinal mucosa and liver. Bioavailability following intramuscular or subcutaneous administration is lower than equivalent intravenous dose.

Distribution—Vd = 3.0±1.9 L/kg (human). Cytarabine is widely distributed throughout the body water. It crosses the blood-brain barrier and attains levels as high as 60% of plasma concentration in the CSF. It crosses the placenta.

Plasma Protein Binding—13%.

Metabolism—Readily metabolized to inactive ara-U (uracil arabinoside) by cytidine deaminase which are abundant in the gastrointestinal mucosa and liver.

Half-life—Human plasma 2.6±0.6 hours; dog plasma, 64-69 minutes; dog CSF, 165 minutes.

Clearance—13 ± 4 ml/min/kg.

Route(s) of Excretion—Urine with 11 ± 8% as unchanged drug in human.

Toxicity and Adverse Effects—Bone marrow depression with prominent leukopenia; anemia, thrombocytopenia, and megaloblastosis are the dose-limiting toxicities of cytarabine. GI disturbances characterized by anorexia, nausea, vomiting, diarrhea, oral ulcerations are also observed. Hepatotoxicity may occur. Toxicity of cytarabine is dependent on dose and rate of administration.

Management of Overdose/Toxicity—There are no specific antidotes. Give symptomatic and supportive therapy.

Contraindications—Hypersensitivity to cytarabine.

Precautions—Use cytarabine with caution in patients with liver impairment.

Drug Interactions—Hydroxyurea increases cellular uptake and activation of cytarabine. Cytarabine reduces the anti-infective potency of gentamicin and flucytosine. It also reduces the rate of oral absorption of digoxin from tablets. The toxicity of cytarabine is increased by alkylating agents, radiation, purine analogs and methotrexate.

Pharmaceutical Formulations—Available as cytarabine hydrochloride in 100 mg, 500 mg, 1 g and 2 g powder for injection. Also available in 20 mg/ml solution for injection.

DACARBAZINE

Dacarbazine

Synonyms—DIC; DTIC; Dimethyl Triazeno Imidazol Carboxamide; Imadazole Carboxamide

Proprietary Names—DTIC-Dome®

Chemical Class—Triazene derivative.

Pharmacological Class—Antimetabolite antineoplastic agent.

Source—Synthetic.

Solubility, Stability and Storage—Dacarbazine is slightly soluble in water and in alcohol. Protect dacarbazine powder for injection from light and heat. Decomposed powder turns pink. The powder and reconstituted products should be refrigerated. Reconstituted solution is stable for 8 hours at room temperature.

Pharmacological Actions—Dacarbazine is slowly cytotoxic. It is cell cycle nonspecific and inhibits RNA and protein synthesis prominently than DNA synthesis. It has high emetogenic potential and moderate myelosuppressive action. Dacarbazine also possesses minimal immunosuppressive activity.

Mechanism of Action—Uncertain, but its active product is known to produce methylcarbonium ions that attack neucleophilic groups in DNA causing cross-linking of strands.

Indications—Treatment of lymphoreticular neoplasms in dogs; adjunctive treatment of malignant melanoma and sarcomas.

Dosages—

Lymphoreticular neoplasm: 200-250 mg/m² daily for 5 days. Repeat treatment every 3 weeks.

For adjunctive treatment in soft tissue sarcomas: 1000 mg/m² intravenously as drip for 6-8 hours. Repeat treatment after 3 weeks.

Route(s) of Administration—The intravenous route is recommended.

Absorption—Dacarbazine is poorly absorbed from oral sites.

Onset of Action—18-24 days (human).

Distribution—Vd=0.6L/kg (human). Dacarbazine probably concentrates in the liver; small amount cross the blood-brain-barrier.

Plasma Protein Binding—5%

Metabolism—Dacarbazine undergoes oxidative N-demethylation to ultimately liberate the active metabolite.

Plasma Half-life—Biphasic; 20-40 minutes (initial) and 5 hours (terminal).

Route(s) of Excretion—Dacarbazine is excreted mainly via urine by active tubular secretion with 30-50% of dose eliminated as unchanged drug. Some part may be excretion through bile.

Toxicity and Adverse Effects—Bone marrow depression characterized by leukopenia, thrombocytopenia and lymphoid depletion is common. Dacarbazine causes pain at injection site and tissue damage following extravasation. Other effects include nausea, vomiting and renal toxicity. Anorexia, malaise and debility have been reported in dogs.

Management of Overdose/Toxicity—There are no known antidotes. Give symptomatic and supportive therapy.

Contraindications—Hypersensitivity to dacarbazine.

Precautions—Use dacarbazine with caution in patients with pre-existing bone marrow depression, infection, hepatic or renal impairment. Use the drug in pregnant animals only when the benefit outweighs the risk of teratogenic effect. Pregnant women should never handle anticancer drugs.

Drug Interactions—The metabolism of dacarbazine may be enhanced by enzyme inducers e.g. phenobarbital. Concurrent use of dacarbazine with other bone marrow depressants may produce additive effects. Solutions of dacarbazine are physically incompatible with those of hydrocortisone and sodium succinate.

Pharmaceutical Formulations—Available in 100 mg, 200 mg and 500 mg powder for injection. Commercially available dacarbazine powder for injection contains anhydrous citric acid and mannitol. Specific veterinary formulations are not available.

DACTINOMYCIN

Synonyms—Actinomycin C_1; Actinomycin D; Meractinomycin; ACT

Proprietary Names—Cosmegen®.

Chemical Class—Chromopeptide.

Pharmacological Class—Antineoplastic antibiotic; Antineoplastic drug; Anticancer drug; Cytotoxic drug; Anticancer antibiotic.

Source—Natural; obtained from *Streptomyces parvulus*.

Solubility, Stability and Storage—Dactinomycin is soluble in water at 10°C but slightly soluble in water at 37°C. It is freely soluble in ethanol and slightly soluble in ether. Protect dactinomycin lyophilized powder from light and store at room temperature. Reconstitute powder with sterile water for injection just before administration. Discard unused solution.

Pharmacological Actions—Dactinomycin has antibacterial action against gram-positive organisms although it is not used therapeutically for this purpose because of toxicity. It also has cytotoxic, hypocalcemic and immunosuppressive actions. Dactinomycin has vesicant properties.

Mechanism of Action—Dactinomycin binds with double helical DNA to block the transcription of DNA by RNA polymerase. It also causes single-stranded breaks in DNA.

Dactinomycin

Indications—The use of dactinomycin in veterinary medicine is still being evaluated. It has been tried in the adjunctive treatment of lymphoreticular neoplasms, malignant melanomas, bone and soft tissue sarcomas in small animals.

Dosages—0.7 mg/m^2 every 7 days.

Route(s) of Administration—The intravenous route is preferred. Dactinomycin adsorbs to glass and plastics, hence it should not be given by infusion.

Absorption—Poor from the oral route.

Distribution—Dactinomycin distributes rapidly and attains high concentration in tumor cells, bone marrow, liver, kidney and submaxillary gland. It cross the placenta but enters the CSF poorly.

Metabolism—It is minimally metabolized.

Plasma Half-life—36 hours.

Route(s) of Excretion—The drug is eliminated via three routes in humans, namely, urine (with 10% as unchanged drug), bile (with 50% as unchanged drug) and feces (with 14% as unchanged drug).

Toxicity and Adverse Effects—Dactinomycin produces life-threatening toxicities. Bone marrow depression (characterized by leukopenia, anemia and thrombocytopenia), gastrointestinal ulceration, and stomatitis are prominent. Increased serum uric acid levels have been observed. Extravasation causes pain, ulceration and tissue necrosis. Its embryotonic and teratogenic actions in laboratory animals have been demonstrated.

Management of Overdose/Toxicity—Give symptomatic and supportive treatment.

Contraindications—Hypersensitivity to dactinomycin; severe bone marrow depression.

Precautions—Dactinomycin is extremely irritating to tissues and, therefore, should not be given IM or subcutaneously. Avoid extravasation during intravenous administration. Use dactinomycin cautiously in patients with pre-existing bone marrow depression, active infection and hepatic impairment. Exposure to dactinomycin during pregnancy should be avoided. It is safer to introduce replacer milk for offspring of nursing animals. Use with caution in patients that have received radiation therapy. Handle dactinomycin products with extreme caution.

Drug Interactions—Dactinomycin may produce additive bone marrow depression with other antineoplastic drugs and bone marrow depressants (e.g. chloramphenicol, flucytosine, amphotericin B, and colchicine. Azathioprine, cyclophosphamide, corticosteroids and other immunodepressants may increase the risk of infection when used concurrently with dactinomycin. Dactinomycin potentiates the effects of radiotherapy. Doxorubicin and dactinomycin may produce additive cardiotoxic effects. Increase the dose of vitamin K in those animals requiring the medication.

Pharmaceutical Formulations—Dactinomycin is available in 0.5 g lyophilized powder with 20 mg mannitol per vial.

DANOFLOXACIN

Proprietary Names—Advocin®; A180™

Chemical Class—Fluorinated 4-quinolone (Fluoroquinolone).

Pharmacological Class—Antimicrobial agent; Antibacterial drug; Antimycoplasma drug.

Source—Synthetic.

Pharmacological Actions—Danofloxacin is effective against organisms causing respiratory tract infections in cattle, pig and poultry. *Pasteurella* spp., *Haemophilus* spp., and *Mycoplasma gallisepticum* are susceptible.

Mechanism of Action—Danofloxacin inhibits gyrase-mediated DNA negative super coiling leading to inability of the bacteria to maintain DNA super helical structure and effect DNA repair.

Indications—Treatment of bovine respiratory disease (BRD) associated with *Mannheimia (Pasteurella) haemolytica* and *Pasteurella multocida*.

Dosages—

Cattle	6 mg/kg SC followed by a second injection in 48 hours.
Pig	1.25 mg/kg per day at 24 hours intervals for 3 days.

Route(s) of Administration—Intramuscular route in pig and subcutaneous route in cattle.

Absorption—Danofloxacin is rapidly absorbed from injection sites. Peak concentrations are attained within 1 hour.

Bioavailability (oral)—Pig, 89%; bioavailability from parenteral route is almost 100% in calves.

Effective Concentration—Minimum Inhibitory Concentration (MIC) for *Pasteurella* spp and *Haemophilus* spp is 0.06 mcg/ml.

Distribution—Vd = 4.3 l/kg. Danofloxacin attains higher concentrations in the lungs than in plasma. High accumulation of free drug occurs in bronchial mucosa and bronchial secretions. It rapidly concentrates in diseased lung tissue.

Metabolism—Partly metabolized to N-desmethyl danofloxacin.

Plasma Half-life—Calf, 7.4 hours; pig, 8.0 hours.

Residue Limit—Maximum residue limit = 0.07 (muscle and liver); 0.4 (kidney). Acceptable Daily Intake = 144 mcg/person/day or 0.024 mg/kg.

Withdrawal Period—7 days.

Route(s) of Excretion—Excreted via urine and feces largely as unchanged drug.

Toxicity and Adverse Effects—Danofloxacin is well tolerated in pigs. Even then, it produces erosions of cartilage in weight-bearing joints and other signs of arthropathy especially in immature rapidly growing animals. Subcutaneous injection can cause a transient local tissue reaction that may result in trim loss of edible tissue at slaughter.

Contraindications—Hypersensitivity to danofloxacin or other fluoroquinolones.

Precautions—Do not use danofloxacin in dairy cows or laying hens. Use cautiously in animals with CNS disorders. Administered volume should not exceed 15 mL per injection site. Quinolones should be used with caution in animals with known or suspected central nervous system (CNS) disorders. In such animals, quinolones have, in rare instances, been associated with CNS stimulation, which may lead to convulsive seizures.

Pharmaceutical Formulations—Available as danofloxacin mesylate in injectable solution containing 180 mg/ml.

DAUNORUBICIN

Daunorubicin

Synonyms—Daunomycin; DNR; Rubidomycin; Leukaemomycin C.

Proprietary Names—Cerubidine®.

Chemical Class—Anthracycline.

Pharmacological Class—Antineoplastic antibiotic; Antineoplastic drug; Anticancer drug; Cytotoxic drug; Anticancer antibiotic.

Source—Natural; obtained from *Streptomyces coeruleorubidus peucetius* var, caesius.

Solubility, Stability and Storage—Daunorubicin hydrochloride is soluble in water but slightly soluble in alcohol. It is unstable if pH of the solution is >8. Protect daunorubicin products from light. Lyophilized powder may be stored at room temperature while solutions are better stored in the refrigerator. Reconstituted powder should be used within 24 hours if kept at room temperature or 48 hours if refrigerated. Daunorubicin is compatible with dextrose saline, normal saline and lactated Ringer's solution. Do not mix daunorubicin with sodium bicarbonate, fluorouracil, or heparin.

Pharmacological Actions—Daunorubicin has activity against a wide variety of tumors although its action against solid tumors appears to be minimal. It is cell-cycle nonspecific but it is most active in the S phase. It inhibits DNA and RNA synthesis. It has antimicrobial and immunosuppressive properties. Its antibacterial action is not utilized therapeutically.

Mechanism of Action—Intercalates and binds to DNA between base pairs on adjacent strands with DNA causing the DNA helix to uncoil. This destroys the DNA template and inhibits RNA and DNA polymerases. It also cause breaks in DNA strands by activating topoisomerase II as well as generating free radicals. It has mutagenic potential resulting from sister chromatid exchange.

Indications—Adjunctive treatment of acute leukemia in humans. Its use in veterinary medicine is not fully established.

Route(s) of Administration—Intravenous; slowly through indwelling catheter. Dilute computed dose with 50 ml 5% dextrose or normal saline.

Absorption—Not absorbed from the GIT.

Bioavailability (oral)—5%.

Distribution—Vd = 40 L/kg. Doxorubicin is cleared rapidly from plasma to the heart, lungs, kidney, liver and spleen. It crosses the placenta but does not cross the blood-brain-barrier.

Plasma Protein Binding—76%.

Metabolism—It is converted to daunorubicinol (an active metabolite).

Plasma Half-life—Multiphasic; first phase, 2 minutes; second phase, 14-20 hours; third phase, 18.5 hours. Half-life of metabolites is 24-48 hours.

Clearance—17 ± 8 ml/min/kg. The drug is rapidly cleared from blood.

Route(s) of Excretion—About 40% of dose is eliminated in bile and feces while about 25% is excreted in urine.

Toxicity and Adverse Effects—Bone marrow depression, cardiomyopathy, alopecia, gastroenteritis and stomatitis are prominent adverse effects. Tissue irritation following extravasation may lead to cellulitis, necrosis and sloughing.

Management of Overdose/Toxicity—Give symptomatic and supportive therapy. Apply cold pack to the site of extravasation in addition to flooding the site with normal saline, sodium bicarbonate solution and topical application of dimethylsulfoxide or corticosteroid.

Contraindications—Hypersensitivity to daunorubicin; severe congestive heart failure; other cardiac impairment; preexisting myelosuppression.

Precautions—Daunorubicin has vesicant properties, hence, subcutaneous extravasation must be avoided. Handle daunorubicin formulations with care. It is recommended that gloves and protective clothing be worn. Wash exposed body parts copiously with soap and water. Reduce the dose in patients with renal impairment. Pretreatment with antihistamine or corticosteroid may be required to prevent hypersensitivity reaction.

Drug Interactions—Daunorubicin may potentiate the cardiotoxic effects of other cardiotoxic drugs, such as doxorubicin and cyclophosphamide. High-dose methotrexate and other hepatotoxic drugs may interfere with the metabolism of daunorubicin, resulting in increased risk of toxicity. Concurrent use with myelosuppressive drugs may produce additive effects.

Pharmaceutical Formulations—Available as daunorubicin hydrochloride in 20 mg lyophilized powder.

DECOQUINATE

Proprietary Names—Deccox®.

Chemical Class—Hydroquinolone.

Pharmacological Class—Anticoccidial agent.

Source—Synthetic.

Solubility, Stability and Storage—Decoquinate is very stable. It is insoluble in water and ethanol; slightly soluble in chloroform and ether and soluble in acetone. Store decoquinate in a cool dry place.

Decoquinate

Pharmacological Actions—Decoquinate prevents the development of *Eimeria* sporozoites. It is ineffective after development of sporozoite has started. Sporozoites can resume development following withdrawal of the drug.

Mechanism of Action—Decoquinate disrupts electron transport in mitochondrial cytochrome of *Eimeria* thereby inhibiting the parasite respiration.

Indications—Prevention of coccidiosis in broiler chickens and ruminants.

Dosages—27.2 g/ton of feed for 28 days.

Route(s) of Administration—Per os.

Absorption—Decoquinate is poorly absorbed from the GIT.

Distribution—It is rapidly cleared from blood and tissues.

Residue Limit—Maximum residue limit is 1.0 ppm in muscles of cattle, goats and chickens.

Withdrawal Period—Not required.

Toxicity and Adverse Effects—Decoquinate is safe. No adverse effects have been reported.

Contraindications—Hypersensitivity to decoquinate.

Precautions—Resistance may develop quickly.

Pharmaceutical Formulations—Available as premix for addition to feed

DEFEROXAMINE

Deferoxamine

Synonyms—DFM; DFOM. Desferrioxamine.

Proprietary Names—Desferal®.

Pharmacological Class—Iron chelator; Chelating agent.

Source—Semi synthetic; deferoxamine is a siderochrome produced as the ferric complex by *Streptomyces pilosus*. The iron is chemically removed and the metal-free ligand is purified for use as the mesylate salt.

Solubility, Stability and Storage—Deferoxamine mesylate is freely soluble in water and soluble in alcohol. Vials of lyophilized deferoxamine mesylate powder should be stored at temperatures less than 25°C. Reconstituted solutions are chemically and physically stable for 1 week at room temperature. However, reconstituted deferoxamine solutions should be used immediately (within 3 hours) for microbiologic safety. When solutions are reconstituted under aseptic conditions, deferoxamine solutions may be stored at room temperature for up to 24 hours before use; the solutions should *not* be refrigerated. Turbid solutions of the drug should not be used.

Pharmacological Actions—Deferoxamine causes easy elimination of iron from the body. The chelation of iron also prevents the production of hydroxyl radical.

Mechanism of Action—Deferoxamine specifically chelates iron by binding ferric ions to the 3 hydroxamic groups of the molecule to form an octahedral iron complex called ferrioxamine in many tissues, but mainly in plasma. Ferrioxamine is stable, water soluble, and readily excreted by the kidneys. Theoretically, 100 mg of deferoxamine can chelate approximately 8.5 mg of iron. The rate of complex formation is most rapid at acid pH.

Indications—Treatment of acute and chronic iron toxicity.

Dosages—Dogs and cats, 15 mg/kg/hour by constant intravenous infusion or 40 mg/kg IM every 4-8 hours.

Route(s) of Administration—Intramuscular, subcutaneous and intravenous.

Absorption—Poorly absorbed after oral administration in the presence of intact mucosa. Absorption of the drug may occur in patients with acute iron intoxication.

Distribution—Widely distributed in body tissues.

Route(s) of Excretion—About 13 to 65% of a dose is excreted in the urine in 24 hours. The octahedral complex, ferrioxamine is also excreted principally in urine. It gives urine a characteristic reddish color which is indicative of elevated iron concentrations in urine.

Dialysis Status—Dialyzable.

Toxicity and Adverse Effects—Deferoxamine may cause allergic reactions, pain and swelling at muscular site. It may also cause GI distress, skeletal abnormalities, and neurotoxicity especially at high dose and prolonged administration. Rapid intravenous infusion may cause tachycardia, convulsion, hypotension, and respiratory distress.

Contraindications—Severe renal failure; hypersensitivity to deferoxamine.

Precautions—Use deferoxamine cautiously during pregnancy.

Drug Interactions—Ascorbic acid enhances the action of deferoxamine by increasing availability of iron for chelation. Hence, ascorbic acid is given as an adjunct to deferoxamine therapy in patients with iron overload. Such patients usually become ascorbic acid deficient, most likely because iron oxidizes vitamin C. Concomitant use of deferoxamine and prochlorperazine may synergistically increase adverse neurologic effects of the drugs.

Pharmaceutical Formulations—Available as deferoxamine mesylate in vials containing 500 mg and 2 g in sterile lyophilized powder.

DEPRENYL

Synonyms—Selegiline.

Proprietary Names—Anipryl`; Eldepryl`.

Pharmacological Class—Monoamine oxidase-B inhibitor.

Source—Synthetic.

Solubility, Stability and Storage—Selegiline is freely soluble in water.

Pharmacological Actions—Selegiline increases the level of dopamine and also prolong its activity. Thus, it reduces the production of cortisone by the adrenal glands and reverses cognitive dysfunction associated with depletion of dopamine. It also enhances and prolongs the effects of levodopa. Selegiline prevents MT (N-methyl-4-phenyl-1,2,3,6-tetrahydropyridine)-induced Parkinsonism due to inhibition of the conversion of MT to the putative toxic product by MAO-B.

Mechanism of Action—Selegiline inhibits monoamine oxidase-B in the brain thereby preventing the breakdown of central neurotransmitters especially dopamine. L-Deprenyl also enhances the production of dopamine. Both actions enhance the action of dopamine on the pituitary thereby reducing the excessive production of ACTH in such situations as tumor of the pituitary. ACTH acts on the adrenal glands to produce cortisone. Selegiline also enhances the scavenging of free radicals.

Indications—Treatment of pituitary dependent Cushing's disease, and senile mental deterioration (canine cognitive dysfunction) in dogs. Deprenyl has been used as an adjunct in the management of Parkinson's disease in humans. It has shown promise in Alzheimer's disease therapy.

Dosages—

127

Dogs: 0.5-1 mg/kg once a day for two months; double the dose and administer for another month if no response is observed. Lack of response after this time is an indication that another treatment be sought.

Cats: 0.25-1.0 mg/kg once or twice daily.

Route(s) of Administration—Per os.

Absorption—Selegiline hydrochloride is rapidly absorbed from the GIT. Peak plasma concentration is attained within 0.5-0.9 hours in fasting humans. The presence of food in the GI tract increases oral bioavailability of selegiline threefold to fivefold. Selegiline is well-absorbed from percutaneous site.

Bioavailability (oral)—10%; undergoes extensive first-pass effect.

Distribution—Vd = 300L for the parent drug and/or metabolites. Selegiline and its metabolites are rapidly and widely distributed into body tissues including brain, liver, kidney, lung, heart, and brown fat.

Plasma Protein Binding—94%.

Metabolism—Selegiline is extensively metabolized to *l*-desmethylselegiline and *l*-methylamphetamine. The latter is further metabolized to *l*-amphetamine.

Plasma Half-life—1.2-2 hours (selegiline); 2 hours (*l*-desmethylselegiline); 20.5 hours (*l*-methamphetamine); 17.7 hours (*l*-amphetamine).

Route(s) of Excretion—The drug is excreted principally in urine with 20-63% as *l*-methamphetamine, 9-26% as *l*-amphetamine, and 1% as *l*-demethylselegiline. Acidic urine enhances excretion of amphetamine metabolites. About 15% of Selegiline dose is excreted in feces within 72 hours following administration.

Toxicity and Adverse Effects—Selegiline is relatively safe. Minor side effects characterized by vomiting, diarrhea, listlessness, disorientation, diminished hearing, or restlessness may be observed in 5% of dogs treated for Cushing's disease. Side effects may not be observed when used to treat cognitive dysfunction as lower doses are used.

Management of Overdose/Toxicity—Give supportive therapy.

Contraindications—Hypersensitivity to selegiline.

Precautions—The concurrent use of selegiline with amitraz should be avoided.

Drug Interactions—Concurrent use of selegiline with tricyclic antidepressants or selective serotonin re-uptake inhibitors may cause serious neurologic side effects. The use of selegiline with phenylpropanolamine, a common medication used in the management of urinary incontinence in older dogs may cause increased blood pressure.

Pharmaceutical Formulations—Available as selegiline hydrochloride in 2 mg, 5 mg, 10 mg, 15 mg, and 30 mg tablets.

DERACOXIB

Proprietary Names—Deramaxx®.

Chemical Class—Diaryl substituted pyrazole compound (related to sulfonamide).

Pharmacological Class—Non Steroidal Anti-inflammatory Drug; Analgesic; Selective cyclo-oxygenase-2 inhibitor.

Source—Synthetic.

Solubility, Stability and Storage—Store deracoxib chewable tablets at room temperature in a tight, childproof container and in a secure area. Note that the chewable tablets are appealing to pets and children.

Pharmacological Actions—Deracoxib has analgesic, and anti-inflammatory properties.

Mechanism of Action—Deracoxib selectively inhibits cyclooxygenase-2. It has no action on cyclooxygenase-1 except at high doses (25 mg/kg).

Deracoxib

Indications—Control of postoperative pain and inflammation associated with osteoarthritis, soft tissue and orthopedic surgery in dogs higher than 1.8 kg body weight.

Dosages—

For musculoskeletal inflammation and pain: 1 to 2 mg/kg body weight every twenty-four hours in dogs.

For postoperative pain: 3 to 4 mg/kg every twenty four hours for up to seven days in dogs of 1.8 kg and above.

Route(s) of Administration—Per os.

Absorption—Deracoxib is readily absorbed following oral administration and plasma concentration reaches its peak in 2 hours. **Bioavailability**—Oral bioavailability is greater than 90% and it is higher when given with food.

Distribution—Vd = 1.5 L/kg (dog).

Plasma Protein Binding—Greater than 90% in dog.

Metabolism—Deracoxib is metabolized in the liver to several inactive metabolites.

Plasma Half-life—3 hours (dog).

Clearance—Approximately 5 ml/min/kg in dog.

Route(s) of Excretion—Deracoxib is eliminated primarily in the feces as parent drug and metabolites. Some metabolites are eliminated via urine.

Toxicity and Adverse Effects—Vomiting and diarrhea are the most common adverse effects reported. Gastrointestinal lesions have been observed at high doses with consequent loss of appetite, vomiting, diarrhea, and dark, tarry or, bloody stools. Renal toxicity may manifest as increased thirst and urination or changes in the color and/or smell of urine. Overdose may cause loss of appetite, vomiting, diarrhea, dark or tarry stools, bloody stools, constipation, increased thirst, increased urination, pale gums, jaundice, lethargy, increased respiration, incoordination, seizures, or behavioral changes.

Management of Overdose/Toxicity—Give general antidotal therapy.

Contraindications—Cats; pre-existing kidney disease or liver disease; hypersensitivity to deracoxib or any sulfonamide.

Precautions—For more effective relief of pain after a surgical procedure, Deracoxib should be administered at least 2 hours prior to surgery since it is always easier to prevent pain than to relieve existing pain. Reduce the dose slightly when the drug is intended for long term use (as in the treatment of arthritis). Deracoxib, like other NSAIDs may increase risk to patients with cardiovascular, hepatic, or renal compromise because the drug has been associated with renal toxicity in certain circumstances. Provide regular drinking water to avoid dehydration which can increase the risk of renal toxicity by deracoxib. Many NSAIDs are known to increase the risk of gastrointestinal disease, particularly ulceration; therefore, the presence of lesions before treatment may put an animal at risk of exacerbation or perforation.

Drug Interactions—Administration of another NSAID or of a corticosteroid concurrently with deracoxib may greatly increase the risk of adverse effects. Concurrent administration of deracoxib with other medications associated with renal toxicity may produce additive effects.

Pharmaceutical Formulations—Deracoxib is available as 25 mg and 100 mg chewable tablets.

DESMOPRESSIN

Synonyms—1-Deamino-8-D-Arginine Vasopressin.

Proprietary Names—DDVAP*; Stimate*.

Chemical Class—Polypeptide.

Pharmacological Class—Antidiuretic hormone.

Source—Synthetic.

Solubility, Stability and Storage—Nasal and injection solutions of desmopressin are better stored in the refrigerator. Products are stable for 2-3 weeks at room temperature.

Pharmacological Actions—Desmopressin promotes water retention in the body by enhancing tubular reabsorption of water at the medullary conducting ducts in the kidney. Thus, it causes increased urine osmolarity and decreased urine output. It has more potent antidiuretic action but less pressor effects than vasopressin. Desmopressin also causes transient increase in the levels of Willebrand factor as a consequence it controls capillary bleeding in animals with Willebrand disease.

Mechanism of Action—Desmopressin activates vasopressin V_2 receptors located on the peritubular (serosal) surface of target cells to cause stimulation of adenylate cyclase with the resultant formation of cAMP. The cAMP formed activates a protein kinase on the luminal membrane resulting in the insertion of protein water channels (aquaporins) and increased permeability of the membrane to water. The water permeability of the cells is increased in proportion to the population of aquaporin channels in the membrane at any given time. It causes release of stored Willebrand factor from endothelial cells and macrophages.

Indications—Treatment of central (pituitary) diabetes insipidus; to control bleeding in mild hemophilia and von Willebrand disease (arising from deficiency of von Willebrand factor in humans, pigs, rabbits and dogs); control of thrombocytopenia; treatment and prevention of post-operative abdominal distention; differential diagnosis of diabetes insipidus.

Dosages—1-2 mcg/kg subcutaneously or 1-2 drops of nasal spray into the conjunctiva once or twice daily for control of diabetes insipidus; 0.4 mcg/kg in dogs for control of Willebrand disease.

Route(s) of Administration—Desmopressin is administered into the conjunctiva or injected subcutaneously in animals. The intranasal route is used in humans.

Absorption—Intraconjunctival administration results in variable absorption and blood levels even in the same animal.

Onset of Action—1.0 hour in dogs following topical application to the conjunctiva.

Peak Action—2-6 hours.

Duration of Action—10-27 hours; 3-4 hours in Willebrand disease.

Distribution—Secreted into milk.

Metabolism—Unknown.

Plasma Half-life—0.4-4 hours (human).

Toxicity and Adverse Effects—Adverse effects are uncommon. It may irritate the eye. Overdose may cause fluid retention and hyponatremia.

Management of Overdose/Toxicity—Reduce dose and restrict fluid intake.

Contraindications—Hypersensitivity to desmopressin.

Precautions—Use cautiously in cases susceptible to thrombotic events.

Drug Interactions—The antidiuretic effect of desmopressin is enhanced by chloropamide, carbamazepine, fludrocortisone and clofibrate. Its antidiuretic effects are reduced by lithium, demeclocycline and high doses of epinephrine.

Pharmaceutical Formulations—The drug is available as desmopressin acetate in 4 mcg/ml solution for injection; 0.1 mg/ml and 1.5 mg/ml solution for nasal spray (preferably applied topically into the conjunctiva in animals). Specific veterinary formulations are not available.

DETOMIDINE

Detomidine HCl

Proprietary Names—Dormosedan*; Domosedan*.

Chemical Class—Imidazoline derivative.

Pharmacological Class—Alpha-$_2$ adrenergic receptor agonist.

Source—Synthetic.

Solubility, Stability and Storage—Detomidine is soluble in water. The solution for injection should be stored at room temperature (15-30°C) and protected from light. Use the product within 28 days following withdrawal of the first dose from the vial.

Pharmacological Actions—Detomidine produces dose-dependent sedative and analgesic effects. It also causes bradycardia, hypotension, and hyperglycemia.

Mechanism of Action—Detomidine acts on central and peripheral α_2 adrenergic receptors to decrease norepinephrine release. Alpha$_2$-adrenergic receptors in the CNS are found on neurons that control blood pressure. The stimulation of these receptors also modulates pain perception.

Indications—Detomidine is used with or without butorphanol as a sedative and analgesic in horses and cattle especially to facilitate handling during diagnostic procedure, minor surgery and other manipulations. The drug is also used with ketamine for general anesthesia required for short surgical procedures such as castration.

Dosages—10-80 mcg/kg.

Route(s) of Administration—Intravenous or intramuscular routes may be used.

Absorption—Detomidine is rapidly absorbed from all routes including oral, but it is administered parenterally for therapeutic purposes.

Bioavailability (oral)—25%.

Onset of Action—2-5 minutes.

Duration of Action—Low doses: 30-90 minutes of sedation; 30-45 minutes of analgesia. High doses: 90-120 minutes of sedation and 45-75 minutes of analgesia.

Distribution—Vd is biphasic (3 and 29 L/kg). Detomidine is rapidly distributed into tissues including the CNS.

Metabolism—The drug is extensively metabolized to inactive metabolites by hydroxylation, dehydrogenation and conjugation with glutathione and glucuronide.

Plasma Half-life—Biphasic (2 and 20 hours).

Clearance (ml/min/kg)—Biphasic (10 and 25).

Route(s) of Excretion—Detomidine is excreted primarily into urine; 60% of the dose appear in urine within the first 24 hours after dosing. Small portion of dose appear in feces due to biliary excretion.

Toxicity and Adverse Effects—Hypertension followed by bradycardia and heart block have been observed at therapeutic doses. Detomidine causes profound lethargy and characteristic lowering of the head with reduced sensitivity to environmental stimuli (sounds, etc.). A short period of incoordination is characteristically followed by immobility and a firm stance with front legs spread. Piloerection, sweating, ataxia, salivation, slight muscle tremors, and penile prolapse may also be observed. Overdose may cause severe and irreversible respiratory and cardiovascular changes and death.

Management of Overdose/Toxicity—Detomidine effects may be reversed with tolazoline. The bradycardia can be prevented or reversed with atropine.

Contraindications—Heart block; severe coronary, cerebrovascular or respiratory disease; chronic renal failure; hypersensitivity to detomidine.

Precautions—Detomidine should be handled with care by a professional as respiratory failure in humans can result from inadvertent injection. Allow the horse to stand quietly for 5 minutes prior to injection and for 10-15 minutes after injection to improve the effect of the drug. Sedated horses may react by very swift kicks to external stimuli. This may be controlled by administering detomidine with opioids (e.g. butorphanol). Use cautiously in animals that are in shock or are stressed due to temperature extremes or fatigue.

Drug Interactions—Other CNS depressants such as barbiturates, narcotics, anesthetics will produce additive effects when used concurrently with detomidine. The doses of such agents must be reduced. The use of detomidine with intravenous potentiated sulfonamides may cause fatal dysrhythmias.

Pharmaceutical Formulations—Available as detomidine hydrochloride in 10 mg/ml solution for injection.

DEXAMETHASONE

Dexamethasone

Synonym—Desamethasone; 9α-Fluoro-16α-methylprednisolone.

Proprietary Names—Decadron˙; Dexone˙; Hexadrol˙; Dexapower˙; Dexacortin˙; Dexafar˙; Cotson˙; Colvasone˙; Dexazone˙; Chlortetrasone˙ (in combination with Prednisolone, lidocaine, oxytetracycline, chloramphenicol, thioglycerol and dimethylsulfoxide); Dexacycline˙ (in combination with oxytetracycline and tripelennamine); Dexacortyl˙ (in combination with sodium methyl hydroxyl benzoate.

Chemical Class—Corticosteroid.

Pharmacological Class—Anti-inflammatory agent; Glucocorticoid.

Source—Synthetic.

Solubility, Stability and Storage—Dexamethasone is insoluble in water but sparingly soluble in alcohol. The sodium phosphate salt is more soluble in water. Products should be stored at room temperature and protected from light.

Pharmacological Actions—Dexamethasone has effects on virtually every cell type and system in mammals. It has high anti-inflammatory potency but devoid of salt-retaining property.

Mechanism of Action—Dexamethasone activates specific glucocorticoid receptors at the cytosol and the hormone-receptor complex is then transported into the cell nucleus where it binds with glucocorticoid response elements (GRE) on various genes and alters their expression. An opposite mechanism is called transrepression in which the activated hormone receptor interacts with specific transcription factors and prevents the transcription of targeted genes. Glucocorticoids are able to prevent the transcription of any of immune genes, including the IL-2 gene.

Indications—Dexamethasone has multiple uses including the control of inflammation associated with conditions like joint pain and itchy skin (as in eczematous conditions, allergic dermatosis, seborrheic dermatitis, and intractable pruritus), suppression of immunity in conditions where the immune system is destructively hyperactive, treatment of cancer especially lymphoma, suppression of scar tissue formation in cornea or ear, improvement of circulation during circulatory shock and treatment of hypercalcemia and adrenal insufficiency. Dexamethasone has also been used to induce parturition in cattle and sheep.

Dosages—

Bird	0.5-2 mg/kg IM, IV once a day
Bovine	5-20 mg IV IM, PO
Cat	0.125-0.5 mg once a day or divided doses IV, IM, PO

Dog	0.25-1.25 mg once a day or divided bid PO
	0.25-1.0 mg once a day IM, IV
Guinea pig	0.1 mg SC
NHP	0.25-1.0 mg/kg PO, IM total dose
Reptile	0.125-0.625 mg/kg IV, IM as needed

Route(s) of Administration—Per os, intramuscular, intravenous and subcutaneous.

Absorption—Dexamethasone is readily absorbed following oral administration and plasma concentration reaches its peak in 1-2 hours.

Duration of Action—Metabolic effect may last up to 72 hours.

Distribution—Vd ~ 1 L/kg.

Plasma Protein Binding—About 67%.

Metabolism—Metabolized in the liver.

Plasma Half-life—About 2 to 5 hours.

Route(s) of Excretion—Up to 65% of a dose is excreted mainly as metabolites in urine within 24 hours. Some are eliminated in bile.

Toxicity and Adverse Effects—Treatment lasting more than 3 months is regarded as long term, and results in the majority of undesirable side effects including Cushing's syndrome.

Contraindications—Systemic fungal infections (unless used for replacement therapy in Addison's disease); hypersensitivity to corticosteroids; pregnancy; diabetes mellitus.

Precautions—Glucocorticoid hormones should not be used in combination with NSAID drugs. Any latent infections can be unmasked by dexamethasone use. Following chronic use, it is important that the dose be tapered to an every third day schedule once the condition is controlled. Patients taking corticosteroids should generally not receive live attenuated-virus vaccines.

Drug Interactions—Concurrent use of dexamethasone with NSAIDs could lead to gastric bleeding and ulceration. Barbiturates and phenytoin may decrease dexamethasone effect. Dexamethasone decreases the effects of salicylates, vaccines and toxoids.

Pharmaceutical Formulations—The drug is available as dexamethasone sodium phosphate or dexamethasone dipropionate in tablets and solution for injection. Note that 4 mg/ml of dexamethasone sodium phosphate injection is approximately equivalent to 3 mg/ml of dexamethasone). Other dosage forms of dexamethasone are cream, drops for eye and ear as well as ointment in combination with antibiotics like neomycin and antimycotic agents e.g. clotrimazole.

DEXTRAN 70

Proprietary Names—Macrodex*.

Chemical Class—Polysaccharide.

Pharmacological Class—Plasma volume expander.

Source—Natural; dextran is synthesized from sucrose by *Leuconostoc mesenteroides* and is also produced by bacteria and yeast.

Solubility, Stability and Storage—Dextran 70 is freely soluble in water and insoluble in alcohol. Use only clear solutions. Dextran flakes can be resolubolized by heating the solution in a boiling water bath until clear, or by autoclaving at 110°C for 15 minutes.

Pharmacological Actions—Dextran 70 increases circulating blood volume by drawing fluid into the vascular lumen from the interstitial spaces through colloidal osmotic effect. Dextran also possesses antithrombotic action.

Mechanism of Action—The antithrombotic effect of dextran is due to its binding of erythrocytes, platelets and vascular endothelium, thus increasing their electronegativity and reducing erythrocyte aggregation and platelet adhesiveness.

Indications—Dextran 70 is useful in the treatment of shock or impending shock when blood or blood products are not available. It is also used to decrease vascular thrombosis.

Dosages—20-40 ml/kg/day; at a rate not faster than 5 ml/kg/hour.

Route(s) of Administration—Intravenous infusion; never administer Dextran 70 by intramuscular route.

Duration of Action—>24 hours.

Distribution—As much as 20-30% of administered dextran remains in the intravascular compartment for up to 24 hours. Dextran 70 may be detected in the blood by 4-6 weeks after dosing.

Metabolism—Dextran 70 is slowly degraded by dextranase usually in the spleen to glucose and then further metabolized to carbon dioxide and water.

Route(s) of Excretion—A small portion of the dose is excreted in feces.

Toxicity and Adverse Effects—Adverse effects can be very serious. These include volume overload, pulmonary edema, cerebral edema, or platelet dysfunction. Anaphylaxis is common in humans but rare in dogs. An uncommon but significant complication of dextran osmotic effect is acute renal failure. It also increases blood sugar levels.

Contraindications—Marked hemostatic defects (thrombocytopenia, hypofibrinogenemia) of all types including those caused by drugs; severe cardiac decompensation; renal disease with severe oliguria or anuria; strict sodium restriction; hypersensitivity to dextran.

Precautions—Use with caution as dextran does not provide necessary electrolytes and can cause hyponatremia or other electrolyte disturbances. Use dextran with caution in patients with fluid overload or active hemorrhage.

Pharmaceutical Formulations—Available as 6% Dextran-70 either in normal saline or 5% dextrose solution.

DIAZEPAM

Diazepam

Proprietary Names—Valium®; Valrelease®; Zentra® injection.

Chemical Class—Benzodiazepine.

Pharmacological Class—CNS depressant; Sedative-hypnotic; Anxiolytic.

Source—Synthetic.

Solubility, Stability and Storage—Diazepam is sparingly soluble in propylene glycol and has solubilities of approximately 3 mg/mL in water and 62.5 mg/mL in alcohol at 25°C. Diazepam is better stored at room temperature in light resistant containers. Do not store in plastic syringes. Administer only clear solutions of diazepam.

Pharmacological Actions—Diazepam causes selective depression of the CNS consequently producing sedation, hypnosis, and stupor with increasing dosage. It decreases anxiety without decreasing alertness or impairing perceptive or cognitive capacities. Also, it decreases nocturnal gastric secretion in humans. It has anticonvulsant and muscle relaxant properties. Diazepam does not cause proper general anesthesia because awareness usually persists following its use even though events cannot be recalled because of retrograde amnesia. It induces taming effects in animals. Intravenous administration produces analgesia.

Mechanism of Action—Diazepam binds to $GABA_A$ receptor/ion channel complex in the presence of GABA and allosterically modulates the action of GABA to produce increase in neuronal chloride conductance resulting in hyperpolarization and reduced neuronal excitability.

Indications—Diazepam is used in preanesthetic medication; as adjuvant in neuroleptanalgesia; to control seizures of different origin; for chemical restraint; and stimulate appetite in cats.

Dosages—

Dog, cat	1 mg/kg up to a maximum of 5 mg in cats and 20 mg in dogs. (0.05-0.4 mg/kg to induce appetite in cats).
Pig	5.5 mg/kg for tranquilization; 8.5 mg/kg for premedication.
Goat	0.9 mg/kg in conjunction with ketamine and atropine to induce sustained analgesia.
Exotic animals	1-3.5 mg/kg to immobilize wild animals

Route(s) of Administration—Per os, intramuscular; intravenous.

Absorption—Diazepam is rapidly absorbed from oral site with peak plasma concentration attained within 30 minutes to 2 hours. It is slowly and incompletely absorbed from muscular site.

Bioavailability—Oral bioavailability in dogs is 74-100%. Bioavailability following intramuscular injection in horses is 93%

Onset of Action. Onset is rapid due to high lipid solubility.

Duration of Action—Brief, due to redistribution from the CNS.

Distribution—Widely distributed; it crosses the blood-brain-barrier readily. It is secreted in milk.

Plasma Protein Binding—Human, 98-99%; horse, 87%.

Metabolism—Metabolized in the liver to several active products such as N-desmethyl diazepam (nordiazepam), temazepam, and oxazepam, which are subsequently conjugated with glucuronic acid.

Plasma Half-Life—Dog, 2.5-3.2 hours; cat, 5.5 hours; horse, 7-22 hours; human, 20-50 hours. Half-life is higher after prolonged use.

Route(s) of Excretion—Urine.

Dialysis Status—Not dialyzable.

Toxicity and Adverse Effects—Diazepam causes phlebitis at the site of injection. Muscle fasciculation, weakness and ataxia have been observed in horses. Behavioral changes such as irritability and depression have been documented in cats. An overdose may cause confusion, coma and decreased reflexes. Hypotension, cardiac arrest and respiratory depression have been reported in humans. There is evidence that it promotes teratogenic and carcinogenic effects in humans. Administration of 0.2 mg/kg IV may produce fixed gaze, muscle tremor and ataxia in horses.

Management of Overdose/Toxicity—Follow general antidotal therapy procedure in addition to adequate supportive measures. Flumazenil will specifically antagonize the CNS depressant effect of diazepam.

Contraindications—Hypersensitivity to diazepam.

Precautions—Diazepam may cause excitement in some dogs. Inject the drug slowly if using intravenous route. Use diazepam cautiously in patients with hepatic or renal diseases, and also in debilitated and old animals.

Drug Interactions—Concurrent administration of diazepam with other CNS depressants will give additive effects. Antacids may slow the rate of absorption from the GIT. Enzyme inducers (e.g. rifampin) may increase diazepam metabolism. Its metabolism may be decreased by cimetidine, erythromycin, isoniazid, ketoconazole, propranolol and valproic acid.

Pharmaceutical Formulations—Only formulations for human use are available in the form of 5 mg/ml injectable solution; 2 mg, 5 mg, and 10 mg tablets; 15 mg sustained release capsules; and 5 mg/ml oral solutions.

DICLAZURIL

Diclazuril

Proprietary Names—Clinicox®.

Chemical Class—Benzeneacetonitrile derivative.

Pharmacological Class—Anticoccidial drug.

Source—Synthetic.

Solubility, Stability and Storage—Diclazuril is almost insoluble in water.

Pharmacological Actions—Diclazuril has potent anticoccidial activity even at low levels. It is effective against second-generation schizonts and sexual stages of *Eimeria tenella, E. necatrix, E. acervulina, E. brunetti,* and *E. mivati.* Diclazuril is effective against *E. maxima* later in its life cycle. It also inhibits sporulation of oocyst. It is effective against *E. tenella* that has become resistant to other anticoccidial drugs.

Mechanism of Action—Unknown

Indications—Prevention of coccidiosis caused by *Eimeria tenella, E. necatrix, E. acervulina, E. brunetti, E. mivati,* and *E. maxima* in broiler birds. Treatment of coccidiosis in rabbits, ruminants and pigs.

Dosages—

Poultry	Administered in a complete feed at 1 ppm that is fed continuously as the sole ration.
Lamb	1 mg/kg once at 6-8 weeks of age or twice at 3-4 weeks and then 3 weeks after.
Calf, piglet	5 mg/kg.

Route(s) of Administration—Per os.

Absorption—The drug is poorly absorbed. Peak plasma concentration is attained within 12 hours in piglets and calves, 24-48 hours in sheep or 6 hours in chicken and turkey.

Bioavailability (oral)—Low.

Distribution—Vd = 100 l/kg (calf). It is poorly distributed.

Metabolism—Metabolized to a limited degree by glucuronide and sulfate conjugation.

Plasma Half-life—53.0 hours (Rabbit); 38 hours (turkey)

Route(s) of Excretion—Mainly in feces as the parent drug.

Residue Limit—0.5 ppm in muscle, 3 ppm in liver, and 1 ppm in skin/fat

Withdrawal Period—Five days in the case of meat.

Toxicity and Adverse Effects—No reports of adverse effects at the recommended dose of 1 ppm in feed. Histopathological changes were observed variously in the liver, lungs or mesenteric lymph nodes of rats fed 250 ppm of diclazuril. LD_{50} in most animals is >5000 mg/kg body weight.

Contraindications—Hypersensitivity to diclazuril.

Precautions—Diclazuril exhibits cross resistance with toltrazuril. Diclazuril should be used in a shuttle program for a period not exceeding 6 months to delay the development of resistance.

Pharmaceutical Formulations—Available as 0.2% premix.

DICLOXACILLIN

Synonyms—Sodium dicloxacillin; Dichlorphenylmethyl isoxazolyl penicillin sodium; Methyldichlorophenyl isoxazolyl penicillin sodium.

Proprietary Names—Dycill˙; Dynapen˙; Pathocil˙.

Chemical Class—6-Aminopenicillinic acid derivative.

Pharmacological Class—Isoxazolyl penicillin; Beta-lactam antibiotic; Penicillinase resistant penicillin.

Source—Semi synthetic.

Solubility, Stability and Storage—Dicloxacillin is readily soluble in water. Store products at room temperature. Reconstituted oral suspension is stable for 7 days at room temperature and 14 days if refrigerated.

Dicloxacillin Sodium

Pharmacological Actions—Dicloxacillin is bactericidal to penicillinase-producing *Staphylococcus aureus* and penicillin G-sensitive Staph and other Gram-positive bacteria. It is less active than penicillin G against penicillin G-sensitive microbes.

Mechanism of Action—Same as for other penicillins.

Indications—Treatment of soft tissue infections, wounds, burns and septicemia due to infections by Gram-positive microbes especially penicillinase-producing staphylococci.

Dosages—Dogs and Cats, 10-50 mg/kg orally every 8 hours.

Route(s) of Administration—Per os.

Absorption—As much as 35-76% is absorbed following oral administration and plasma concentration reaches its peak in 30-60 minutes in the dog. The rate and extent of absorption decrease with food intake. It is acid-resistant.

Bioavailability—Oral bioavailability is 50-85%.

Distribution—Dicloxacillin is widely distributed to body fluids and bones but it penetrates into cells, eye, and CSF poorly but it appears in milk and crosses the placenta. Vd in humans = 0.086 ± 0.017 L/kg (higher in uremia). Vd in dog = 0.20 L/kg.

Plasma Protein Binding. 95.8 ± 0.2 %.

Metabolism—Dicloxacillin is partially metabolized to active and inactive products.

Plasma Half-Life—Human, 0.70 ± 0.07 hours; dog, 0.67 hours. Values are higher in uremia.

Clearance—(ml/min/kg)—Human, 1.6 ± o.3 (higher in uremia); Dog, 3.5.

Route(s) of Excretion—Urine (56-70% as unchanged drug) and bile.

Dialysis Status—Dialyzable.

Toxicity and Adverse Effects—Hypersensitivity reaction ranging from skin rash to serum sickness-like reactions. Nausea, vomiting, diarrhea, hematologic disorders, hepatotoxicity and hematuria have been observed at therapeutic doses. Overdose may cause electrolyte imbalance, renal failure and neuromuscular hypersensitivity in humans (characterized by agitation, hallucinations, seizures and confusion).

Management of Overdose/Toxicity—Set up hemodialysis. Give supportive and symptomatic treatment.

Contraindications—Hypersensitivity to dicloxacillin or other penicillins, or their products and components.

Precautions—Administer dicloxacillin one hour before, or two hours after food. Use cautiously in patients with history of cephalosporin use.

Drug Interactions—Effects of anticoagulants may be increased by dicloxacillin. Probenecid and disulfiram increase dicloxacillin plasma concentration.

Pharmaceutical Formulations—Available as dicloxacillin sodium in 125mg, 250mg, and 500 mg capsules. Also available as powder for oral suspension containing 62.5 mg/5ml. No specific veterinary formulations are available.

DIETHYLCARBAMAZINE

Diethylcarbamazine

Synonym—DEC.

Proprietary Names—Banocide˚; Caricide˚; Dirocide˚; Filaricide˚; Filaribits˚; Hetrazan˚; Notézine˚.

Chemical Class—Methylpiperazine derivative.

Pharmacological Class—Anthelmintic; Filaricide.

Source—Synthetic.

Solubility, Stability and Storage. Diethylcarbamazine is freely soluble in water; soluble 1 in 35 of ethanol; practically insoluble in acetone, benzene, chloroform, and ether.

Pharmacological Actions—DEC is effective against mosquito-borne infective larvae and microfilariae of *Dirofilaria immitis* in dogs as well as the immature forms of *Dictyocaulus* species in cattle and sheep. In humans, it causes rapid disappearance of microfilariae of *Wuchereria bancrofti*, *W (Brugia) malaya* and Loa loa from blood and microfilariae of *Onchocerca volvulus* from skin.

Mechanism of Action—Uncertain; DEC is known to cause two types of actions, namely paralysis of the organism apparently due to hyper polarization caused by the piperazine moiety; and alteration in the microfilaria surface membrane which renders them more susceptible to host defense mechanism.

Indications—Prophylaxis of heart worm (*Dirofilaria immitis*) disease in dogs and treatment of parasitic bronchitis in cattle and sheep.

Dosages—

Dogs:	5.5mg/kg in dry or wet food, or immediately after food daily for 3-5 weeks for the prophylaxis of *Dirofilaria immitis*.
Cattle and sheep:	22mg/kg/day for 3 days in *Dictyocaulus* infection.

Route(s) of Administration—Per os, intramuscular (in cattle and sheep)

Absorption—DEC is rapidly absorbed following oral administration. Peak plasma concentration is attained within 1-3 hours.

Distribution—DEC is widely distributed to organs and tissues except fat.

Plasma Protein Binding—Not significantly bound—

Metabolism—Rapidly metabolized.

Plasma Half-Life—10-12 hours.

Route(s) of Excretion—Eliminated via urine with 10-25% of dose excreted as unchanged drug.

Toxicity and Adverse Effects—DEC is relatively nontoxic; therapeutic index in calves is 20. Gastric irritation is a major disadvantage especially with large doses. Anaphylactic type of reaction in microfilaria-positive dogs can be fatal. Major adverse effect in humans is linked to the destruction of parasites. In onchocerciasis, this produces the Mazzotti-reaction. Direct adverse reactions are mild and include anorexia, nausea, vomiting and headache.

Management of Overdose/Toxicity—Give supportive therapy.

Contraindications—Hypersensitivity to diethylcarbamazine or its components; microfilaria-positive dogs.

Precautions—Obtain a negative heartworm test before DEC therapy in dogs. Omission of one or two doses of this daily medication can allow infection to take hold.

Pharmaceutical Formulations—Available as diethylcarbamazine citrate in 50 mg chewable or nonchewable tablets; and 120 mg/5 ml syrup. Powder formulations are also available. Solutions containing the equivalent of 40% w/v of the acid citrate is available for cattle and sheep.

DIETHYLSTILBESTROL

Diethylstilboestrol

Synonyms—Stilbestrol; Stilbol; Diethylstilboestrol; DES.

Proprietary Names—Stiphostrol*.

Chemical Class—Stilbene.

Pharmacological Class—Estrogen.

Source—Synthetic.

Solubility, Stability and Storage—DES is practically insoluble in water; soluble 1 in 5 of ethanol, 1 in 200 of chloroform and 1 in 3 of ether. It is soluble in acetone, methanol and fatty oils. The dipropionate and diphosphate salts are slightly soluble in water.

Pharmacological Actions—DES stimulates growth and development of the tubular reproductive tract and accessory reproductive organs including the mammary glands. It maintains normal contractility of the uterus and enhances its response to oxytocin. DES increases blood fat and calcium in birds, improves weight gain, inhibits bone growth, induces sexual receptivity (estrus, heat) in animals, causes hyperemia and hypertrophy of the female reproductive tract and induces development of secondary sexual characteristics. In laboratory animals, low doses re-establishes normal estrous cycle in an anestrous female. It increases the plasma concentration of growth hormone and insulin which stimulate amino acid uptake into muscles.

Mechanism of Action—DES binds to estrogen receptors in the nuclei of cells in responsive tissues to regulate the transcription of a limited number of genes resulting in *de novo* synthesis of proteins. These functional proteins express the actions of the steroid in the cell.

Indications—DES is useful mainly but not exclusively in gynecological conditions. It is used to control a number of conditions such as anestrus or subestrus in mares and cows, vaginal discharges associated with 'bunch of grapes ovaries', irregular cycles in mare, anal adenomata, prostatic hypertrophy, excessive libido in dogs and urinary incontinence in spayed bitches. DES is also used to aid the expulsion of mummified fetus or removal of retained placenta, promote growth in fattening steers, induce estrus in sheep, and prevent pregnancy in bitches following mismating (postcoital contraception).

Dosages—

Dog	Postcoital contraception. 0.1-1 mg/day PO for 5 days if animal is presented 24-48 hours post-coitus.
	Urinary incontinence. 0.1-1 mg/day PO for 3-5 days, then 1 mg PO per week.
	Anal adenoma and prostatic hypertrophy. 0.1-1 mg/day PO q24-48h.
Steer	Growth promotion. 50-60 mg SC implant at base of ear 120 days before slaughter (implant discarded with the ear at the time of slaughter).
Beef cattle	Growth promotion. 10 mg/head/day PO followed by a 14-day withdrawal period.
Mare	5-15mg injection once, or 500 mg—2×500mg subcutaneous implants.
Bird	0.03-0.1 ml of 0.25 mg/ml stock/30 g BW IM or 1 drop of 0.25 mg/ml stock/30 ml drinking water.
Cat	0.05-0.1 mg/day PO
Sheep, goat	0.25 mg
Sow	5-10mg

Route(s) of Administration—Per os, intramuscular, intravenous and subcutaneous implant.

Absorption—DES is promptly and completely absorbed from the oral route.

Metabolism—It undergoes sulfate and glucuronide conjugation.

Route(s) of Excretion—Excreted in urine and bile.

Toxicity and Adverse Effects—Gastrointestinal upset resulting in nausea, vomiting, anorexia and mild diarrhea are common. Large and prolonged doses may cause post parturient straining with vaginal or uterine prolapse in cows. Subcutaneous implants in animals may cause pelvic fragility. Ovarian suppression and hypoplasia may be followed by development of ovarian cysts in prolonged and excessive administration. DES causes feminization in the male. In humans, it produces vaginal tumors in the female offsprings of women who took the drug during pregnancy. Genital erythema, irritation, polydipsia and polyuria are features of chronic overdose in animals.

Contraindications—Pregnancy; mammary tumors.

Precautions—A large dose of DES for long periods is not recommended in dogs. Use cautiously in humans with history of jaundice. Contact with the skin or inhalation should be avoided.

Pharmaceutical Formulations—Available as diethylstilbestrol dipropionate or diethylstilbestrol diphosphate in tablets, cutaneous implants and solutions for injection.

DIFLOXACIN

Proprietary Names—Dicural®.

Chemical Class—Fluorinated 4-quinolone (Fluoroquinolone).

Pharmacological Class—Antimicrobial agent.

Source—Synthetic.

Solubility, Stability and Storage—Store at 15-30⁰C; protect from excessive heat.

Pharmacological Actions—Difloxacin has bactericidal action against many Gram-negative and some Gram-positive bacilli and cocci. Most species and strains of *E. coli, Shigella, Enterobacter, Campylobacter, Staphylococci, Klebsiella, Proteus* and *Pasteurella* are susceptible. Some strains of *Pseudomonas aeruginosa* are resistant. It has poor activity against anaerobic organisms.

Mechanism of Action—Difloxacin inhibits gyrase-mediated DNA negative super coiling leading to inability of the bacteria to maintain DNA super helical structure and effect DNA repair.

Indications—Treatment of wounds, abscesses and urinary tract infections in dogs and cats.

Dosages—5-10 mg/kg orally once a day.

Route(s) of Administration—Per os.

Absorption—Difloxacin is well absorbed after oral dose. Peak plasma concentration is attained within 3 hours.

Distribution—Vd = 2.8 L/kg. Difloxacin is well distributed.

Plasma Protein Binding—16-25%.

Plasma Half-Life—9 hours in dogs

Route(s) of Excretion—A high proportion of the dose is eliminated unchanged in urine. Therapeutic levels may appear in urine even 24 hours after dosing.

Toxicity and Adverse Effects—Like other fluoroquinolones, difloxacin causes arthropathy in immature growing animals particularly in dogs. Otherwise, it is very well tolerated. Gastrointestinal effects (vomiting, diarrhea and anorexia) are most common adverse effects even with overdose. Difloxacin tend to always cause inappetence and vomiting in cats.

Management of Overdose/Toxicity—Give supportive measures.

Contraindications—Small and medium breeds of dogs less than 8 months; large breeds less than 12 months; giant breeds less than 18 months; patients with suspected CNS disorders; hypersensitivity to difloxacin or any other quinolone.

Precautions—Continue treatment for 2-3 days after symptoms have disappeared. Administer the drug 2 hours before or after the administration of sucralfate and antacids containing magnesium, calcium and aluminium. Use difloxacin with extreme caution in cats, especially those with pre-existing kidney failure.

Drug Interactions—Difloxacin has been used concurrently with ectoparasiticides, antiepileptics, anesthetics, antihistamines, and topical anti-inflammatory drugs without adverse effects. The drug inhibits the metabolism of theophylline, caffeine, cyclosporine, and warfarin. Azlocillin, cimetidine, and probenecid increase quinolone blood levels. The absorption of difloxacin is reduced if co-administered with sucralfate and antacids containing magnesium, calcium, and aluminium. Probenecid blocks tubular secretion of difloxacin and increases its half-life. Nitrofurantoin may antagonize difloxacin antimicrobial activity but synergism may occur when difloxacin is used with aminoglycoside antibiotics, third generation cephalosporins and extended spectrum penicillins against some bacteria such as *Pseudomonas*. Flouroquinolones may enhance the nephrotoxic effect of cyclosporine.

Pharmaceutical Formulations—Available as difloxacin hydrochloride in 11.4 mg, 45.4 mg and 136 mg tablets.

DIGOXIN

Proprietary Names—Cardoxin˚; Digoxin˚; Lanoxin˚; Lanoxicaps˚.

Chemical Class—Cardiac glycoside; Digitalis.

Pharmacological Class—Cardiac stimulant; Antiarrhythmic drug; Inotropic Agent.

Source—Natural; contained in the leaf of *Digitalis lanata*.

Solubility, Stability and Storage—Digoxin is practically insoluble in water, slightly soluble in dilute alcohol, and very slightly soluble in 40% propylene glycol solution. Store digoxin dosage forms in light resistant containers at room temperature (15-30°C).

Pharmacological Actions—Cardiac glycosides cause increased force of contraction (positive inotropic affect) and slowing of the heart rate (negative chronotropic effect). The consequences of digoxin actions are strong heartbeat, increased cardiac output and efficiency. These are followed by decreased venous pressure and diuresis. In normal heart, cardiac glycosides have little effect on heart rate.

Mechanism of Action—The positive inotropic action may be due to inhibition of the membrane bound Na^+—K^+-ATPase enzyme which supplies the energy for the transmembrane transport of Na and K. Inhibition of the enzyme is thought to increase the intracellular sodium which in turn may exchange with extracellular calcium. It is also possible that the enzyme inhibition decreases the outward pumping of both Na^+ and Ca^{++}, thus increasing the Ca^{++} pool available for excitation-contraction coupling. Its positive chronotropic action is due to suppression of AV node conduction to increase effective refractory period and decrease conduction velocity.

Digoxin

Indications—Treatment of congestive heart failure, atrial fibrillation or flutter, and supraventricular tachycardia.

Dosages—

Horse	0.06-0.08 mg/kg PO every 8 hours for 5-6 doses to digitalize, then 0.01-0.02 mg/kg PO for maintenance.
Dog	0.022-0.044 mg/kg PO every 12 hours for 48 hours to digitalize, then 0.011 mg/kg PO every 12 hours for maintenance.
Cattle	0.0088 mg/kg IV for digitalization
Cat	0.0075-0.015 mg/kg PO on alternate days for digitalization; 0.003-0.004 mg/kg/day or 0.005-0.010 mg/kg PO, every 24-48 hours for maintenance.

Route(s) of Administration—Per os and intravenous.

Absorption—Absorption is variable depending upon the oral dosage form used; food may delay, but does not alter the extent of absorption. Peak plasma concentration is attained within 45-60 minutes after oral elixir, and about 90 minutes after oral tablet administration.

Bioavailability (oral)—Bioavailability is formulation-dependent (about 70% from tablets, 80% from elixirs, and over 90% from liquid-filled soft gelatin capsules).

Effective Concentration—>0.8 ng/ml (inotropic effect).

Onset of Action—1-2 hours (oral); 5-30 minutes (IV).

Peak Action—6-8 hours following initial oral dose; 1-4 hours (IV).

Duration of Action—3-4 days (human).

Distribution—Digoxin is widely distributed with highest levels found in kidneys, heart, intestine, stomach, liver and skeletal muscle. Lowest concentrations are found in the brain and plasma. Only small amounts are found in fat. It crosses the placenta.

Plasma Protein Binding—Digoxin is tightly bound to tissues.

Metabolism—Digoxin is slightly metabolized by stepwise removal of the sugar moieties to form digoxigenin, which is further inactivated to inactive metabolites.

Plasma Half-life—Dog, 14.4-56 hours; Cats, 33.3±9.5 hours; Sheep, 7.15 hours; Horses, 16.9-23.2 hours; Cattle, 7.8 hours; Humans, 39 ± 13 hours.

Clearance—1 to 4 ml/min/kg.

Route(s) of Excretion—60±11% excreted in urine by glomerular filtration and tubular secretion.

Dialysis Status—Not dialyzable.

Toxicity and Adverse Effects—Digoxin, like other cardiac glycosides has narrow safety margin. A serious arrhythmia may be the first indication of toxicity. Intermittent anorexia and nausea, extra-systoles and bradycardia are often the early signs. Cats are relatively sensitive to digoxin while dogs are relatively tolerant of high serum digoxin levels.

Management of Overdose/Toxicity—Give general antidotal therapy.

Contraindications—Ventricular fibrillation; hypersensitivity to digoxin.

Precautions—Adjust dosage in patients with significant renal disease and in those receiving thyroid replacement therapy. Also, digoxin should be used with extreme caution in cases with heart failure, severe pulmonary disease, hypoxia, acute myocarditis, myxedema, or acute myocardial infarction. Reduce the dose in hypernatremic, hypokalemic, hypercalcemic, hyper—or hypo-thyroid animals.

Drug Interactions—Digitalis and calcium act synergistically. Sudden deaths have been reported following the rapid administration of calcium salts to digitalised patients. The levels of oral absorption and effect of digoxin may be reduced by antacids containing magnesium and aluminum, and other drugs such as metoclopramide, cimetidine, neomycin (oral), cyclophosphamide, doxorubicin, vinca alkaloids, and cytarabine. Diazepam, quinidine, anticholinergic drugs, succinylcholine, non depolarizing muscle relaxants, potassium losing diuretics, verapamil, tetracycline and erythromycin may increase the serum level, effectiveness and toxicity of digoxin. Penicillamine may decrease serum levels of digoxin independent of route of digoxin dosing. Drugs that affect electrolyte (especially potassium) balance e.g. diuretics (furosemide, thiazides), amphotericin B, glucocorticoids, ACTH, laxatives, sodium polystyrene sulfonate, glucagon, high dose IV dextrose, dextrose/insulin infusions may predispose the patient to digitalis toxicity.

Pharmaceutical Formulations—Available in 0.15 mg/ml and 0.05 mg/ml elixir; 0.1 mg/ml and 0.25 mg/ml solution for injection; 0.05 mg, 0.1 mg, and 0.2 mg capsules; 0.125 mg, 0.25 mg and 0.5 mg tablets.

DIMERCAPROL

Synonyms—BAL; British anti-lewisite;Dimercaptopropanol;Dithioglycerol.

Proprietary Names—BAL in oil*; Sulfactin*.

Chemical Class—A dithiol.

Pharmacological Class—Chelating agent.

Source—Synthesis.

Solubility, Stability and Storage—BAL is soluble in alcohol, vegetable oils, and water. It is unstable in aqueous solutions. Solutions which are turbid or contain sediments may still be potent. Store solutions for injection preferably at room temperature (15-30°C).

HS⌒SH⌒OH

Dimercaprol

Pharmacological Actions—BAL chelates heavy metals, principally arsenic, lead, mercury and gold. It is relatively ineffective in chelating some metals (*e.g.,* selenium). Chelation to dimercaprol may become irreversible in an acidic environment, as dimercaprol concentrations decrease or if oxidized. The dimercaprol-metal chelate is excreted via renal and fecal routes thus reducing the levels of the heavy metal in the body.

Mechanism of Action—The—SH group in BAL has higher affinity for metals than the—SH groups in sulfhydryl-dependent enzymes. Thus, BAL readily forms chelate complexes with metals; and spares the binding of the—SH groups of sulfhydryl-dependent enzymes by heavy metals.

Indications—Primarily for the treatment of arsenic poisoning. Dimercaprol is also used occasionally to treat mercury and gold poisoning and in combination with $CaNa_2EDTA$ to treat lead poisoning.

Dosages—Horses, 5 mg/kg IM immediately, followed by 3 mg/kg IM every 6 hours for the remainder of the first day, then 1 mg/kg IM every 6 hours for two or more additional days, as needed.

Route(s) of Administration—Intramuscular.

Absorption—Dimercaprol is well absorbed from muscular site; peak blood levels occur in 30-60 minutes. BAL is slowly absorbed through the skin after topical administration.

Duration of Action—4 hours in humans.

Distribution—BAL is widely distributed throughout the body, including the brain. It attains the highest levels in the liver and kidneys.

Metabolism—Free BAL is rapidly metabolized to inactive compounds and is completely eliminated within 6-24 hours.

Plasma Half-life—Short; degradation and excretion is complete within 4 hours.

Route(s) of Excretion—Urine, bile and feces.

Toxicity and Adverse Effects—Adverse effects are mostly transient. BAL causes pain at the point of IM injection. Systemic adverse effects include vomiting and seizures especially at high doses. Transient tachycardia and hypertension has been reported. BAL may cause nephrotoxicity.

Management of Overdose/Toxicity—Give symptomatic and supportive therapy.

Contraindications—Impaired hepatic function, unless secondary to acute arsenic toxicity; iron, cadmium, and selenium poisoning; hypersensitivity to BAL.

Precautions—Allow at least 24 hours after the last dimercaprol dose before administering iron or selenium medications. Use cautiously in patients with impaired renal function. Alkalinize urine to prevent the chelate from dissociating in the urine. Adjust the dosage or discontinue therapy in animals with diminished renal function prior to or during therapy. Maintain excess of dimercaprol in plasma.

Drug Interactions—BAL forms toxic complexes with cadmium, selenium, uranium and iron.

Pharmaceutical Formulations—Available in 100 mg/ml solution for injection in peanut oil and benzyl benzoate.

DIMETHYL SULFOXIDE

Dimethyl sulfoxide

Synonyms—Dimethyl Sulphoxide; Dimexide; DMSO; Methyl Sulfoxide.

Proprietary Names—Deltan˙; Dolicur˙; Dolmoso˙; Kemsol˙; Rheumabene˙; Rimso-50˙.

Chemical Class—Dipolar organic compound.

Pharmacological Class—Antioxidant; Anti-inflammatory; Analgesic.

Source—Natural; derived from wood pulp.

Solubility, Stability and Storage—DMSO is soluble in water, ethanol, acetone, benzene, chloroform, ether, and most organic solvents. DMSO products are better stored in glass containers. Protect its products from light and moisture because DMSO is highly hygroscopic. DMSO is compatible with most compounds but since it can enhance the cutaneous absorption of other compounds, care must be taken in mixing DMSO with other drugs to avoid unintended percutaneous absorption of a potentially toxic compound.

Pharmacological Actions—DMSO has diverse pharmacological actions. It has anti-inflammatory (scavenges reactive oxygen species), analgesic (controls acute and chronic musculoskeletal and postoperative pains), immunomodulatory (inhibits leukocyte migration, antibody production, and fibroblast proliferation), radioprotective, cryopreservative, diuretic, sedative (in some species), anti-ischemic and antimicrobial properties. Acute inflammation responds better to DMSO than chronic one. Its analgesic effect is comparable to those of narcotic analgesics. DMSO dilates blood vessels and inhibits platelet aggregation. It enhances cutaneous absorption and membrane penetration by other drugs. It also inhibits alcohol dehydrogenase and cholinesterase enzymes. DMSO liberates histamine.

Mechanism of Action—DMSO and its metabolite, dimethyl sulfide scavenge reactive oxygen species. This is thought to be responsible for its anti-inflammatory properties. It causes vasodilation apparently due to histamine release. The mechanisms by which DMSO causes most other pharmacological actions are poorly understood.

Indications—DMSO is purportedly used to treat a wide variety of conditions including

- Reduction of acute swelling due to trauma; adjunctive treatment in ischemic conditions; control of severe musculoskeletal pain.
- Boosting of antimicrobial agent penetration in cases of mastitis in cattle,
- Limitation of tissue damage that may result from extravasation of an irritant drug.
- Reduction of cerebral edema and CNS trauma. Reduction of engorged mammary glands in bitches.
- Treatment of urinary tract obstruction in male cats.
- Treatment of acute and chronic otitis.
- Facilitation of wound healing.

- Treatment of ethylene glycol poisoning.
- DMSO may also be used to treat burns, cancer, colitis, lupus, muscle pain, cystitis, gallstones, herpes, pancreas infection and ulcers.

Dosages—Apply DMSO topically over affected area 2-4 times daily for a maximum of 14 days or 1 g/kg body weight as a 10% solution by slow intravenous administration.

Route(s) of Administration—Per os, topical, and intravenous.

Absorption—DMSO is readily absorbed after injection or after oral or percutaneous administration. Peak serum concentration is attained within 1 to 4 hours after an oral dose of 1 g/kg. DMSO penetrates the skin rapidly. Peak plasma concentration is attained 2 hours after topical administration.

Distribution—Widely distributed throughout the body including the CNS. DMSO does not penetrate tooth enamel and keratin.

Metabolism—Partially degraded in the liver to an active dimethyl sulfide.

Plasma Half-life—10 to 20 hours for the parent compound; about 70 hours for the sulfone metabolite.

Route(s) of Excretion—30 to 70% is excreted in the urine unchanged and about 20% as the sulfone following oral dose; 13% is excreted unchanged and about 18% as the sulfone after percutaneous administration; 3% of a dose is eliminated through the lungs as dimethyl sulfide.

Dialysis Status—Dialyzable.

Toxicity and Adverse Effects—DMSO is well tolerated. The LD_{50} in dog is 2.5 grams/kg. However, topical application may cause transient erythema, dry skin, cutaneous allergy, and bad breath. Intravenous overdose causes hemolysis, hematuria, sedation, diuresis, hypotension, convulsion, and respiratory distress. Hepatotoxicity and ocular lesions resulting in myopia have been reported following chronic use.

Contraindications—Severe dehydration; mastocytoma; shock; hypersensitivity to DMSO.

Precautions—Adequate care must be taken to avoid contamination by potentially harmful compounds during topical application. It is advisable to wear rubber gloves and apply with clean cotton wool. Use with caution in pregnant animals since DMSO is teratogenic in chicks. Intravenous injection should be made slowly and a 10% concentration or less is recommended.

Drug Interactions—DMSO enhances the percutaneous absorption of other drugs. Drugs such as insulin, heparin, phenylbutazone, and sulfonamide may attain effective concentration in plasma if mixed with DMSO and applied topically. DMSO may cause additive effects if used with anticholinesterase agents. It may prolong the effect of alcohol and potentiates the actions of insulin, corticosteroids and atropine.

Pharmaceutical Formulations—Available as 90% gel for topical application, and 90% solution for intravenous injection. DMSO (60%) is also available in combination with 0.01% fluocinolone acetonide for the treatment of otitis.

DIMINAZENE

Diminazene

Proprietary Names—Berenil˚; Ganaseg˚; Veriben˚; Nozomil˚; Samorenil˚; Ebenil˚; Dimenil˚; Trypadim˚.

Chemical Class—Diamidine.

Pharmacological Class—Antitrypanosomal drug; Trypanocide; Antibabesial drug.

Source—Synthetic.

Solubility, Stability and Storage—Diminazene is soluble in 14 parts of water at 20°C, slightly soluble in alcohol, very soluble in ether and chloroform. Administer diminazene solution within 5 days of preparation if stored at room temperature or 14 days, if stored in a refrigerator.

Pharmacological Actions—Diminazene is effective against *T. vivax* and *T. congolense* but less so against *T. brucei* hence there is the necessity to double the dose in such cases. Diminazene is also effective against *Babesia* species and bacteria (mainly *Brucella* and *Streptococcus* species).

Mechanism of Action—Diminazene distorts DNA structure especially at the kinetoplast of the parasite. Other possible sites of action are modification of cytoplasmic membranes and lysosomes; inhibition of phospholipid synthesis and basic amino acid transport.

Indications—Treatment of trypanosomosis in cattle, sheep, goats, and dogs; treatment of babesial infections.

Dosages—

Cattle, Sheep, Goat. 3.5 mg/kg in *T. congolense* and *T. vivax* infections.

Dog. 3.5 mg/kg in *Babesia canis* infection; 7 mg/kg in *T. brucei* infection.

Horse. 6-12 mg/kg in *Babesia equi* infection.

Route(s) of Administration—Intramuscular

Absorption—Diminazene is well absorbed from intramuscular site. Peak plasma concentration is attained within 18.00 ± 6.71 to 36.00 ± 8.22 minutes.

Distribution—Vd = 1.93-2.60 L/kg (goat); 1.91 ± 0.42 L/kg (cattle); Diminazene accumulates in the liver and kidneys; concentration in CSF is 3-4 times lower than concentration in plasma.

Plasma Protein Binding—38.01-91.10% (cattle).

Metabolism—Extensively metabolized to p-aminobenzamidine and p-amino-benzamide in cattle.

Plasma Half-life—31.7 hours (cattle).

Clearance—1.7 ± 0.40 ml/min/kg in cattle.

Route(s) of Excretion—Mainly urine where about 80% of the dose is excreted within 20 days and 8.26% as unchanged drug within the first 24 hours.

Withdrawal Period—21days (meat); 5 days (milk).

Toxicity and Adverse Effects—Local reactions at the site of administration may be severe in horses. At high doses, toxicity may involve the CNS. This may manifest as ataxia and convulsions. Diminazene aceturate is toxic to camels.

Contraindications—Camels; hypersensitivity to diminazene.

Precautions—Administer by deep intramuscular injection into the muscle of the mid-neck in cattle. It may be injected subcutaneously in dogs.

Pharmaceutical Formulations—Available as diminazene aceturate or diaceturate in granules for reconstitution for injection. It is formulated with antipyrine.

DINOPROST

Synonyms—Dinoprost trometamol; PGF_2 alpha THAM; prostaglandin F_2 alpha tromethamine.
Proprietary Names—Lutalyse*.

Chemical Class—Prostaglandin F_2 alpha.

Pharmacological Class—Luteolytic agent.

Source—Synthetic.

Solubility, Stability and Storage—One gram of dinoprost is soluble in about 5 ml of water. Dinoprost injection may be stored at room temperature (15-30°C) in airtight containers but storage in the refrigerator is preferred.

Pharmacological Actions—Dinoprost causes functional and morphologic regression of the corpus luteum. It stimulates myometrial activity, and relaxes the cervix.

Indications—Dinoprost is also used to synchronize oestrus, induce parturition in sows and to terminate early pregnancy either alone, or in combination with corticosteroids (in cattle and sheep) or dopaminergic agents (in dogs). It is also used to treat pyometra and expel mummified fetus.

Dosages—

Horse	5 mg IM
Cattle	25-35 mg IM
Pig	10 mg IM
Sheep, goat	5-10 mg IM
Dog	For pyometra: 0.25 mg/kg SC once a day for 5 days. Give bactericidal antibiotics concurrently. As abortifacient: 1. During the first half of gestation: 0.25 mg/kg SC every 12 hours for 4 days. 2. During the second half of gestation: 0.25 mg/kg SC every 12 hours until abortion is complete.

Cat	For pyometra: initially 0.1 mg/kg SC, then 0.25 mg/kg SC once a day for 5 days. Give bactericidal antibiotics concurrently. As abortifacient after day 40 of gestation: 0.5-1 mg/kg SC initially and then 24 hours later.

Route(s) of Administration—Intramuscular.

Distribution—Dinoprost distributes very rapidly to tissues after injection.

Plasma Half-life—Short; only minutes in cattle.

Withdrawal Period—No preslaughter withdrawal or milk withdrawal is required.

Toxicity and Adverse Effects—Colic, placental retention, dystocia, broncho-constriction, tachycardia, tachypnea, sweating, and salivation have been reported in most species. Decreased rectal temperature in mares and increased temperature in cattle have been observed. Erythema and pruritus, urination, defecation, slight ataxia, hyperpnoea, dyspnea have been reported in sows. Abdominal pain, emesis, defecation, urination, pupillary dilation followed by constriction, tachycardia, restlessness and anxiety, fever, hypersalivation, dyspnea and panting have been reported in dogs. Dogs are sensitive to overdose. Cats may exhibit increased vocalization and intense grooming behavior.

Management of Overdose/Toxicity—Give supportive therapy.

Contraindications. Pregnancy (unless used as an abortifacient or parturition inducer); animals with bronchoconstrictive respiratory disease (e.g. asthma, "heavy" horses); mares with acute or sub acute disorders of the vascular system, GI tract, respiratory system or reproductive tract.

Precautions—Do not administer dinoprost intravenously. Use dinoprost cautiously in dogs or cats greater than 8 years old, or with pre-existing cardiopulmonary or other serious disease (liver, kidney, etc.). Do not administer before three days of expected farrowing in sows to avoid increased neonatal mortality. Dinoprost should be handled with extreme caution by pregnant women, asthmatics or other persons with bronchial diseases. Any accidental exposure to skin should be washed off immediately.

Drug Interactions—Dinoprost activity may be enhanced by oxytocic agents. Its effects may be reduced by concomitant administration of progestins.

Pharmaceutical Formulations—Available as dinoprost tromethamine in solution for injection equivalent to 5 mg/ml of dinoprost.

DIPHENHYDRAMINE

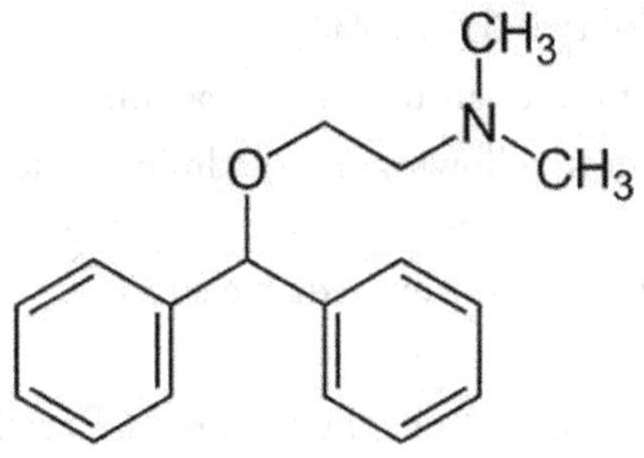

Diphenhydramine

Proprietary Names—Benadryl®.

Chemical Class—Ethanolamine.

Pharmacological Class—Antihistamine; H_1 antagonist; Anti-allergic drug.

Source—Synthetic.

Solubility, Stability and Storage—Diphenhydramine is soluble in water and alcohol. It is photosensitive; it darkens when exposed to light. Store products in tight and light-resistant containers at room temperature.

Pharmacological Actions—Diphenhydramine blocks the actions of histamine at the H_1 receptor sites. Hence, the histamine released during allergic conditions is unable to constrict smooth muscle, make exocrine glands secrete, or increase capillary permeability. Diphenhydramine possesses some anticholinergic, sedative, antiemetic, antitussive, and local anesthetic actions.

Mechanism of Action—Competitively excludes histamine from H_1 receptor sites.

Indications—Symptomatic control of allergic conditions involving histamine release; treatment or prevention of motion sickness; prevention of emesis; relief of cough; control of extrapyramidal effects associated with phenothiazines; control of pruritus. H_1 blockers such as diphenhydramine and H_2 blockers such as ranitidine or cimetidine are used in dogs prior to surgical excision of mast cell tumors in order to prevent some of the effects of massive histamine release due to mast cell de-granulation. These drugs are generally continued during the recovery period in order to improve wound healing.

Dosages—

Bird	2-4 mg/kg every 12 hours.
Cat	4 mg/kg every 8hours.
Dog	4 mg/kg every 8hours.
Guinea pig	5 mg/kg SC; 12.5 mg/kg IP.
Non Human Primate	5 mg/kg.
Rat	10 mg/kg SC.

Route(s) of Administration—Per os, intramuscular, intravenous and topical.

Absorption—Diphenhydramine is readily absorbed from the gastrointestinal tract of monogastric animals. Peak plasma concentrations are reached within 1-4 hours. Diphenhydramine can be absorbed from the skin following topical administration.

Bioavailability—Oral bioavailability is 61 ± 25%.

Effective Concentration: >25 ng/ml for antihistaminic action; 30-40 ng/ml for sedation.

Onset of Action: 20-45 minutes following oral administration; 3-5 minutes following IV administration.

Peak Action—It takes 1-3 hours for maximum sedative effect.

Duration of Action—4-7 hours.

Distribution—Vd = 4.5 ± 2.8 L/kg. Diphenhydramine attains high concentrations in spleen, lungs, and brain. It crosses the placenta and is secreted in milk.

Plasma Protein Binding—78 ± 3%.

Metabolism—Diphenhydramine is excessively degraded in the liver.

Plasma Half-life—8.5 ± 3.2 hours in humans.

Clearance (ml/min/kg)—6.2 ± 1.7 in humans.

Route(s) of Excretion—Urine with 1.9 ± 0.8% as unchanged drug.

Toxicity and Adverse Effects—CNS depression (characterized by somnolence and lethargy) and anticholinergic effects (characterized by dry mouth, urinary retention) are most common. Overdose is characterized by more prominent anticholinergic effects, CNS depression, respiratory depression, and death.

Management of Overdose/Toxicity—Undertake general antidotal therapy procedures. Control CNS excitement with phenytoin. Anticholinergic effects may be controlled with physostigmine.

Contraindications—Angle closure glaucoma; hypersensitivity to diphenhydramine or other antihistamines belonging to the ethanolamine group; bladder neck obstruction; pyloroduodenal obstruction; asthma. Antihistamines should not be used within a week of skin testing for allergies.

Precautions—Do not mix diphenhydramine with barbiturates, promethazine, tetracycline, heparin, hydrocortisone, amphotericin B, cephalothin, phenytoin and promazine in the same syringe. Use antihistamines such as diphenhydramine in combination with smaller doses of corticosteroids if antihistamines alone are unable to control all the allergic signs. For control of motion sickness, give the drug 30 to 60 minutes before travelling.

Drug Interactions—Concurrent use of diphenhydramine with other CNS depressants may cause additive effect.

Pharmaceutical Formulations—Available as diphenhydramine hydrochloride in 25 mg, 50 mg capsules; 1% and 2% cream; 25 mg and 50 mg tablets; 12.5 mg/ml elixir; 10 mg/ml and 50 mg/ml solution for injection; 12.5 mg/ml syrup.

DIPHENOXYLATE

Diphenoxylate

Proprietary Names—Lomotil˙; Logen˙; Lonox˙; Diphenatol˙; Lofene˙; Lomanate˙; Lomodix˙; Low-Quel˙; Lomocot˙; Vi-Atro˙

Chemical Class—Piperidine opioid derivative.

Pharmacological Class—Antidiarrheal agent. Antiperistaltic agent.

Source—Synthetic.

Solubility, Stability and Storage—Diphenoxylate is sparingly soluble in water; soluble 1 in 50 of ethanol and 1 in 2.5 of chloroform. It is soluble in methanol but practically insoluble in ether. Store diphenoxylate products in a tightly sealed container in a dry place away from heat, moisture, and direct light. Freeze the liquid form.

Pharmacological Actions—Diphenoxylate inhibits GI motility and excessive peristalsis thus causing increase in intestinal transit time. It reduces fecal volume and viscosity and also decreases fluid and electrolyte loss. Thus, diphenoxylate reduces the amount of fluid presented to the large intestine by the small intestine. It also has antisecretory action. High doses produce typical opioid activities such as euphoria, physical dependence and suppression of morphine withdrawal syndrome.

Mechanism of Action—Diphenoxylate activates mu-opioid receptors in the gastrointestinal tract. Opioids are also known to inhibit acetylcholine release in the GIT and modulates the effects of already released acetylcholine. These actions may be due to increased calcium-dependent potassium conductance and hyperpolarization. Opioids reduce calcium entry during action potential and deplete the neurons of calcium.

Indications—Diphenoxylate is used to control severe acute and chronic diarrhea and intestinal cramps.

Dosages—0.1-0.2 mg/kg in dogs.

Route(s) of Administration—Per os.

Absorption—Diphenoxylate is absorbed following oral administration and plasma concentration reaches its peak in 2 hours.

Bioavailability—Bioavailability for tablet is 90% that of oral liquid.

Onset of Action: 45-60 minutes (humans).

Peak Action—Within 2-4 hours.

Duration of Action: 3-4 hours.

Distribution—Appears in milk.

Plasma Protein Binding: 74-95%.

Metabolism—Diphenoxylate is de-esterified in the liver to the active difenoxin (diphenoxylic acid).

Plasma Half-Life: 2.5 hours for parent compound and about 4.5 hours for active metabolite.

Route(s) of Excretion—Feces (via bile) mainly; 14 % of dose is excreted in urine with 1 % as unchanged drug.

Toxicity and Adverse Effects—Normal therapeutic dose may produce nervousness, urinary retention, and difficulty in urination. Dry mouth and miosis may also be experienced due to the presence of atropine in the formulation. Nausea, emesis and abdominal discomfort have been reported in few cases. In dogs, constipation and bloat with potential occurrence of paralytic ileus are common. Overdose may cause drowsiness, blurred vision, hypotension, dry mouth, miosis, and delayed or prolonged GI absorption.

Management of Overdose/Toxicity—Reduce bioavailability by administering activated charcoal. Administer naloxone to reverse the action of diphynoxylate. Administration of physostigmine will reverse the action of atropine in the formulation.

Contraindications—Hypersensitivity to diphenoxylate, atropine, or any other component; severe hepatic disease; diarrhea caused by toxic ingestion; cats.

Precautions—The use of diphenoxylate at high doses and for prolonged period may cause physical and psychological dependence. Diphenoxylate should be used cautiously in severely debilitated animals and those with hypothyroidism, renal insufficiency, adrenocortical insufficiency, increased intracranial pressure, respiratory disease, and abdominal conditions. Do not use diphenoxylate in diarrhea caused by poisoning, until toxic material has been eliminated from the gastrointestinal tract. Acute dysentery characterized by bloody feces and elevated temperature may require additional antibiotic therapy.

Drug Interactions—Other CNS depressants may potentiate the actions of diphenoxylate. Concomitant use of the drug with MAO inhibitors may precipitate hypertensive crises. Use of the formulation with antimuscarinics may cause paralytic ileus. Naltrexone blocks the therapeutic effects of opioids, including the antidiarrheal effects. Concurrent use of opioid (narcotic) analgesics with diphenoxylate may result in increased risk of severe constipation and additive CNS depressant effects.

Pharmaceutical Formulations—Diphenoxylate is available in oral solution and tablets containing 2.5 mg diphenoxylate hydrochloride and 0.025 mg atropine sulfate. Excipients in the dosage forms include lactose (monohydrate), magnesium stearate, microcrystalline cellulose, and pregelatinized starch (corn). Atropine is included in the preparation in doses below the therapeutic level in an attempt to prevent abuse in humans by deliberate overdosage. No specific veterinary formulation is available.

DIPYRONE

Dipyrone

Synonyms—Metamizol; Methampyrone; Aminopyrine-sulfonate Sodium.

Proprietary Names—Analgin˚ Novalgin˚; lagalgin˚; Algopyrin˚.

Chemical Class—Parazolone (pyrrazolone; pyrazolone) derivative.

Pharmacological Class—Nonsteroidal Anti-inflammatory Drug (NSAID); Simple analgesic; Non-narcotic analgesic; Analgesic-antipyretic.

Sources—Synthetic.

Solubility, Stability and Storage—Dipyrone is soluble 1 in 1.5 of water and 1 in 30 of ethanol. It is practically insoluble in ether, acetone, benzene, and chloroform. Store dipyrone at room temperature in tightly closed containers.

Pharmacological Actions—Dipyrone possesses analgesic, antipyretic and anti-inflammatory actions. It inhibits kinin-induced muscle spasm.

Mechanism of Action—It irreversibly blocks cyclooxygenase.

Indications—The antipyretic, analgesic, and anti-inflammatory properties are utilized in colic condition in horses (usually in combination with antispasmodic agents), control of mild pain associated with smooth muscle spasm or mild colon impaction and control of GI hypermotility or spasm.

Dosages—10-11 mg/kg in horses; 25 mg/ kg in dogs.

Route(s) of Administration—Formulations are available for oral, intramuscular, subcutaneous and intravenous administration.

Metabolism—Dipyrone is rapidly hydrolyzed in gastric juice after oral administration to an active metabolite which is further metabolized following absorption.

Plasma Half-Life—This varies with the metabolite; e.g. 10.6 hours for 4-acetylamino-phenazone; 5 hours for 4-amino-phenazone; 10 hours for 4-formylamino-phenazone, and 3.3 hours for 4-methylamino-phenazone.

Route(s) of Excretion—About 70% of a dose is excreted in the urine in 24 hours as metabolites. Dipyrone metabolites are excreted in breast milk.

Withdrawal Period—5 days in race horses.

Toxicity and Adverse Effects—The most common side effect for dipyrone is injection site reactions. Others are anorexia, oral ulcers, depression, decreased plasma protein, increased creatinine, anemia, and leukopenia. Agranulocytosis and leukopenia with prolonged use is the most serious adverse effect in humans. Agranulocytosis is not a serious problem in animals. Dipyrone also causes increased bleeding time. Overdose may cause convulsive seizure.

Management of Overdose—Therapy should be stopped at the first sign of any adverse reaction. Give symptomatic and supportive therapy. Injection site reactions usually respond to hot compresses and NSAIDs.

Contraindications—Hypersensitivity to dipyrone or other pyrazolone derivatives; cats; dogs treated with phenothiazine compounds; food animals; racing animals for at least five days prior to a race.

Precautions—Use dipyrone cautiously in animals with liver, kidney or GI dysfunction. Dipyrone should be given slowly when administered intravenously to avoid seizure. Use the drug with caution in older or debilitated animals particularly those with cardiac disease. Do not use dipyrone in animals with history of blood or bone marrow abnormalities.

Drug Interactions—Barbiturates and phenylbutazone will induce the enzyme system involved in the metabolism of dipyrone. Dipyrone causes severe hypothermia when used in combination with chlorpromazine.

Pharmaceutical Formulations—Available in 500 mg tablets; 500 mg/ml drops; 250 mg/5 ml syrup; 1 g and 300 mg suppositories; and 500 mg/ml solution for injection.

DOBUTAMINE

Proprietary Names—Dopastat®; Intropin®; Dubutrex®.

Chemical Class—Catecholamine.

Pharmacological Class—β-adrenergic agonist; Sympathomimetic drug; Inotropic agent.

Source—Synthetic.

Solubility, Stability and Storage—Dobutamine is sparingly soluble in water and ethanol but soluble in methanol. Dobutamine hydrochloride for injection should be stored at 15-30°C; solutions in 5% dextrose should be stored at room temperature (25°C) and protected from freezing or excessive heat for long periods.

Dobutamine

Pharmacological Actions—Dobutamine selectively increases cardiac contractility with little effect on heart rate, rhythm, and peripheral vascular resistance. The net cardiovascular response to dobutamine is due to different actions of its stereoisomers, which act to different intensity on alpha—and beta-adrenergic receptors. Dobutamine produces more prominent inotropic than chronotropic effects on the heart. It increases cardiac output and produces a relatively constant peripheral resistance due to balancing of the opposing $alpha_1$ and $beta_2$-mediated vascular actions.

Mechanism of Action—Dobutamine interacts directly with alpha and beta adrenergic receptors but acts mainly on cardiac β_1 receptors.

Indications—Short term treatment of heart failure.

Dosages—Small animals, 2-20 mcg/kg/min—Large animals; 1-10 mcg/kg/min.

Route(s) of Administration—Intravenous (constant IV infusion). Dobutamine is usually added to infusion fluids.

Bioavailability—Zero, (following oral administration).

Effective Concentration: >35 mcg/ml (threshold for change in cardiac output); >50 mcg/ml (threshold for change in heart rate). These figures were obtained in humans.

Onset of Action: 1-10 minutes.

Peak Effect: 10-20 minutes.

Duration of Action—The effects decline rapidly after stoppage of infusion.

Distribution—Vd = 0.20 ± 0.08 (human).

Metabolism—Dobutamine is rapidly inactivated in the gut. It is metabolized in the liver and other tissues to 3-O-methyl dobutamine, and conjugated products.

Plasma Half-Life: 2.4 ± 0.7 minutes (human). This may be higher in cats due to deficiency of glucuronyl transferase.

Clearance: 59 ± 22 ml/min/kg in human.

Route(s) of Excretion—Eliminated via urine, and to a minor extent in feces.

Toxicity and Adverse Effects—Adverse effects are documented in humans. Dobutamine may cause increase in heart rate and blood pressure to warrant reduction in dose. Other adverse effects include headache, nausea, vomiting, dyspnea and hyperesthesia. Overdose may cause palpitation, nervousness, fatigue and increased blood pressure. Extravasation may cause dermal necrosis.

Management of Overdose/Toxicity—Reduce the dose—

Contraindications—Idiopathic, hypertrophic subaortic stenosis; hypersensitivity to dobutamine or any component, e.g., sodium bisulfite.

Precautions—Dilute proprietary preparation to at least 5 mg/ml before use—Use dobutamine with caution in cats because one of the metabolic pathways of dobutamine is glucuronidation, which is deficient in cats. Use cautiously after myocardial infarction as it may increase oxygen demand. Correct hypovolemic states before administration of dobutamine. Administer digitalis in animals that have atrial fibrillation before dobutamine is administered. Because of potential physical incompatibilities, it is recommended that dobutamine solutions not be admixed with other drugs.

Drug Interactions—Beta-adrenergic blockers will cause preponderance of dobutamine alpha-adrenergic effects. Concurrent administration with halothane and cyclopropane will cause ventricular arrhythmia. Concurrent use with sodium nitroprusside will result in enhanced effect of dobutamine. Concurrent use with oxytocic drugs may cause severe hypertension.

Pharmaceutical Formulations—Available as dobutamine hydrochloride in vials containing 250 mg/20 ml solution.

DOCUSATES

Synonyms—Docusate sodium (Dioctyl sodium succinate, Dioctyl sodium sulfosuccinate, DSS, or DOSS); Docusate calcium (Dioctyl calcium succinate, Dioctyl Calcium Sulfosuccinate); Docusate potassium (Dioctyl potassium succinate).

Proprietary Names—Docusate Sodium (Colace*; Dioctyl*; Docusoft*; Docusol*); Docusate Calcium (Surfak*); Docusate Potassium (Kasof*).

Chemical Class—Anionic surface-active agents.

Pharmacological Class—Fecal softeners; Laxatives.

Source—Synthetic.

Solubility, Stability and Storage—One gram of DOSS is soluble in approximately 70 ml of water and it is freely soluble in alcohol and glycerin. Docusate calcium is very slightly soluble in water, but freely soluble in alcohol. Docusate potassium is sparingly soluble in water and soluble in alcohol. Capsules of salts of docusate should be stored in tight containers at room temperature. Docusate sodium solutions should be stored in tight containers and the syrup stored in tight, light-resistant containers.

Docusate sodium

Pharmacological Actions—Docusates possess wetting and emulsifying properties. They produce modest softening of feces within 24-48hrs after administration.

Mechanism of Action—Their laxative effect is attributed to their physical property of lowering surface tension which is thought to facilitate the penetration of feces by fat and water. Docusates also increase cAMP concentrations in colonic mucosal cells which may increase both ion secretion and fluid permeability from these cells into the colon lumen.

Indications—Treatment of constipation in small animals. Docusates are used alone and in combination with mineral oil in treating fecal impactions in horses.

Dosages—

Horses. 10-20 mg/kg diluted in 2 liters of warm water PO; may repeat in 48 hours.

Route(s) of Administration—Per os.

Absorption—Some docusate is absorbed from the small intestine and is then excreted into the bile.

Onset of Action—1-3 days.

Route(s) of Excretion—Bile.

Toxicity and Adverse Effects—At therapeutic doses, clinically significant adverse effects are rare. Cramping, diarrhea and intestinal mucosal damage are possible. The liquid preparations may cause throat irritation if administered by mouth. High dose docusate produce secretory effects that can cause dehydration and altered electrolyte status. Overdose causes anorexia, vomiting, diarrhea and colic. In the horse, overdose has caused dehydration, intestinal mucosal damage, and death.

Contraindications—Docusates should not be used concurrently with mineral oils in small animals as they may enhance the absorption of the oils.

Precautions—Use docusates with caution in patients with pre-existing fluid or electrolyte abnormalities. Do not administer concurrently with oral drugs having low therapeutic indices.

Drug Interactions—Docusate sodium increases the extent of mineral oil and phenolphthalein absorption. Concomitant administration of aspirin and docusate sodium may cause greater intestinal mucosal damage than occurs with aspirin alone.

Pharmaceutical Formulations—Available as sodium, potassium, and calcium salts in powder, liquid-filled capsules, solutions, syrup, suspensions and tablets.

DOPAMINE

Synonyms—3,4-dihydroxyphenylethylamine.

Proprietary Names—Dopamex˙; Dopaminex˙; Docard˙; Dopmin˙; Dynatra˙; Dynos˙; Inopin˙; Inovan˙; Intropin˙; Medopa˙; Dopastat®; Dopamine HCl®.

Chemical Class—Catecholamine.

Pharmacological Class—Autonomic-acting drug; Adrenergic agonist.

Source—Endogenous.

Solubility, Stability and Storage—Dopamine is freely soluble in water, soluble in methanol and ethanol but practically insoluble in ether. Solutions of dopamine oxidizes readily on exposure to light or heat to inactive product. Oxidized solution turns pink, yellow, brown or purple. Hence, solutions should be stored in tight containers and protected from light.

Pharmacological Actions—Dopamine activates different catecholaminergic receptors at different doses. At low doses, it causes renal and mesenteric, coronary and intracerebral vasodilatation resulting in decreased total peripheral and renal vascular resistance, increase in renal and mesenteric blood flow and cardiac output. These actions are of advantage in the treatment of shock. Large doses increase cardiovascular pressure and pronounced increase in myocardial contraction partly through $alpha_1$–adrenergic receptor mediated vasoconstriction. The vasodilatation effects are blocked by haloperidol, a dopamine antagonist while alpha-adrenergic blockers block the pressor effects. The cardiostimulatory effects are blocked by propranolol, a beta-adrenergic blocker.

Mechanism of Action—Dopamine predominantly activates D1 dopaminergic receptors at low doses, $beta_1$ adrenergic and dopaminergic receptors at moderate doses and alpha-adrenergic receptors at high doses. Its actions are mediated through activation of adenylyl cyclase leading to increases in intracellular cyclic AMP. It also acts indirectly by releasing norepinephrine.

Indications—Dopamine is effectively used to correct hemodynamic imbalances in circulatory shock after adequate fluid replacement and to treat oliguric renal failure. It has been used to terminate atrio-ventricular heart block in foals and control of Parkinson's disease in humans.

Dosages—

Oliguric renal failure: 2-5 mcg/kg/min by IV infusion in conjunction with a diuretic e.g. furosemide.

Acute heart failure: 1-10 mcg/kg/min.

Circulatory shock: 1-20 mcg/kg/min.

Route(s) of Administration—Intravenous infusion.

Onset of Action—5 minutes.

Duration of Action—< 10 minutes. This is increased to about 1 hour in patients receiving MAO inhibitors.

Distribution—Dopamine is widely distributed but it does not cross the blood-brain barrier in appreciable quantities.

Metabolism—Dopamine is rapidly metabolized in the gut. It is metabolized in the liver, kidney and plasma by MAO and COMT to inactive metabolites. A portion of administered dose is converted to norepinephrine.

Plasma Half-Life—~2 minutes.

Route(s) of Excretion—Urine.

Toxicity and Adverse Effects—These have been better documented in humans. They include headache, nausea, vomiting, tachycardia, angina pain and arrhythmias, which are due to excessive sympathomimetic activity. Extravasation into the tissue during infusion may cause ischaemic necrosis and sloughing. Overdose can cause severe hypertension, cardiac arrhythmia and acute renal failure.

Management of Overdose/Toxicity—Instill saline solution with phentolamine in the tissue where extravasation had occurred.

Contraindications—Pheochromocytoma; tachyarrhythmia; ischaemic heart disease; occlusive vascular disease; hypersensitivity to dopamine or any component.

Precautions—Hypovolemic shock must be corrected by fluid or blood replacement before dopamine infusion. Monitor blood pressure and renal function during infusion. Reduce the dose in patients receiving MAO inhibitors. Reduce the dose or terminate infusion if blood circulation to the heart and extremities decreases or if arrhythmia occurs.

Drug Interactions—MAO inhibitors, alpha—and beta-adrenergic blockers, general anesthetic agents and phenytoin increase the duration and effects of dopamine.

Pharmaceutical Formulations—Available as dopamine hydrochloride in solutions for injection containing 40 mg/ml, 80 mg/ml and 160 mg/ml in 5, 10, and 20 ml vials or 5 and 10 ml syringes. A formulation in dextrose for intravenous infusion is also available. Veterinary formulations are not available.

DORAMECTIN

Proprietary Names—Dectomax*.

Chemical Class—Macrocyclic lactone.

Pharmacological Class—Endectocide; Anthelmintic; Ectoparasiticide.

Source—Semisynthetic; obtained from products of *Streptomyces avermitilis*.

Solubility, Stability and Storage—Store doramectin products at temperatures not higher than 30⁰C.

Pharmacological Actions—Doramectin, like other macrocyclic lactones is an endectocide. It is active against a wide variety of nematodes of the gastrointestinal tract and lungs of cattle. It is also active against eye worms, screw worms, and several ectoparasites like sucking lice, grubs, ticks, and mites that plaque cattle. Doramectin is highly effective against adult and larvae of *Ostertagia, Haemonchus, Trichostrongylus, Cooperia, Oesophagostonum, Trichuris, Nematodirus, Bunostonum* and *Dictyocaulus* species. Doramectin is effective against eye worms (Thelazia). Arthropods such as *Psoroptes bovis, Sarcoptes scabei, and Hypoderma bovis* are susceptible. Doramectin is particularly effective against screw worms unlike other macrocyclic lactones.

Mechanism of Action—Doramectin increases neuronal chloride conductance by opening glutamate-gated chloride channels and also by potentiating the release and binding of GABA at certain synapses in invertebrates. This results in hyperpolarization and reduced neuronal excitability thereby causing tonic paralysis of the peripheral musculature of susceptible parasites.

Mechanism of Selective Toxicity—High affinity avermectin receptors are absent in cestodes and trematodes. The sensitivity of avermectin receptors in nematodes and arthropods is 100-fold higher than those in mammals.

Indications—Control of gastrointestinal nematodes, eye worms, lungworms, screw worms, and ectoparasites in cattle.

Dosages—200 mcg/kg.

Route(s) of Administration—Subcutaneous.

Absorption—The sesame oil/ethyl oleate vehicle used in formulation delays absorption from subcutaneous site of administration. Peak plasma concentration is attained within 5 days. Therapeutic plasma concentration is high and prolonged.

Duration of Action—At least 12 days and up to 35 days. Protection against some arthropods for up to 35 days has been reported.

Withdrawal Period—35 days before slaughter.

Route(s) of Excretion—Mainly feces.

Toxicity and Adverse Effects—Doramectin is very well tolerated. Twenty five times the recommended dose in cattle did not cause any adverse effects. It may cause tissue reaction if injected intramuscularly. Three times the recommended dose in breeding animals did not affect reproductive performance.

Contraindications—Animal species other than cattle; hypersensitivity to doramectin or other macrocyclic lactones.

Precautions—Do not use doramectin in dairy cow of 20 months or older.

Drug Interactions—No known adverse interaction.

Pharmaceutical Formulations—Available in sesame oil/ethyl oleate (90:10 v/v). Each ml of vehicle contains 10 mg of doramectin.

DOXAPRAM

Proprietary Names—Dopram-V®.

Chemical Class—Pyrrolidine derivative.

Pharmacological Class—Analeptic; Respiratory stimulant.

Source—Synthetic.

Stability And Storage—Doxapram solution is better stored at room temperature. Avoid mixing the solution with alkaline solutions. It is compatible with normal saline.

Pharmacological Actions—Doxapram stimulates respiration. It acts on the medulla and directly on the chemoreceptors of the carotid and aortic regions leading to increase in tidal volume and respiratory frequency. Doxapram has been observed to aid recovery from anesthesia. It is reputed to be the most effective antagonist of thiopental-acepromazine anesthesia in dogs.

Doxapram

Mechanism of Action—It is a general CNS stimulant. Its exact mechanisms are unknown.

Indications—Doxapram is effective in reversing drug-induced central respiratory depression during anesthesia or post anesthetic recovery in man and animals. It is also used to initiate or stimulate respiration in neonates following caesarian section or dystocia, reverse the effects of xylazine and facilitate endoscopic examination of laryngeal motion in the horse.

Dosages—

Bird	5-10 mg/kg once.
Dog, Cat	1-5 mg/kg IV in adults; 1-2 drops under the tongue or 0.1 ml in umbilical vein for neonates.
Goat	2-10 mg/kg.
Guinea pig	5 mg/kg.
Mouse	5-10 mg/kg.
NHP	2 mg/kg.
Rat	5-10 mg/kg.
Rabbit	2-5 mg/kg.
Sheep	2-10 mg/kg
Pig	2-10 mg/kg
Horse	0.5-1 mg/kg every 5 minutes in adults; 0.02-0.05 mg/kg/min in foals; 100-160 mg for endoscopic examination.
Cattle	5-10 mg/kg.

Doses can be repeated in 15-20 minutes after initial administration. Repeat doses can be increased or decreased depending on the response obtained—

Route(s) of Administration—Intravenous, subcutaneous (in rabbits and rodents) and intramuscular (in birds) are used for therapeutic purposes.

Absorption—Doxapram is readily absorbed from the oral route but is not administered by this route for therapeutic purposes.

Bioavailability. About 60%.

Onset of Action—Within 20-40 seconds (following intravenous injection).

Peak Effect: 1-2 minutes.

Duration of Action—Doxapram acts for 5-12 minutes.

Distribution—Vd, about 3 L/kg. It distributes well into tissues.

Metabolism—Metabolized in the liver.

Plasma Half-Life: 3.4 hours (adult human); ~ 7-10 hours (human neonates).

Clearance—Plasma clearance is about 5 mL/min/kg.

Route(s) of Excretion. Urine.

Dialysis Status—Not dialyzable.

Toxicity and Adverse Effects—Doxapram has narrow therapeutic index especially in humans. Therapeutic doses may produce hypertension, cardiac arrhythmia and hyperventilation. High or repeated doses may cause generalized CNS hyper-stimulation, seizure, muscular hyperactivity and tachycardia. It also causes hyperventilation resulting in respiratory alkalosis.

Management of Overdose/Toxicology—Give supportive therapy. A short-acting barbiturate may be needed to reduce CNS hyperactivity. Consider oxygen therapy.

Contraindications. Cardiorespiratory impairment; seizure; cerebral edema; head injury; pheochrocytoma; hypersensitivity to doxapram—

Precautions. Use cautiously in pregnancy. Allow at least 10 minutes between discontinuation of halothane, cyclopropane and enflurane anesthesia and administration of doxapram.

Drug Interactions—Sympathomimetic agents may enhance the hypertensive effect of doxapram. Doxapram enhances the release of epinephrine, a catecholamine. Inhalational anesthetic agents like cyclopropane, halothane and enflurane sensitize the myocardium to the actions of catecholamines. Doxapram may reduce the effects of muscle relaxants.

Pharmaceutical Formulations—Available as doxapram hydrochloride in 20 mg/ml solution for injection.

DOXORUBICIN

Synonyms—ADR; Hydroxydaunomycin.

Proprietary Names—Adriamycin®; Rubex®; Doxil®, Doxorubicin HCL®.

Chemical Class—Anthracycline.

Pharmacological Class—Antineoplastic antibiotic; Antineoplastic drug; Anticancer drug; Cytotoxic drug; Anticancer antibiotic.

Source—Natural; obtained from *Streptomyces peucetius* var, *caesius.*

Solubility, Stability and Storage—Doxorubicin is soluble in water and methanol but insoluble in organic solvents. It is unstable in pH <3 and >7. The drug is photolabile; thus, its dosage forms must be protected from light. Lyophilized powder may be stored at room temperature while solutions are better stored in the refrigerator. Reconstituted powder should be used within 24 hours if kept at room temperature or 48 hours if refrigerated. Doxorubicin is compatible with dextrose saline, normal saline and lactated Ringer's solution. Do not mix doxorubicin with hydrocortisone, dexamethasone, fluorouracil, aminophylline, furosemide, cephalothin or heparin.

Doxorubicin

Pharmacological Actions—Doxorubicin has activity against a wide variety of tumors. It is cell-cycle nonspecific although it is most active in the S phase. It inhibits DNA and RNA synthesis and chelates iron. It has antimicrobial action that is not utilized therapeutically. It possesses some immunosuppressant properties. Doxorubicin has teratogenic and embryotoxic effect in laboratory animals.

Mechanism of Action—Doxorubicin intercalates with DNA to inhibit DNA-dependent RNA synthesis. It also causes breaks in DNA strands by activating topoisomerase II as well as generating free radicals. It has mutagenic potential resulting from sister chromatid exchange.

Indications—Doxorubicin is a useful adjunct in the treatment of wide variety of carcinomas and sarcomas in dogs and cats.

Dosages—30 mg/m^2 every 3 weeks up to a cumulative maximum of 240 mg/m^2.

Route(s) of Administration—Intravenous, slowly through indwelling catheter. Dilute computed dose with 50 ml 5% dextrose or normal saline.

Absorption—Doxorubicin is not absorbed from the gastrointestinal tract.

Bioavailability—Oral bioavailability is 5%.

Distribution—Vd = 17 ± 11 L/kg. Doxorubicin is cleared rapidly from plasma to the heart, lungs, kidney, liver and spleen. It does not cross the blood-brain-barrier but is distributed into milk.

Plasma Protein Binding—76%.

Metabolism—Doxorubicin is converted to doxorubicinol (an active metabolite), aglycones and other metabolites.

Plasma Half-life—Multiphasic; first phase = 0.6 hours; second phase = 3.3 hours; third phase = 17 hours. Half-life of metabolites = 32 hours.

Clearance (ml/min/kg)—17 ± 8. Rapidly cleared from blood.

Route(s) of Excretion—Primarily in bile and feces; <7% excreted in urine.

Toxicity and Adverse Effects—Bone marrow depression, cardiomyopathy, alopecia, gastroenteritis and stomatitis are prominent adverse effects. Tissue irritation following extravasation may lead to cellulitis, necrosis and sloughing. Hypersensitivity reaction following rapid injection may be observed. This is due to histamine release. Doxorubicin tints urine orange to red.

Management of Overdose—Give symptomatic and supportive therapy. Apply cold pack to site of tissue extravasation in addition to flooding the site with normal saline, sodium bicarbonate solution and topical application of dimethylsulfoxide or corticosteroid.

Contraindications—Hypersensitivity to doxorubicin; severe congestive heart failure; other cardiac impairment; pre-existing myelosuppression.

Precautions—Doxorubicin has vesicant properties hence subcutaneous extravasation must be avoided. Handle doxorubicin formulations with care. It is recommended that gloves and protective clothing be worn. Wash exposed body parts copiously with soap and water. Reduce the dose in patients with renal impairment. Pretreatment with antihistamine or corticosteroid may be required to prevent hypersensitivity reaction.

Drug Interactions—Cyclophosphamide causes additive cardiotoxic effect with doxorubicin. Mercaptopurine, streptozocin and verapamil increase the toxicity of doxorubicin. Allopurinol may enhance its antitumor activity. Doxorubicin decreases the plasma levels and excretion of digoxin.

Pharmaceutical Formulations—Available as doxorubicin hydrochloride in 10 mg, 20 mg, 50 mg, 100 mg and 150 mg lyophilized powder. Also available in normal saline or preservative free solution for injection containing 2 mg/ml.

DOXYCYCLINE

Doxycycline

Proprietary Names—Vibramycin˚; Vibra—tabs˚, Doxychel˚, Doryx˚; Doxy˚; Vibravet˚; Doxylag˚; Radox˚; Zadorin˚; Duocycline LA®; Doxysol®; Colidox® (doxycycline hydrochloride in combination with colistin sulfate).

Chemical Class—Polycyclic naphthacenecarboxamide derivative; tetracycline.

Pharmacological Class—Broad spectrum bacteriostatic antibiotic.

Source—Semisynthetic; derived from oxytetracycline or methacycline.

Solubility, Stability and Storage—Doxycycline is soluble in water and slightly soluble in alcohol. Doxycycline hydrochloride capsules and film-coated tablets should be stored in tight, light-resistant containers at room temperature.

Pharmacological Actions—Doxycycline has prolonged action and is twice as active as tetracycline against a wide spectrum of organisms including Gram-positive and Gram-negative bacteria. Rickettsia, Chlamydia, Mycoplasma and some protozoa like Plasmodium are susceptible. Certain spirochaetes such as *Treponema* and *Leptospira* species are also susceptible.

Mechanism of Action—Doxycycline inhibits protein synthesis by binding principally to the 30s subunit of bacterial ribosome to prevent access of aminoacyl tRNA to the acceptor site of the mRNA-ribosome complex thereby preventing the addition of amino acids to the growing peptide chain.

Indications—Doxycycline is used to treat infections caused by susceptible organisms such as rickettsia, chlamydia, mycoplasma and bacteria. It is effective in the treatment and prevention of chronic respiratory disease, other respiratory diseases and diseases caused by *E. coli. Ehrlichia canis* infection in dogs, psittacosis in birds and mycoplasma infection in tortoise respond to doxycycline treatment.

Dosages—

Bird	18-26 mg/kg PO twice a day in psittacines
	or 25-50 mg/kg IV once to get peak dose in critical cases.
Dog, cat	5-10 mg/kg PO or IV every 12 hours.
NHP	5 mg/kg PO in two divided doses on day 1; 2.5 mg/kg the following days.
Rabbit	2.5 mg/kg PO twice a day.
Reptile	5-10 mg/kg PO once a day for 10-45 days.

Route(s) of Administration—Oral, intramuscular and intravenous routes are appropriate.

Absorption—About 95% of administered dose is absorbed from the GIT. Peak plasma concentration is attained within 2 hours. Absorption is not significantly impaired by food.

Bioavailability—93%

Distribution—Vd = 1.5 L /kg in dogs. Doxycycline is more lipid soluble and penetrates body tissues and fluids better than tetracycline and oxytetracycline. It undergoes enterohepatic circulation. Doxycycline is distributed into milk.

Plasma Protein Binding—88 ± 5% in humans (lower in uremia); 75-86% in dogs; 93% in cattle and pigs.

Metabolism—Doxycycline appears not to be significantly metabolized—

Plasma Half-Life—16 ± 6 hours (human), 10-12 hours (dog); 4.5 hours (cats); 4.04 hours (pigs); 9.5 hours (calves); 16.7 hours (goats).

Clearance (ml/min/kg)—0.5±0.18 in humans (lower in hyperlipoproteinemia and the aged); 1.7 in dogs, pigs; 1.2 in calves; 6.91 in goats.

Withholding Period—24 hours (chicken).

Route(s) of Excretion—Urine (25% as unchanged drug in dogs); feces (75% as inactive conjugate or chelate in dogs); and bile (5% in dogs). Doxycycline can be used in patients with renal insufficiency.

Dialysis Status—Not dialyzable.

Toxicity and Adverse Effects—Doxycycline causes cutaneous rash and phototoxicity. Discoloration of teeth in growing subjects, pigmentation of the nails, nausea, diarrhea, neutropenia, eosinophilia, phlebitis, hepatotoxicity, and eosophagitis are other notable adverse effects. It causes cardiac arrhythmias, collapse and death in horses following IV injection of even low doses.

Management of Overdose/Toxicity—Give symptomatic and supportive therapy—

Contraindications—Hypersensitivity to tetracyclines; pregnancy; growing animals; parenteral administration in horses.

Precautions—The use of tetracyclines during tooth development or in latter half of pregnancy may cause discoloration of teeth of the offspring. Prolonged administration may produce superinfection. Do not use in commercial layer from point of lay. Withdraw medication from birds 24 hours prior to slaughter. Administer doxycycline with food in dogs and cats to avoid emesis.

Drug Interactions—The half-life of doxycycline may be shortened to seven hours in animals on long-term treatment with barbiturates, phenytoin or carbamazepine. Doxycycline increases the effect of warfarin. Absorption of doxycycline is impaired by concurrent administration of dairy products and aluminum hydroxide gel. Bismuth subsalicylate and salts of Ca, Mg and Fe also hinder oral absorption of doxycycline. It may increase the bioavailability of digoxin.

Pharmaceutical Formulations—The drug is available as doxycycline hyclate (hydrochloride hemiethanolate hemihydrate) in 50 mg and 100 mg capsules; 100 mg and 200 mg powder for injection; 5% powder for administration in drinking water for animals; 50 mg and 100 mg tablets. It is also available as doxycycline monohydrate in 25 mg/5 ml powder for oral suspension and as doxycycline calcium in 50 mg/5 ml syrup.

DROPERIDOL

Proprietary Names—Inapsine˙; Paxical˙. It is an ingredient of Innovar vet˙ and Thalamonal˙.

Chemical Class—Butyrophenone derivative.

Pharmacological Class—Antipsychotic; Tranquillizer; Neuroleptic agent.

Source—Synthetic.

Solubility, Stability and Storage—The level of solubility of droperidol is 0.1 mg/mL in water and 7.14 mg/mL in alcohol at 25°C. Droperidol injection should be protected from light and stored at room temperature. It is physically and/or chemically incompatible with parenteral barbiturates.

Pharmacological Actions—Droperidol has sedative and potent antiemetic actions. In animals, droperidol produces catalepsy and reverses the behavioral effects caused by amphetamine and apomorphine. It also causes reduction in the sensitivity to epinephrine and norepinephrine. Droperidol attenuates the cardiovascular response to sympathomimetic amines and produces direct peripheral vasodilation, which alone or in conjunction with its α-adrenergic blocking activity may cause hypotension and decreased peripheral vascular resistance.

Droperidol

Mechanism of Action—Droperidol blocks the action of dopamine by binding to dopamine receptors in the CNS. It also produces peripheral α_1-adrenergic receptor blockade.

Indications—Droperidol is used primarily in combination with fentanyl to produce a calm state of neuroleptanalgesia (characterized by enhanced CNS depression, reduced tendency to voluntary motion, and reduced pain) to facilitate minor surgical, dental, and orthopaedic procedures. The combination is also used to immobilize game animals. Droperidol is used singly as a tranquilizer and anesthetic premedicant.

Dosages—

Fentanyl/droperidol (Innovar-Vet')

Dog	1 ml/7-10 kg IM; 1 ml/12-30 kg IV.
Guinea pig	0.22 ml/kg IM.
Mouse	0.5 ml/kg IM.
NHP	0.3 ml/kg IM.
Rat	0.5 ml/kg IM.
Rabbit	0.17 ml/kg IM.
Pig	0.07 ml/kg IM.

A preanesthetic dose of atropine or glycopyrrolate may be necessary to prevent bradycardia and excess salivation.

Route(s) of Administration—Intramuscular and intravenous.

Absorption—Droperidol is absorbed after oral administration but the oral route is not used clinically.

Onset of Action—Droperidol action may become evident in 3-10 minutes.

Peak Action—30 minutes.

Duration of Action—Sedative and tranquilizing effects last 2-4 hours following IM or IV administration of a single dose. Alteration of consciousness may persist for up to 12 hours.

Distribution—Droperidol is reported to cross the blood-brain barrier and distributes into the CSF. It is also reported to cross the placenta.

Plasma Protein Binding—85 to 90%.

Metabolism—The butyrophenone moiety is metabolized to p-fluorophenylacetic acid, which is then conjugated with glycine. The nitrogenous moiety appears to be metabolized to benzimidazolone and p-hydroxypiperidine. Metabolism takes place in the liver.

Plasma Half-life—2 to 3 hours.

Route(s) of Excretion—About 75% of a dose is excreted in urine with less than 10% as unchanged drug; about 22% of a dose is eliminated in faeces.

Toxicity and Adverse Effects—Transient, mild to moderate hypotension and occasionally tachycardia, defaecation, and flatulence are common adverse effects. Transient personality changes characterized by aggression, dysphoria, restlessness, or hyperactivity have been observed. Persistent head-bobbing is a frequent nervous effect. Overdosage of droperidol produces effects that are extensions of its pharmacologic actions and may include QT prolongation and severe cardiac arrhythmias.

Management of Overdose/Toxicity—Give symptomatic and supportive therapy.

Contraindications—Hypersensitivity to droperidol.

Precautions—Droperidol should be used with caution in patients with impaired hepatic and renal function. Reduce the doses of droperidol and other CNS depressants if both drugs must be used concomitantly. Droperidol should be used with extreme caution in patients with congestive heart failure, bradycardia, cardiac hypertrophy, hypokalemia, hypomagnesaemia, or on diuretic therapy.

Drug Interactions—Droperidol may produce additive effect or potentiate, the action of other CNS depressants such as opioid analgesics, barbiturates or other sedatives, and anesthetics.

Pharmaceutical Formulations—Droperidol is available alone and in combination with fentanyl citrate in parenteral solution.

EDROPHONIUM

Proprietary Names—Tensilon⁺; Enlon⁺; Reversol⁺.

Chemical Class—Quaternary ammonium compound.

Pharmacological Class—Reversible cholinesterase inhibitor; Indirect-acting cholinomimetic drug; Anticholinesterase.

Source—Synthetic.

Solubility, Stability and Storage—Edrophonium is soluble 1 in 0.5 of water and 1 in 5 of ethanol. Store products at room temperature.

Pharmacological Actions—Edrophonium initiates and increases GI motility. It also stimulates other smooth muscles such as those of respiration and bladder. At low doses, edrophonium and other anticholinesterase agents augment the nervous stimulation of secretory glands including bronchial, lacrimal, sweat, salivary, gastric, and intestinal glands. Higher doses produce increased secretion of these glands. Edrophonium may cause twitching of skeletal muscle at high doses as a result of direct nicotinic receptor activation. It causes persistent depolarization of the motor end plate if acetylcholinesterase is sufficiently inhibited resulting in neuromuscular blockade. The CNS is stimulated at low doses but depressed at high doses of edrophonium and other anticholinesterases. Anticholinesterase agents cause miosis, blockade of accommodation reflex and conjunctiva hyperemia if applied directly to the conjunctiva. They also reduce intraocular pressure.

Edrophonium

Mechanism of Action—Edrophonium competes with acetylcholine for acetylcholinesterase enzyme. It is less rapidly hydrolyzed than acetylcholine. This allows acetylcholine to accumulate leading to prolongation and exaggeration of its effect.

Indications—Edrophonium is used in the diagnosis of myasthenia gravis, reversal of curare (and other non-depolarizing neuromuscular blockers) muscle paralysis and treatment of curare overdose. Edrophonium is most suitable for the diagnosis of myasthenia gravis because of it short duration of action. It is used in humans to differentiate between myasthenia and cholinergic crises.

Dosages—Cats and dogs. 0.5 mg/kg IV: 0.1-0.2 mg/kg IV for diagnosis of myasthenia gravis.

Route(s) of Administration—Intramuscular and intravenous routes are preferred.

Absorption—Poorly and incompletely absorbed from the GIT.

Onset of Action—Within 1 minute (IV); 2-5 minutes (IM).

Duration of Action—10 minutes (IV); 5-30 minutes (IM).

Distribution—Vd = 1.1 ± 0.2 (human). Edrophonium crosses plasma membranes poorly because of its quaternary ammonium constituent.

Plasma Protein Binding—15-25%.

Metabolism—Hydrolyzed by cholinesterase to weakly active metabolite.

Plasma Half-life—1.8 ± 0.6 hours in human; prolonged in patients with renal impairment.

Clearance (ml/min/kg)—9.2 ± 3.2 in humans.

Route(s) of Excretion—Edrophonium is excreted mainly via urine with > 50% of dose as unchanged drug.

Dialysis Status—Nondialyzable.

Toxicity and Adverse Effects—Nausea, vomiting, miosis, and dyspnea are most common adverse effects caused by edrophonium at therapeutic doses. Overdose produce signs characteristic of excessive cholinergic stimulation. Signs include excessive salivation, sweating, miosis, lacrimation, bronchial secretion, bronchospasm, hypotension, and muscle weakness.

Management of Overdose/Toxicity—Atropine is an antidote.

Contraindications—Hypersensitivity to edrophonium; intestinal or urinary tract obstruction; late pregnancy; asthma; concurrent treatment with other anticholinesterase.

Precautions—Edrophonium should be used by an experienced professional in a controlled setting. Use cautiously in patients with cardiac irregularities. Administer edrophonium with atropine when used to reverse curare muscle relaxation.

Drug Interactions—Edrophonium reverses the actions of competitive neuromuscular blockers and augments those of depolarizing neuromuscular blockers. Atropine obliterates the muscarinic effects of edrophonium because edrophonium effects are attributed to the unhydrolyzed acetylcholine. Edrophonium may produce pronounced bradycardia in patients receiving digoxin. The effect of edrophonium may be reduced by drugs that have neuromuscular blocking actions (e.g. aminoglycoside antibiotics and anesthetics).

Pharmaceutical Formulations—The drug is available as edrophonium chloride in 10 mg/ml parenteral solution. Formulation containing 0.14 mg/ml of atropine is also available.

ENROFLOXACIN

Enrofloxacin

Proprietary Name—Baytril®; Enprotil˚; Conflox˚.

Chemical Class—Fluorinated 4-quinolone (Fluoroquinolone).

Pharmacological Class—Antimicrobial agent.

Source—Synthetic.

Stability and Storage—Store in tight containers at less than 30°C.

Pharmacological Actions—Enrofloxacin is rapidly bactericidal to several bacteria including *E. coli*, various species of *Salmonella, Shigella, Enterobacter, Campylobacter, Neisseria, Chlamydia, Mycoplasma, Legionella, Brucella, Staphylococci, Klebsiella, Pseudomonas aeruginosa, Haemophilus, Proteus, Yesinia, Serratia, Vibrio, Salmonella,* and *Aeromonas*. It is weakly active against anaerobic organisms.

Mechanism of Action—Enrofloxacin inhibits gyrase-mediated DNA negative super coiling leading to inability of the bacteria to maintain DNA super helical structure and effect DNA repair.

Indications—Enrofloxacin is used to treat infections caused by susceptible aerobic organisms in dogs, cats, chickens, turkeys, beef cattle and exotic species.

Dosages—

Dog, cat	5-20 mg/kg orally every 12 hours for 10-30 days.
Cattle	2.5-5 mg/kg SC once daily for 3-5 days or 7.5-12.5 mg/kg once.
Bird	20-40 mg/kg orally or 250 mg/L of drinking water.
Exotic species	5-15 mg/kg orally every 12 hours.

Route(s) of Administration—Oral, intramuscular, intravenous and subcutaneous routes are appropriate.

Absorption—Enrofloxacin is well absorbed from the GIT. Peak plasma concentration is attained within one hour. The rate, but not extent of absorption is delayed by the presence of food in the stomach.

Bioavailability—Oral bioavailability is 80% in dog—

Distribution—Vd = 2.8 L/kg in dog. Enrofloxacin is widely distributed in tissues and body fluids. The highest concentrations are attained in kidney, liver, lungs, spleen, bile and prostate glands. It attains lower but therapeutic concentrations in poorly perfused tissues like bone, skin and muscle but concentrations in the CSF are low. Enrofloxacin tends to accumulate in serum following multiple administrations.

Plasma Protein Binding—27% in dog.

Metabolism—30-40% is metabolized to ciprofloxacin. It is also converted to other less active products.

Plasma Half-Life—4 to 5 hours (dogs); 6 hours (cats); 1.7 hours (subcutaneous) to 7.7 hours (per os) in rabbits.

Withholding Period—28 days in cattle meant for slaughter.

Route(s) of Excretion—Enrofloxacin is eliminated in urine (15-50% of dose as unchanged drug) and feces.

Dialysis Status—Non dialyzable.

Toxicity and Adverse Effects—Enrofloxacin is highly tolerated. Gastrointestinal effects (vomiting and anorexia) are most common adverse effects. It causes bubble-like abnormalities in articular cartilage at high doses especially in growing animals. Overdose may not cause serious effects beyond vomition. It causes severe CNS effects in humans.

Management of Toxicity/Overdose—Give supportive therapy.

Contraindications—Small and medium breeds of dogs less than 8 months; large breeds of dogs less than 12 months; giant breeds of dogs less than 18 months; pregnancy; dairy cattle; hypersensitivity to enrofloxacin or any other quinolone.

Precautions—Avoid dehydration during therapy to prevent crystalluria. Adjust the dose in patients with hepatic or renal impairment. Administer the drug 2 hours before or after the administration of sucralfate or antacids containing magnesium, calcium and aluminium. Do not administer concurrently with nitrofurantoin.

Drug Interactions—Enrofloxacin inhibits the metabolism of theophylline, caffeine, cyclosporine, and warfarin. Azlocillin, cimetidine, and probenecid increase quinolone blood levels. The absorption of enrofloxacin is reduced if co-administered with sucralfate and antacids containing magnesium, calcium and aluminum. Probenecid blocks tubular secretion of enrofloxacin and increases its half-life. Nitrofurantoin may antagonize its antimicrobial activity but synergism may occur when enrofloxacin is used with aminoglycoside antibiotics, 3rd generation cephalosporins and extended spectrum penicillins against some bacteria such as *Pseudomonas*. Flouroquinolones may enhance the nephrotoxic effect of cyclosporine.

Pharmaceutical Formulations—Enrofloxacin is available as 10% soluble liquid; 22.7 mg, 68 mg, and 500 mg oral tablets; 22.7 mg/ml parenteral solution for injection.

EPHEDRINE

Ephedrine

Proprietary Names—Ectasule®; Efedron®; Ephedson®; Vicks Vatrronol®.

Chemical Class—Alkaloid.

Pharmacological Class—Sympathomimetic drug.

Source—Originally isolated from *Ma huang* (ephedra), a Chinese shrub. Now obtained by synthesis.

Solubility, Stability and Storage—Ephedrine sulfate is soluble 1 in 1.3 of water and 1 in 90 of ethanol.

Pharmacological Actions—Ephedrine stimulates heart rate and cardiac output; increases peripheral resistance and blood pressure. It causes bronchodilation; stimulates the CNS; activates the respiratory center; causes mydriasis following local or systemic administration; and causes resistance to urine flow due to stimulation of smooth muscle cells at the base of the bladder. Frequent dosing or prolonged administration results in tachyphylaxis.

Mechanism of Action—Ephedrine activates adrenergic receptors directly and also enhances release of endogenous norepinephrine.

174

Indications—Ephedrine is used to treat urethral sphincter hypotonus in dogs and cats, decongest mucous membrane and maintain of blood pressure following initial administration of epinephrine.

Route(s) of Administration—Ephedrine may be administered per os, intramuscularly or intravenously.

Absorption—The drug is rapidly absorbed from the GIT.

Onset of Action—0.25 to1 hour.

Duration of Action—3 to 6 hours.

Distribution—Ephedrine is widely distributed. It crosses the placenta and is distributed into milk.

Metabolism—Small portion of administered dose is metabolized in the liver.

Plasma Half-Life—3 to 6 hours.

Route(s) of Excretion—Ephedrine is eliminated via urine with 60-77% of dose as unchanged drug.

Toxicity and Adverse Effects—Ephedrine causes anorexia in some animals. It may also cause restlessness, hypertension, and insomnia at therapeutic doses. Overdose may cause excitement, anxiety and muscular tremor.

Management of Overdose/Toxicity—Give symptomatic and supportive therapy.

Contraindications—Cardiovascular diseases; hypersensitivity to ephedrine or its components.

Precautions—Use ephedrine cautiously in cases with glaucoma, prostatic hypertrophy, hyperthyroidism, and diabetes mellitus. Do not administer ephedrine with other sympathomimetic drugs or within two weeks of giving MAO inhibitors.

Drug Interactions—Adrenergic receptor blockers will reduce ephedrine's vasopressor effect. Sympathomimetic drugs and MAO inhibitors (which prevents metabolism of sympathomimetic drugs) will enhance the effect of ephedrine. Concurrent administration with NSAIDs, reserpine, tricyclic antidepressants or ganglion blocking drugs may enhance the potential for hypertension. Concurrent administration with theophylline, cardiac glycosides and general anesthetics will cause increased cardiac stimulation.

Pharmaceutical Formulations—The drug is available as ephedrine sulfate in 25 mg and 50 mg oral capsules; 25 mg/ml and 50 mg/ml parenteral solution. It is sometimes incorporated in cough suppressant preparations. No specific formulation is available for veterinary use.

ERGOMETRINE

Ergometrine

Synonyms—Ergonovine; Ergobasine.

Proprietary Names—Ergotrate˚. It is an ingredient of syntometrine˚.

Chemical Class—Amine ergot alkaloid; Lysergic acid derivative.

Pharmacological Class—Ecbolic.

Source—Natural; found in *Claviceps purpurea*.

Solubility, Stability and Storage—Ergometrine is sparingly soluble in water and slightly soluble in alcohol. Ergonovine maleate darkens with age and on exposure to light. Injections of ergonovine maleate should be stored at temperatures below 8°C and protected from light. Solutions may be stored at 15-30°C for 60-90 days. Discolored solutions should not be used. Ergometrine may be incompatible with solutions containing adrenaline hydrochloride, amylobarbitone sodium, ampicillin sodium, cephalothin sodium, chloramphenicol sodium succinate, heparin sodium, chlortetracycline hydrochloride, metaraminol tartrate, methicillin sodium, nitrofurantoin sodium, pentobarbitone sodium, sulphadiazine sodium, thiopentone sodium, vitamin B complex with C, and warfarin sodium.

Pharmacological Actions—Ergometrine causes prolonged contraction of smooth muscles, including the myometrium and blood vessels. Therapeutic doses of ergonovine causes intense contractions of the uterus usually followed by periods of relaxation. Larger doses of the drug produce sustained, forceful contractions followed by only short or no periods of relaxation. Increases in the amplitude and frequency of uterine contractions and uterine tone in turn impede uterine blood flow. Contraction of the uterine wall around bleeding vessels at the placental site produces hemostasis. Ergometrine also increases contractions of the cervix. It produces vasoconstriction, mainly of capacitance vessels causing increased central venous pressure, elevated blood pressure, and rarely, peripheral ischemia and gangrene.

Mechanism of Action—Ergometrine acts mainly by stimulating alpha-adrenergic and serotonin receptors and inhibiting the release of endothelial-derived relaxation factor.

Indications—Ergometrine is used to control postpartum hemorrhage, remove fluid from atonic uteri, prevent prolapsed uteri, induce uterine involution and expel retained placenta particularly in cows and bitches.

Dosages—

Cow, mare	2 to 5 mg/animal IM or IV
Ewe, doe, sow	0.5-1 mg/animal IM
Bitch	0.2-1 mg IM
Queen	0.125 mg IM

Route(s) of Administration—Per os, intramuscular and intravenous (recommended only for emergencies; in which case dilute solution should be injected slowly).

Absorption—Ergometrine is rapidly absorbed after oral or IM administration. Peak plasma concentrations are attained within 60 to 90 minutes following oral administration.

Bioavailability—Average = 80.7%. There is a wide individual variation.

Onset of Action—Uterine contractions are usually initiated within 5–15 minutes following oral administration; 2-5 minutes after IM injection, and immediately following IV injection.

Duration of Action—Uterine contractions persist for 3 hours or longer after oral or IM administration and for 45 minutes after IV injection.

Distribution—Not certain; the drug appears to be rapidly distributed into tissues.

Metabolism—Ergometrine is metabolized in the liver by hydroxylation and glucuronic acid conjugation and possibly *N*-demethylation.

Route(s) of Excretion. Ergometrine is mainly excreted in bile as 12-hydroxyergometrine glucuronide.

Toxicity and Adverse Effects—CNS excitation, vomiting, hypertension; muscle weakness, coronary and other vascular spasms are common. Ergometrine may cause agalactia through inhibition of prolactin release. Overdose may cause convulsion and gangrene.

Management of Overdose/Toxicity—If the drug was given orally, the stomach should be evacuated immediately by inducing emesis or by gastric lavage, followed by administration of activated charcoal and catharsis. Supportive and symptomatic treatment should be initiated.

Contraindications. Induction or augmentation of labour; concurrent use of sympathomimetics; severe or persistent sepsis; retained placenta; peripheral vascular disease or heart disease; impaired hepatic or renal function; hypersensitivity to ergometrine.

Precautions—Use ergometrine with caution in patients with sepsis or with hepatic or renal impairment. Prolonged use of the drug should be avoided. Dilute the formulation and administer slowly if the choice of route is IV.

Drug Interactions—Ergot alkaloids interact with beta-adrenergic blockers resulting in excessive, additive peripheral vasoconstriction. The drugs also interact with dopamine resulting in excessive peripheral vasoconstriction. Concurrent use of general anesthetics and ergometrine may potentiate peripheral vasoconstriction. Halothane in concentrations greater than 1% may interfere with the oxytocic actions of ergometrine, resulting in severe uterine hemorrhage. The pressor effect of sympathomimetic pressor amines may be potentiated by ergometrine.

Pharmaceutical Formulations—It is available as ergometrine maleate in 0.2 mg tablets and 0.2 mg/ml parenteral solution. Ergometrine Injection consists of ergometrine maleate BP 500 mcg/ml and maleic acid BP in water for injections.

ERYTHROMYCIN

Proprietary Names—Erythromycin (E-mycin*, Ilotycin*). Erythromycin stearate (Emu-V*, Eritrolag*, Erolin*, Erylan*, Erythrocin*). Erythromycin estolate (Ilosone*). Erythromycin ethylsuccinate (E.E.S*, Pediamycin*, Erythroped*). Erythromycin glucceptate (Ilotycin glucceptate®). Erythromycin esters are also components of Keproceryl*, Neoceryl*, Coryl SP*, Doseryl*, Mirth-O-Ceryl*, Ladseryl*; Aseryl*.

Chemical Class—Macrolide.

Pharmacological Class—Macrolide antibiotic; Narrow spectrum antibiotic.

Sources—Natural; (elaborated by a strain of *Streptomyces erythreus*).

Erythromycin

Solubility, Stability and Storage—Erythromycin base is slightly soluble in water but soluble in organic solvents. Store erythromycin capsules, tablets, and powder at room temperature protected from light. Erythromycin oral suspension should be refrigerated. Reconstituted oral suspension is stable for 14 days at room temperature. Reconstituted powder for injection is stable for 24 hours at room temperature and 7-14 days when refrigerated depending on the ester form.

Pharmacological Actions—Erythromycin has either bacteriostatic or bactericidal action against most Gram-positive organisms. Bactericidal action predominates against small number of rapidly dividing organisms over a pH range of 5.5-8.5. Some Gram-negative organisms such as *Neisseria gonorrhoeae* are inhibited. It has activity against mycoplasmas.

Mechanism of Action—Erythromycin inhibits protein synthesis by binding reversibly to the 23s rRNA on the 50s ribosomal subunit causing blockade of the translocation steps involving newly synthesized peptide tRNA. It is accumulated about 100 times more in Gram-positive than in Gram-negative bacteria.

Indications—Erythromycin is effective in the treatment of chronic respiratory disease, mastitis caused by penicillin-resistant staphylococcus and other infections (e.g. sinusitis, synovitis) caused by susceptible organisms. It is also used to treat streptococci infections (as alternative to penicillins) and control PPLO in poultry.

Dosages—4.5-11 mg/kg 3 or 4 times daily orally; 2-4.5 mg/kg IM or IV followed by oral medication; 92.5 g/ton of feed or 0.5 g/3.8 liters of drinking water.

Route(s) of Administration—Oral, intravenous and intramammary routes are preferred.

Absorption—Adequately but incompletely (18-45%) absorbed from the upper small intestine. Food delays absorption. Peak plasma concentration is attained within 4 hours for the base and 0.5-2.5 hours for the ethylsuccinate ester.

Bioavailability—35 ± 25% in human (lower in pregnancy).

Distribution—Vd = 0.78 ± 0.44 L/kg. Erythromycin attains high concentration in the liver, kidneys, lungs and submaxillary gland. Erythromycin penetrates the ICF, pleural, peritoneal, and prostatic fluids. It crosses the placenta, appears in milk and attains trace amounts in the CSF.

Plasma Protein Binding—84 ± 3%.

Metabolism—Erythromycin is partly demethylated in the liver.

Plasma Half-Life—1.6 ± 0.7 hours in humans (higher in cirrhosis and anuria). Half-life of 8-9 hours has been reported in animals after IM injection.

Clearance—9.1 ± 4.1(ml/min/kg).

Residue Limit—Tolerance level in eggs is 0.025ppm.

Withdrawal Period—Slaughter: 14 days (cattle); 3 days (sheep and goat); 7 days (pig); 1-2 days (chicken). Milk: 72 hours.

Route(s) of Excretion—Erythromycin is eliminated via urine, bile and feces with $12 \pm 7\%$ of the dose excreted as active drug in urine.

Dialysis Status—Nondialyzable.

Toxicity and Adverse Effects—Anorexia, nausea, vomiting and diarrhea may accompany oral administration especially of large doses. Intravenous administration may occasionally cause these symptoms. The most striking adverse effects especially of the estolate ester are cholestatic hepatitis characterized by fever, jaundice, and impaired liver function. It also causes allergic reactions observed as fever, eosinophilia, and rashes. It causes pain and irritation with intramuscular injection and thrombophlebitis with intravenous injection.

Management of Overdose/Toxicity—Give supportive and symptomatic therapy.

Contraindications—Hypersensitivity to erythromycin or its components; impaired hepatic function.

Precautions—Discontinue use of Erythromycin if it causes hepatic impairment. Avoid IM injection. Do not use the lactobionate form in new born animals. Do not use topically. Do not use in egg-laying birds.

Drug Interactions—Erythromycin potentiates the effects of carbamazepine, corticosteroids, cyclosporine, digoxin and warfarin by inhibiting their metabolic enzymes. Concomitant administration with theophylline decreases the clearance of theophylline.

Pharmaceutical Formulations—Available as stearate, estolate, and ethylsuccinate esters in a wide variety of preparations for oral use. Erythromycin is also available as the lactobionate and gluceptate forms in sterile powders for reconstitution into parenteral solution; as the thiocyanate form for administration in drinking water for poultry and as the base in various preparations. Intramammary formulations for use in lactating cows are also available.

ESTRADIOL

Proprietary Names—Primogyn*; progynoval*; Estrace* (micronised estradiol); Delestrogen*; Estraderm* (for trans cutaneous patches).

Chemical Class—Steroid.

Pharmacological Class—Estrogen.

Sources—Naturally occurring; may be obtained from natural sources or prepared synthetically.

Solubility, Stability and Storage—Estradiol is practically insoluble in water. Solubility in alcohol is approximately 35.7 mg/mL at 25°C. Estradiol tablets and injections should be stored in tight, light-resistant containers at a temperature less than 40°C, preferably between 15–30°C.

Estradiol

Pharmacological Actions—Estradiol stimulates growth and development of the tubular reproductive tract and accessory reproductive organs including the duct of the mammary glands. It maintains normal contractility of the uterus and enhances its response to oxytocin. Estradiol increases blood fat and calcium in birds, improves weight gain, inhibits bone growth, induces sexual receptivity (estrus, heat) in animals, causes hyperemia and hypertrophy of the female reproductive tract and induces development of secondary sexual characteristics. In laboratory animals, low doses of estradiol re-establish a normal estrous cycle in an anestrous female.

Mechanism of Action—Estradiol binds to estrogen receptors in the nuclei of cells of the responsive tissues to regulate the transcription of a limited number of genes resulting in the *de novo* synthesis of proteins. These functional proteins express the actions of steroids in the cell. It increases the plasma concentration of growth hormone and insulin which stimulates amino acid uptake into muscles.

Indications—Estradiol is used to control anestrus or subestrus in mares and cows. It also controls vaginal discharges associated with 'bunch of grapes ovaries', anal adenomata, prostatic hypertrophy, excessive libido in dogs, urinary incontinence in spayed bitches and irregular cycles in mare. Estradiol is also used to aid expulsion of mummified fetus or removal of retained placenta, promote growth in fattening steers, induce estrus in sheep and prevent pregnancy in bitches following mismating (postcoital contraception).

Dosages—0.5-2 mg IM within 5 days of mating (for post coital contraception). 1-5 mg in mares.

Route(s) of Administration—Per os; intramuscular.

Absorption—Estradiol is promptly and completely absorbed from the GIT but the natural hormone is highly susceptible to hepatic degradation. The alkyl derivatives are suitable for oral administration.

Metabolism—Estradiol is conjugated with sulfate and glucuronic acid.

Toxicity and Adverse Effects—Nausea is most frequent in humans. There may be anorexia, emesis and mild diarrhea following large doses. Large and prolonged doses may cause post parturient straining with vaginal or uterine prolapse in the cow. Subcutaneous implants in animals may cause pelvic fragility. Ovarian suppression and hypoplasia followed by development of ovarian cysts is observed in prolonged or excessive administration. Estradiol causes feminization in the male. It produces vaginal tumors in the female offsprings of women who took the drug during pregnancy.

Contraindications—Pregnancy.

Precautions—Large doses for long periods is not recommended in dogs. Do not use estradiol in food animals.

Pharmaceutical Formulations—Estradiol is available in 1 mg and 2 mg tablets of micronised estradiol; and 1-40 mg/ml oil preparations of estradiol valerate and cypionate for slow release after intramuscular injection. Preparations for administration as transcutaneous patches with 4 mg or 8 mg of the hormones are also available.

ETHACRYNIC ACID

Ethacrynic acid

Proprietary Names—Edecrin®; Hydromedin®; Edecril®.

Chemical Class—Phenoxyacetic acid derivative.

Pharmacological Class—High-ceiling diuretic; Loop diuretic.

Source—Synthetic.

Solubility, Stability and Storage—Ethacrynic acid is slightly soluble in water and freely soluble in alcohol. Ethacrynate sodium for injection has a solubility of about 70 mg/mL in water at 25°C. Ethacrynic acid tablets and ethacrynate sodium powder for injection should be stored at 15-30°C. The tablets should be stored in tight containers. Solutions of ethacrynate sodium should be used within 24 hours of their preparation.

Pharmacological Actions—Ethacrynic acid causes increased urinary excretion of water and electrolytes particularly sodium, chloride, calcium, and magnesium ions. It also causes increased renal blood flow, albeit, short-lived. Ethacrynic acid inhibits several enzymes and biochemical systems such as Na^+, K^+-ATPase, adenylyl cyclase, phosphodiesterase, prostaglandin dehydrogenase, glycolysis, and mitochondrial respiration. It blocks the excretion of uric acid.

Mechanism of Action—Ethacrynic acid inhibits the Na^+ K^+-$2Cl^-$cotransport mechanism at the luminal membrane of the epithelial cells of the ascending limb of the loop of Henle by attaching to the chloride-binding site of the glycoprotein transporter. The excretion of Ca, K, Mg, Na and Cl are thus enhanced.

Indications—Ethacrynic acid is used to mobilize edema fluid, induce diuresis during poisoning and remove excess water from show animals. It is also used for prophylaxis for epistaxis in race horses, management of hypercalcemia and renal calcium stones.

Dosages—5 mg/kg in dogs and cats.

Route(s) of Administration—Ethacrynic acid is administered orally and intravenously.

Absorption—It is rapidly and almost completely absorbed from gastrointestinal sites.

Onset of Action—5 minutes (IV), 30 minutes (oral).

Peak Effect—30 minutes (IV), 2 hours (oral).

Duration of Action—2 hours (IV), 12 hours (oral).

Distribution—Ethacrynic acid accumulates in the liver. It is excluded from the CNS.

Plasma Protein Binding—> 90%.

Metabolism—35%-40% of dose is metabolized in the liver.

Plasma Half–Life—0.5-1 hour.

Route(s) of Excretion—Ethacrynic acid is excreted in urine and bile with 65% of dose appearing in urine as unchanged drug. It is secreted actively by the organic acid transport system in the renal proximal tubule. profile

Dialysis Status—Nondialyzable.

Toxicity and Adverse Effects—Abnormalities of fluid and electrolyte balance manifesting as hypokalemia, hypochloremic alkalosis, hyperuricemia, and magnesium wasting are common. Ethacrynic acid causes gastrointestinal disturbances characterized by emesis, diarrhea and gastrointestinal bleeding especially following oral administration. Ototoxicity is a potential adverse effect especially following high IV dose in humans and cats. Less common adverse effects include skin rashes, photosensitivity, bone marrow depression and restlessness. Overdose causes electrolyte depletion, dehydration and circulatory collapse.

Management of Overdose/Toxicity—Reduce GI absorption and give supportive therapy.

Contraindications—Hypersensitivity to ethacrynic acid; severe water and sodium depletion; metabolic alkalosis; anuria.

Precautions—Ethacrynic acid should be used cautiously in the following conditions—patients with diarrhea or are vomiting, severe hepatic and renal dysfunction, diabetes mellitus, patients with pre-existing water and electrolyte imbalance, concurrent administration of warfarin, digitalis and cephalosporin. Do not administer ethacrynic acid with aminoglycoside antibiotic. Potassium supplement may be required.

Drug Interactions—The effects of ethacrynic acid are additive to those of hypotensive agents, drugs affected by or causing K^+ depletion, and aminoglycoside antibiotics (both drugs cause ototoxicity). Concurrent use with cardiac glycosides increases the risk of digitalis-induced arrhythmias. Ethacrynic acid increases the blood levels of lithium and propranolol. It competes for protein binding sites with warfarin and clofibrate. It decreases the effectiveness of antidiabetic drugs. Its effects are reduced by NSAIDs and probenecid.

Pharmaceutical Formulations—Available in tablets of 25 mg and 50 mg and as ethacrynate sodium in 50 mg powder for injection. Ethacrynate sodium contains 0.17 mEq of sodium, and 62.5 mg of mannitol in each vial containing the equivalent of 50 mg of ethacrynic acid.

ETORPHINE

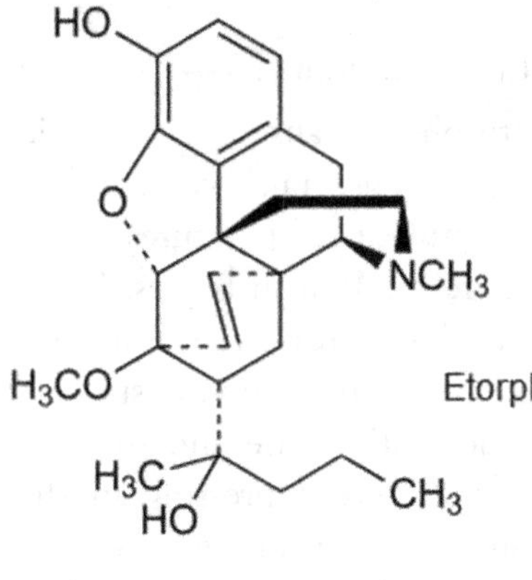

Etorphine

Proprietary Names—Oripavine*; M99*; Immobilon* (Etorphine+ acepromazine).

Chemical Class—Oripavine derivative of thebaine.

Pharmacological Class—Narcotic analgesic; Neuroleptanalgesic; Opioid analgesic.

Sources—Semisynthetic; derived from thebaine.

Solubility, Stability and Storage—Etorphine is soluble 1 in 30,000 of water. It is freely soluble in ethanol, chloroform, and ether.

Pharmacological Actions—Etorphine has actions similar to those of morphine but it is 10,000 times as potent as morphine. It causes analgesia, sedation and immobilization. A 2,000 kg rhinoceros has been immobilized with just 1 mg and a 5,000 kg African elephant by 4 mg.

Mechanism of Action—Etorphine activates opioid receptors.

Indications—Etorphine is used alone or in a neuroleptanalgesic combination (usually with acepromazine) for the immobilization of various domestic, wild, and exotic animals for the purpose of diagnosis and/or treatment particularly in animals difficult or dangerous to approach. It is found particularly useful in very large ungulates and sub-ungulates such as African elephant (*Loxodonta africana*), black rhino (*Diceros bicornis*), white rhino (*Ceratotherium simum*), African buffalo (*Syncerus caffer*), Burchell's zebra (*Equus burchelli*), eland (*Taurotragus oryx*) etc. It is generally not suitable for use in primates or felids.

Dosages—

Exotic animals.	1-2 mg (total dose).
Elephant.	5-6 mg (total dose).
Camels.	4 mg for adults and 0.5-2 mg for juvenile (total dose).
Domestic animals.	24.5 mcg/kg in combination with acepromazine at 100 mcg/kg.

Route(s) of Administration—Etorphine may be given intramuscularly or intravenously. The intravenous route is contraindicated in camels.

Onset of Action—2-3 minutes for etorphine alone. (Less than 1 minute for etorphine-acepromazine mixture given IV).

Duration of Action—30-60 minutes (etorphine alone).

Metabolism—Etorphine is conjugated with glucuronic acid. The glucuronide is secreted into bile hydrolyzed in the caecum; the etorphine thus released is partially reabsorbed.

Route(s) of Excretion—19 % of etorphine is eliminated via kidney; 42 % is eliminated in feces via the bile.

Withdrawal Period—30 days (meat in game animals)—

Toxicity and Adverse Effects—Etorphine causes hypertension, tachycardia, muscle spasm and tremor in horses; bradycardia in dogs, rats, cats and monkeys. Etorphine may cause hyperexcitability if underdosed. High ambient temperatures increase its toxicity. A combination of etorphine and acepromazine depresses respiration in horses. Etorphine has been reported to cause pronounced tachycardia and increased blood pressure in Grevy's zebra (*Equus grevyi*), and African elephants (*Loxodonta africana*). Muscular tremors, mydriasis, teeth grinding, bellowing, bleating, hyperpyrexia have been observed in domestic cattle and sheep. Opisthotonus is a common side effect amongst Giraffidae and Camelidae. Head pressing in rhinoceros has been noted. Other possible effects of etorphine include stoppage of ruminal movements.

Management of Overdose/Toxicity—Diprenorphine is an antagonist.

Contraindications—Animals meant for human consumption.

Precautions—It is recommended to dose animals heavily with etorphine and then reverse its action as soon as possible with diprenorphine, an antagonist of etorphine—For veterinarians, it is wise to have a loaded syringe with nalorphine or naloxone before administration of etorphine in case of accidental self-injection. Avoid intraperitoneal or abdominal injection. Do not administer etorphine when environmental temperature is above 37⁰C. It is dangerous to smell or taste the product.

Drug Interactions—Etorphine actions are reversed by diprenorphine.

Pharmaceutical Formulations—Available as etorphine hydrochloride in 4.9 mg/ml and 9.8 mg/ml solutions for injection. A fixed-dose combination of 2.45 mg/ml of etorphine and 10 mg/ml acepromazine is also available.

FENBENDAZOLE

Proprietary Names—Panacur®.

Chemical Class—Benzimidazole compound.

Pharmacological Class—Anthelmintic.

Source—Synthetic.

Pharmacological Actions—Fenbendazole is effective against cattle lungworms and the major gastrointestinal nematodes of cattle, sheep, goats and pigs. Large and small strongyles, oxyuris, pin worms and ascaris of horses are also susceptible. It is active against liver flukes. It is also effective against ascarids, tapeworms, whipworms and hookworms of dogs except *Dipylidium caninum*.

Fenbendazole

Mechanism of Action—Fenbendazole inhibits microtubule polymerization in susceptible helminthes by binding to β-tubulin. This action results in progressive energy depletion and degenerative alteration in the integument and intestinal cells of the parasite.

Mechanism of Selective Toxicity—Binding of fenbendazole and other benzimidazole anthelmintics to parasite tubulin takes place at a lower concentration than does the binding to mammalian tubulin.

Indications—Treatment and prophylaxis of susceptible parasitic helminthes especially gastrointestinal parasites of horses, cattle, sheep, goats and pigs; treatment of lungworm infection in cattle; control of gastrointestinal nematodes in wild birds and reptiles.

Dosages—

Pig	3-6 mg/kg or 3 mg in feed for 3 days.
Horse, cattle, sheep and goat	5 mg/kg
Dog	50 mg/kg for 10-14 days
Cat	20-50 mg/kg for 10-14 days.
Bird	10-15 mg/kg.
Reptile	50-100 mg/kg, repeat in 2-3 weeks.

Route(s) of Administration—Per os.

Absorption—Fenbendazole is poorly absorbed. Peak blood levels of 0.11 mcg/ml and 0.07 mcg are attained in calves and horses respectively.

Bioavailability—Plasma level is about 1% of administered dose.

Metabolism—Fenbendazole is activated to oxfendazole.

Withdrawal Period—8-16 days for beef cattle depending on the formulation.

Route(s) of Excretion—Feces (44-50% as unchanged drug in cattle, sheep and pigs); less than 1% in urine.

Toxicity and Adverse Effects—Fenbendazole is a safe drug. 100 times the recommended dose can be tolerated. However, vomition may occur frequently in dogs and cats.

Contraindications—Lactating dairy cattle; horses intended for food; breeding season and molting period in wild birds.

Precautions—Do not administer concurrently with bromsalan trematocides. Dying parasites may induce secondary antigen release.

Drug Interactions—Concurrent administration with dibromsalan and tribromsalan has caused abortion in cattle and death in sheep.

Pharmaceutical Formulations—Fenbendazole is available as oral suspension containing 25 mg, and 100 mg per ml in 250 ml bottle. Also available in oral bolus containing 250 mg per bolus.

FENTANYL

Fentanyl

Proprietary Names—Sublimaze˙; Durogesic˙; Innovar˙ (fentanyl citrate, 0.05 mg/ml and droperidol, 2.5 mg/ml) or Innovar Vet˙ (for veterinary use).

Chemical Class—Phenylpiperidine derivative.

Pharmacological Class—Narcotic analgesic; Opioid analgesic.

Source—Synthetic.

Solubility, Stability and Storage—Fentanyl is sparingly soluble in water. Protect injection products from light; store at controlled room temperature. Fentanyl is incompatible with phenobarbital in the same syringe.

Pharmacological Actions—Fentanyl has analgesic potency of about 80 times that of morphine. It causes respiratory depression which may be of long duration and biphasic (due apparently to redistribution). Fentanyl reduces heart rate and cardiac output.

Mechanism of Action—It interacts with opioid receptors.

Indications—Used as a neuroleptanalgesic usually in combination with a butyrophenone like droperidol for immobilization of game animals, minor surgical operations (e.g. orthopedic and dental manipulations) and diagnosis.

Dosages—

Dog: 1 ml of innovar-Vet˙ per 6.8-9 kg IM; or 1 ml per 11.4-27.3 kg IV. Two mcg/kg IM is recommended for preanesthetic medication.

Cat: 1 ml/9 kg SC.

Route(s) of Administration—Fentanyl is given intravenous (in humans), intramuscular (in animals) and subcutaneous.

Absorption—Absorption from the muscular site is rapid. Maximum effect is achieved in 15 minutes.

Onset of Action—Rapid.

Duration of Action—1 to 1.5 hours.

Distribution—Vd = 4.0 ± 0.4 L/kg. Fentanyl undergoes significant tissue redistribution because of its high lipid solubility. It crosses the placenta and small amounts may be found in milk.

Plasma Protein Binding—84 ± 2%.

Metabolism—Fentanyl is rapidly hydroxylated and dealkylated in the liver.

Plasma Half-Life—3.7 ± 0.4 hours.

Clearance (ml/min/kg)—13 ± 2%.

Route(s) of Excretion—In humans, about 70% of a dose is excreted via urine in 72 hours, mostly as metabolites, with about 10 to 20% of a dose being excreted as unchanged drug in 48 hours. About 9% of a dose is eliminated in faeces.

Toxicity and Adverse Effects—Muscular rigidity, bradycardia, and respiratory depression are common—

Management of Overdose/Toxicity—Naloxone antagonizes the action of fentanyl.

Contraindications—Hypersensitivity to fentanyl.

Precautions—Abrupt changes in posture may precipitate marked hypotension in humans receiving fentanyl/droperidol. Avoid contact with skin and the inhalation of particles of fentanyl citrate.

Drug Interactions—Fentanyl effects are easily terminated by intravenous narcotic antagonist e.g. naloxone.

Pharmaceutical Formulations—Available as fentanyl citrate in parenteral solution and in a fixed dose combination with droperidol. Innovar-Vet˙ contains 20 mg droperidol and 0.4 mg fentanyl per milliliter.

FLUCONAZOLE

Proprietary Names—Diflucan˙.

Chemical Class—Triazole compound.

Pharmacological Class—Antimycotic drug.

Source—Synthetic.

Solubility, Stability and Storage—Fluconazole is slightly soluble in water and saline. Store tablets in a dry place at 20-25° C (68-77° F).

Pharmacological Actions—Fluconazole is active against infections with strains of *Candida, Cryptococcus, Aspergillus, Blastomyces, Coccidioides* and *Histoplasma*. Its action could be fungistatic or fungicidal depending on the susceptibility of the strain and the dose used.

Fluconazole

Mechanism of Action—Fluconazole inhibits the fungal P450-enzyme which converts lanosterol to ergosterol, an essential part of the fungal membrane. This deficit alters the permeability of the membrane and eventually disrupts fungal growth.

Indications—Treatment of yeast and other fungal infections.

Dosages—Non human primates: 2-3 mg/kg.

Route(s) of Administration—Per os and intravenous.

Absorption. Fluconazole is almost completely absorbed from the GIT within two hours. Absorption is not significantly reduced by concomitant intake of meals and co-medication with H_2-antagonists (e.g. cimetidine, ranitidine).

Bioavailability—Oral bioavailability is over 90%. Do not expect rapid results because one to two weeks are needed to get a stable blood level of fluconazole.

Distribution—Fluconazole is widely distributed. Concentrations in urine, saliva, sputum and vaginal secretions are approximately equal to the plasma concentration. Fluconazole also attains high concentrations in milk. It penetrates the blood-brain-barrier.

Plasma Half-life—Approximately 30 hours (higher in patients with impaired renal function).

Route(s) of Excretion—Primarily excreted in the urine with 80% as unchanged drug.

Toxicity and Adverse Effects—The incidence of side effects is relatively high (up to 25%) but much less than with ketoconazole. GI tract effects characterized by nausea, dyspepsia, abdominal pain, vomiting, diarrhea, and flatulence have been reported. Severe skin rash may occur but is uncommon. In rare cases, fluconazole may cause serious cardiac arrhythmias. Electrolyte imbalance such as hypokalemia, low serum level of magnesium and hypocalcemia may predispose a patient to this heart condition. Fluconazole may infrequently cause severe or lethal hepatotoxicity. It is an experimental fetotoxic agent.

Management of Overdose/Toxicity—If an adverse side effect occurs, it is expected to resolve with discontinuation of the medication. After recovery, fluconazole can usually be restarted at a lower dose.

Contraindications—Pregnancy; hypersensitivity to fluconazole. The drug may be given to patients already pregnant, if the severity of the disease outweighs the potential harm to the fetus.

Precautions—Use with caution in patients with electrolyte imbalance. Any electrolyte imbalance should be corrected before therapy is initiated. Liver function studies should be obtained regularly. The drug should be immediately withdrawn from patients showing clinical signs of liver damage. Patients with pre-existing liver disease should be treated with particular care.

Drug Interactions—Fluconazole may enhance the actions of rifampin, digoxin, warfarin, glipizide and cyclosporine.

Pharmaceutical Formulations—Available in 50 mg, 100 mg, 150 mg, 200 mg tablets.

FLUMAZENIL

Flumazenil

Proprietary Names—Romazicon®.

Chemical Class—Imidazobenzodiazepine.

Pharmacological Class—Benzodiazepine antagonist.

Source—Synthetic.

Solubility, Stability and Storage—Flumazenil is insoluble in water but slightly soluble in dilute acidic solutions. Discard injection solution after 24 hours if it was already mixed with normal saline or Ringer's solution and drawn into a syringe.

Pharmacological Actions—Flumazenil reverses the cardiovascular, respiratory and anticonvulsant effects of benzodiazepines. The reversal of amnesic effects of benzodiazepines is inconsistent. Its intrinsic pharmacological actions are subtle. At high doses, these actions resemble those of benzodiazepines. Flumazenil increases the anthelmintic effectiveness of 3-methylclonazepam, a benzodiazepine used for the treatment of schistosomiasis in humans. In this condition, flumazenil prevents sedation without interfering with the antiparasitic action of 3-methylclonazepam as it does not combine with the benzodiazepine receptor in the parasite. Flumazenil does not reverse the actions of other CNS depressants like ethanol, barbiturates or opioids.

Mechanism of Action—Flumazenil has high affinity for benzodiazepine receptors to which it binds and competitively antagonizes the binding and allosteric effects of benzodiazepines.

Indications—Flumazenil is effective in benzodiazepine overdose or reversing benzodiazepine sedation.

Dosages—Dogs and Cats: 2-5 mg with slow intravenous administration.

Route(s) of Administration—Intravenous.

Absorption—Flumazenil is rapidly absorbed after oral administration, but this route is not used therapeutically.

Bioavailability—< 25% (oral).

Effective Concentration—>5 ng/ml.

Onset of Action—1-3 minutes (human).

Peak Effect—6-10 minutes (human).

Duration of Action—Dose-related; sedation may recur especially with long acting benzodiazepines. Thus, a second dose may be required after 20-30 minutes.

Distribution—Flumazenil has variable volume of distribution. Initial V_d is 0.5 L/kg in humans while V_d at steady state (V_{dss}) is 0.77-1.6L/kg.

Plasma Protein Binding—40-50%.

Metabolism—Flumazenil undergoes hepatic metabolism to inactive products.

Plasma Half-Life—1 hour.

Clearance—(ml/min/kg)—17 ± 3 (lower in hepatitis).

Route(s) of Excretion—The drug is excreted in urine with 0.2% as unchanged drug.

Toxicity and Adverse Effects—Flumazenil causes nausea, vomiting and dizziness in more than 10% of human patients. Its use may precipitate seizure especially in patients on prolonged medication with benzodiazepines or tricyclic antidepressants. Adverse effects in animals have not been fully documented. It has caused teratogenic effects at high doses.

Management of Toxicity/Overdose—Treat seizure with barbiturates or phenytoin.

Contraindications—Hypersensitivity to flumazenil or benzodiazepines; life-threatening cases that are being treated with benzodiazepines (e.g. status epilepticus); cases with serious tricyclic antidepressant overdose.

Precautions—Use flumazenil with caution during pregnancy. Reduce the dose in patients with liver disease if the need for repeat administration arises. Use cautiously in patients with mixed drug overdose. Sedation may reoccur in cases where large doses of benzodiazepines were administered with neuromuscular blockers and multiple anesthetic agents.

Drug Interactions—Long-acting benzodiazepines may elicit their effects after the action of flumazenil subsides.

Pharmaceutical Formulations—Flumazenil is available in 0.1 mg/ml parenteral solution. No specific veterinary formulation is available.

FLUMEQUINE

Proprietary Names—Flumesol*; Flumisol*; Flumeq* Q-50SP; Flumequine*; Flumicof* ; It is a component of Imequyl*.

Chemical Class—Fluoroquinolone.

Pharmacological Class—Broad-spectrum bactericidal agent.

Source—Synthetic.

Pharmacological Actions—Flumequine is active against Gram-positive and Gram-negative bacteria, mycoplasmas, and chlamydia. It has exceptional activity against coliform bacteria and salmonella.

Mechanism of Action—Flumequine inhibits gyrase-mediated DNA negative super coiling leading to inability of the bacteria to maintain DNA super helical structure and effect DNA repair.

Indications—Control of intestinal infections especially those of coliform or salmonella origin.

Dosages—

Cattle, sheep, goat	12-15 mg/kg every 12h
Pig	12-20 mg/kg every12h
Dog, cat	12-15 mg/kg every12h

Route(s) of Administration—Per os.

Absorption—Flumequine is rapidly absorbed after oral administration. **Bioavailability**—Oral bioavailability is dose-dependent. In calves, it is 55.7% for 5 mg/kg dose and 92.5% for 20 mg/kg dose.

Distribution—Apparent area volume of distribution, Vd = 1.48 l/kg.

Plasma Protein Binding—Flumequine is 74.5% bound in serum.

Metabolism—It is metabolized to 7-hydroxyflumequine.

Plasma Half-life—11.5 hours in calf.

Toxicity and Adverse Effects—Flumequine causes erosion of load-bearing articular cartilage in young dogs and horses. It also causes neurotoxicity and convulsions at high doses.

Management of Overdose/Toxicity—Give general antidotal therapy and symptomatic treatment.

Contraindications—Growing dogs or cats; dogs under 8 (small breeds) to 18 (large breeds) months of age, and cats under 8 weeks of age; concurrent use with trimethoprim, nitrofurantoin, theophylline or copper sulfate in drinking water.

Drug Interactions—Concomitant intramuscular or oral administration of probenecid may slightly decrease the elimination rate of flumequine.

Pharmaceutical Formulations—Flumequine is available as oral solution and water soluble powder.

FLUNIXIN

Proprietary Names—Banamine®; Finadyne®; Flumeglumine®.

Chemical Class—Amino nicotinic acid derivative.

Pharmacological Class—Nonsteroidal Anti-inflammatory Drug; Analgesic.

Source—Synthetic—

Solubility, Stability and Storage—Flunixin is soluble in water. Its products may be stored in the refrigerator or at room temperature. Do not mix flunixin injection product with other drugs in the same syringe.

Pharmacological Actions—Flunixin possesses analgesic and anti-inflammatory properties. It suppresses but does not abolish acute inflammatory responses. In the horse, it is about four times as potent in its anti-inflammatory action as phenylbutazone. Flunixin has potent analgesic action and is particularly effective in visceral pain. It also has antipyretic and anti endotoxic properties.

Flunixin

Mechanism of Action—Flunixin inhibits cyclooxygenase and prevents the synthesis of prostaglandins and thromboxanes.

Indications—Treatment of equine spasmodic colic and pain associated with musculoskeletal disorders. Treatment of endotoxic shock, acute mastitis, and acute pulmonary emphysema in cattle.

Dosages—

Horse	1.1 mg/kg/day IV or IM for up to 5 days.
Dog	1 mg/kg once a day for not more than 3 days.
Cattle	1.1 mg/kg IV once a day or divided into two doses every 12 hours for 3 days.

Route(s) of Administration—Oral, intramuscular or intravenous routes may be used.

Absorption—Flunixin is rapidly absorbed from the GIT. Peak plasma concentration is reached within 30 minutes.

Bioavailability—Oral bioavailability is 80% in horses.

Onset of Action—Within 2 hours in horses.

Peak Action—2-16 hours in horses.

Duration of Action—30 hours.

Distribution—Vd = 0.2-0.3 L/kg (horse); 0.18 ± 0.08 L/kg (dog).

Metabolism—Flunixin is conjugated in the liver.

Plasma Half-Life—8.12 hours (cow); 1.6-2.5 hours (horse); 3.67 ± 1.2 hours (dog).

Clearance (ml/min/kg)—0.76-0.98.

Withdrawal Period—4 days before slaughter (cattle).

Route(s) of Excretion—Flunixin is eliminated in urine.

Toxicity and Adverse Effects—The drug is well tolerated. However, gastrointestinal erosion or ulceration has been reported in horses. GI ulceration has been observed in dogs following high doses or chronic use. Gastrointestinal upset characterized by emesis and diarrhea is commonly observed in the dog.

Management of Overdose/Toxicity—Give general antidotal therapy—

Contraindications—Food producing animals; hypersensitivity to flunixin.

Precautions—Use flunixin cautiously in patients with pre-existing ulcer, severe cardiac failure and in cats.

Drug Interactions—Flunixin may produce additive effects with other ulcerogenic drugs such as salicylates.

Pharmaceutical Formulations—Available as flunixin meglumine in 250 mg and 500 mg oral granules, 1500 mg/syringe oral paste, and 15 mg/ml solution for injection.

FLUOROURACIL

Synonyms—5-Fluorouracil; 5-FU.

Proprietary Names—Adrucil®; Efudex®; Fluoroplex®.

Chemical Class—Pyrimidine analogue.

Pharmacological Class—Antineoplastic drug; Anticancer agent; Antimetabolite; Fluorinated pyrimidine antagonist.

Source. Synthetic.

Solubility, Stability and Storage—Fluorouracil is sparingly soluble in water and slightly soluble in alcohol. Protect fluorouracil products from light. Fluorouracil injection should be stored at 15-30°C; freezing and exposure to light should be avoided. Solution may become discolored on storage without loss of potency but dark yellow solutions must be discarded. The drug can be made to redissolve by heating to 60°C if precipitates have formed in a solution.

Fluorouracil

Pharmacological Actions—Fluorouracil inhibits DNA and RNA synthesis. It is cell-cycle specific. It has low to moderate emetogenic potential and myelosuppressive actions.

Mechanism of Action—The activated products of fluorouracil (and its analogs), 5'-fluorodeoxyuridine monophosphate (FdUMP) inhibit thymidylate synthetase and block the conversion of deoxyuridilic acid to deoxythymidylic acid and consequently inhibits DNA and RNA synthesis.

Indications—Treatment of mammary and gastrointestinal carcinomas, actinic keratosis and superficial basal cell carcinoma in humans. The drug has been tried in dogs.

Dosages—200 mg/m^2.

Route(s) of Administration—Intravenous and topical.

Absorption—Oral absorption is unpredictable.

Distribution—Vd = 0.25 ± 0.12 (human). Fluorouracil distributes readily into the CSF, ECF, pleural effusions and ascitic fluids.

Plasma Protein Binding—8-12%.

Metabolism—Fluorouracil is highly metabolized in the liver to 5'-fluorouridine monophosphate (FUMP) and then to 5'-fluorodeoxyuridine monophosphate (FdUMP). It undergoes saturable first pass effect.

Plasma Half-life—11 ± 4 minutes. Its metabolites have longer half-lives.

Clearance—16 ± 7 ml/min/kg in human.

Route(s) of Excretion—The drug is eliminated in urine (< 10% as unchanged drug) and lungs (as carbon dioxide).

Toxicity and Adverse Effects—Bone marrow depression characterized by anemia, leukopenia, and thrombocytopenia are most prominent. Oral and gastrointestinal toxicities manifesting as anorexia, nausea, vomiting, diarrhea, and stomatitis have been reported. CNS toxicity has been observed in animals.

Management of Overdose—Give supportive therapy; no specific antidote.

Contraindications—Hypersensitivity to fluorouracil; severe renal or hepatic impairment; severe pre-existing bone marrow depression.

Precautions—Use fluorouracil with caution in patients with renal or hepatic impairment. Fluorouracil is an irritant; avoid contact with skin and mucous membranes. Handle products with gloves or wash hands almost immediately after handling. Pregnant women must avoid handling antineoplastic agents. Closely monitor blood cells, hepatic, and renal functions regularly during therapy. Discontinue when vomition or diarrhea become intractable.

Drug Interactions—In an intermittent combination therapy, fluorouracil should not be given prior to methotrexate. Leucovorin, given before or with fluorouracil, primes the cells and increases the efficacy of fluorouracil. It is advisable to administer both drugs separately as concentrations more than 25 mg/ml and 2 mg/ml of fluorouracil and leucovorin respectively may form precipitates. Allopurinol increases the toxicity of fluorouracil. Cimetidine increases the blood levels of fluorouracil by reducing blood flow to the liver and inhibiting fluorouracil metabolism. Fluorouracil is incompatible with cytarabine, diazepam, and doxorubicin.

Pharmaceutical Formulations—The drug is available in 50 mg/ml solution for injection; 1% and 2% solution as well as 1% and 5% cream for topical application.

FLUOXETINE

Proprietary Names—Prozac`.

Chemical Class—Phenylpropylamine.

Pharmacological Class—Antidepressant; Selective serotonin re-uptake inhibitor.

Source—Synthetic.

Solubility, Stability and Storage—Fluoxetine is slightly soluble in water but soluble in alcohol. Store fluoxetine tablets and capsules at room temperature, away from excess heat, light and humidity.

Pharmacological Actions—Fluoxetine potentiates the pharmacological actions of serotonin.

Mechanism of Action—It selectively inhibits serotonin re-uptake in the CNS.

Fluoxetine

Indications—Treatment of canine aggression and obsessive compulsive disorders; treatment of aggression, refractory urine spraying, inappropriate urination, compulsive behaviors, such as psychogenic alopecia and fabric chewing in cats.

Dosages—The usual dose in dogs and cats is dependent on the condition being treated and the animal's response to treatment. It may take up to 3 or 4 weeks before the medication becomes effective. Duration of treatment depends on the reason for treatment and response to treatment. The medication should be discontinued gradually over a 2-3 week period.

Cat	0.5 to 1 mg/kg once daily.
Dog	1 mg/kg once daily.

Route(s) of Administration—Per os.

Absorption—Fluoxetine is readily absorbed after oral administration.

Bioavailability—Oral absorption is approximately 60%.

Effective Concentration—Therapeutic serum concentrations are 0.15 to 0.5 mg/L for fluoxetine and 0.1 to 0.5 mg/L for norfluoxetine, a fluoxetin active metabolite.

Distribution—27 L/kg (between 20 and 42 L/kg for both fluoxetine and norfluoxetine). Fluoxetine is widely distributed throughout the body and secreted into milk.

Plasma Protein Binding—About 94.5%.

Metabolism—Fluoxetine is extensively metabolized in the liver by demethylation primarily to an active metabolite, norfluoxetine.

Plasma Half-life—4 to 6 days (fluoxetine); 4 to16 days (norfluoxetine).

Route(s) of Excretion—80% of a drug dose is excreted in urine with less than 10% as the unchanged parent drug and 15% excreted in faeces.

Toxicity and Adverse Effects—Not well documented in animals. Side effects of fluoxetine that may occur include loss of appetite, stomach upset, lethargy, anxiety, restlessness, panting and irritability. Vomiting and jaundice may also occur. Symptoms of overdose may include seizures or liver disease with symptoms of jaundice or vomiting.

Contraindications—Concurrent use with ephedrine and monoamine oxidase inhibitors (MAOI's) such as selegiline or amitraz; known hypersensitivity to fluoxetine; lactating females.

Precautions—Use fluoxetine with caution in animals with diabetes, liver disease and those that have had seizures. Use with caution when given with warfarin, phenylbutazone, digoxin, diazepam, buspirone, clomipramine and other tricyclic antidepressants such as amitriptyline. Do not abruptly discontinue therapy with fluoxetine.

Drug Interactions—Higher blood levels of alprazolam may occur and its effects may be increased if used concurrently with fluoxetine. Taking NSADs with fluoxetine may cause bleeding problems.

Pharmaceutical Formulations—The drug is available as fluoxetine hydrochloride in capsules, tablets and oral liquid.

FUROSEMIDE

Synonyms—Frusemide.

Proprietary Names—Lasix®; Oedemex®; Trofurit®; Diuresal®; Dryptal®.

Chemical Class—Orthochlorosulfonamide.

Pharmacological Class—High-ceiling diuretic; Loop diuretic.

Source—Synthetic.

Furosemide

Solubility, Stability and Storage—Furosemide is insoluble in dilute acids, practically insoluble in water, sparingly soluble in alcohol, and freely soluble in alkali hydroxides. Furosemide injection and tablets should be stored at 15-30°C and protected from light. Injections having a yellow color should not be used; discolored tablets should not be dispensed. To avoid precipitation, furosemide injection should not be mixed with strongly acidic solutions (i.e., pH less than 5.5), such as those containing ascorbic acid, tetracycline, epinephrine, or norepinephrine. In addition, furosemide should not be mixed with most salts of organic bases including local anesthetics, alkaloids, antihistamines, hypnotics, meperidine, morphine, ciprofloxacin, labetalol, and milrinone.

Pharmacological Actions—Furosemide causes increased urinary excretion of water and electrolytes particularly sodium, chloride, calcium, and magnesium ions. It also causes increased renal blood flow, albeit short-lived. Furosemide inhibits several enzymes and biochemical systems such as Na⁺, K⁺-ATPase, glycolysis, mitochondrial respiration, the mitochondrial Ca^{2+}, adenylyl cyclase, phosphodiesterase, and prostaglandin dehydrogenase.

Mechanism of Action—Furosemide inhibits the reabsorption of sodium and water in the ascending limb of the loop of Henle by interfering with the chloride binding site of the Na⁺, K⁺, 2Cl⁻cotransport system. The excretion of Ca, K, Mg, Na, and Cl are enhanced. It lowers blood pressure initially by reducing plasma and extracellular fluid volume; cardiac output also decreases. Eventually, cardiac output returns to normal with an accompanying decrease in peripheral resistance.

Indications—To mobilize edema fluid as in udder edema, hydrothorax, ascites, cerebral edema and edema associated with cardiovascular, pulmonary, hepatic or renal dysfunction. It is also used in the symptomatic treatment of hypercalcaemia and hypercalcuric nephropathy; prevention of exercise-induced pulmonary haemorrhage and epistaxis in race horses.

Dosages—

Bird	0.15-2 mg/kg IM, IV every 12-24 hours
Cat	2 mg/kg IV every12 hours to a maximum total dose of 5 mg or 2-4 mg/ kg PO every 8-12 hours.
Dog	2 mg/kg IV every 12 hours to a maximum total dose of 40 mg or 2-4 mg/kg PO every 8-12 hours.
Pig	5 mg/kg IM or IV
NHP	2 mg/kg PO.
Horse	1.5-3 mg/kg/day PO or 0.5-1 mg/kg IM or IV, 1-2 times daily.
Cattle	2-5 mg/kg PO or 0.5-1 mg/kg IM or IV, 1-2 times daily
Reptile	5 mg/kg IM, IV once or twice a day.

Route(s) of Administration—Oral, intramuscular and intravenous routes are appropriate.

Absorption—Furosemide is readily absorbed from the GIT; 40-70% of administered dose is absorbed. Food reduces the rate but not extent of absorption. practical

Bioavailability—61 ± 17% (human); 77% (dog).

Onset of Action—30-60 minutes (oral); 30 minutes (IM); 5 minutes (IV).

Peak Effect—1-2 hours (oral); 30 minutes (IV).

Duration of Action—6-8 hours (oral); 2 hours (IV).

Distribution—Vd = 0.11 ± 0.02 L/kg (human). Furosemide is secreted into milk and inhibits lactation.

Plasma Protein Binding—98.8 ± 0.2% (almost totally to albumin) in humans (lower in uremia, nephrotic syndrome, cirrhosis, hypoalbuminemia and the aged).

Metabolism—Furosemide is metabolized in the liver.

Plasma Half-Life—1.5 ± 0.12 hours in humans; 1-1.5 hours in dogs. Values are higher in renal failure, uremia and congestive heart failure.

Clearance—2.0 ± 0.4 (ml/min/kg).

Route(s) of Excretion—Excreted in urine (66 ± 7% as unchanged drug), bile, and feces.

Dialysis Status—Not dialyzable.

Toxicity and Adverse Effects—Abnormalities of fluid and electrolyte balance manifesting as hypokalemia, hypochloremic alkalosis, hyperuricemia, and magnesium wasting are common. Furosemide causes gastrointestinal disturbances characterized by vomition, diarrhea and gastrointestinal bleeding especially following oral administration. Ototoxicity is a potential adverse effect especially following high IV dose in humans and cats. Less common adverse effects include skin rashes, photosensitivity, bone marrow depression and restlessness. Overdose causes electrolyte depletion, dehydration and circulatory collapse.

Management of Overdose—Reduce GI absorption and give supportive therapy.

Contraindications—Hypersensitivity to furosemide; severe water and sodium depletion; metabolic alkalosis; anuria; history of watery diarrhea from furosemide.

Precautions—Use furosemide only for short periods if it is strictly indicated in a pregnant animal. Furosemide should be used cautiously in the following conditions—patients with diarrhea, patients that are vomiting, severe hepatic and renal dysfunction, diabetes mellitus, patients with pre-existing water and electrolyte imbalance, concurrent administration of warfarin, digitalis and cephalosporin. Do not administer furosemide with aminoglycoside antibiotic. Potassium supplement may be required.

Drug Interactions—The effects of furosemide are additive to those of hypotensive agents, drugs which cause or are affected by K^+ depletion and aminoglycoside antibiotics (both drugs cause ototoxicity). Concurrent use with cardiac glycosides increases the risk of digitalis-induced arrhythmias. Furosemide increases the blood levels of lithium and propranolol. It decreases the effectiveness of antidiabetic drugs. Its effects are reduced by NSAIDs, and sucralfate. Probenecid inhibits its tubular secretion.

Pharmaceutical Formulations—Furosemide is available in tablets of 10 mg, 40 mg and 80 mg as well as 20 mg/2 ml solution for human use. It is also available in 12.5 mg and 50 mg tablets as well as 5% injectable solution for veterinary use.

GALLAMINE

Gallamine triethiodide

Synonyms—Bencurine iodide.

Proprietary Names—Flaxedil`.

Chemical Class—Amine.

Pharmacological Class—Non-depolarizing muscle relaxant; Competitive neuromuscular blocker; Muscle relaxant.

Source. Synthetic.

Solubility, Stability and Storage—Gallamine is soluble 1 in 0.6 of water, and 1 in 115 of ethanol. Store gallamine injection below preferably between 15 and 30 °C (59 and 86 °F); protect from light and freezing.

Pharmacological Actions—Gallamine causes paralysis of skeletal muscle. It has parasympatholytic effect on the cardiac vagus nerve thereby causing tachycardia, and occasionally, hypertension. Very high doses may cause histamine release.

Mechanism of Action—Gallamine acts by competing with acetylcholine for nicotinic receptors at the motor end plate of skeletal muscle. Because it has higher affinity for the receptors gallamine is able to exclude acetylcholine from the receptor sites but it is unable to activate the receptors since gallamine has no intrinsic activity. The receptors are therefore blocked and the muscle becomes paralysed. **Indications**—Gallamine is used with general anaesthetic agent to induce skeletal muscle relaxation. Its use results in reduction in the dose of the anaesthetic agent, easy access to difficult anatomic regions and orthopaedic manipulations, particularly, fracture reduction. It is also used to facilitate tracheal intubation (succinylcholine is particularly useful in this respect); to control convulsions and trauma during electroconvulsive therapy, tetanus and status epilepticus. Intramuscular injection of neuromuscular blocking agents is occasionally used to immobilize non domestic animals.

Dosages—

Dog, Cat	1 mg/kg
Goat	4 mg/kg
Sheep	1 mg/kg
Pig	2 mg/kg

Route(s) of Administration—Intravenous.

Absorption—Gallamine is slowly and incompletely absorbed after oral administration. It is absorbed after IM administration but is generally given by the IV route.

Onset of Action—Dose dependent; generally 1 to 2 minutes.

Peak Action—It is dose dependent and is generally 3-5 minutes.

Duration of Action—Dose dependent; generally 15–30 minutes; duration is increased by repeated dosing.

Distribution—Vd = 0.3 L/kg. Gallamine crosses the placenta. Small amounts enter the CSF.

Metabolism—20% is metabolized.

Plasma Half-life—2 to 3 hours; greatly increased in renal failure.

Clearance—Plasma clearance is about 1.4 mL/min/kg in humans.

Route(s) of Excretion—Gallamine is excreted mainly in urine with 80% as unchanged drug. Negligible amounts are excreted in the bile.

Toxicity and Adverse Effects—Gallamine causes tachycardia and hypertension due to vagolytic activity.

Management of Overdose/Toxicity—Administer anticholinesterase agents, e.g. edrophonium, neostigmine or pyridostigmine to antagonize the action of gallamine. Atropine or another suitable anticholinergic agent should be administered prior to or concurrently with the anticholinesterase to control its cholinergic side effects.

Contraindications. Known hypersensitivity to gallamine or iodide.

Precautions. Use gallamine with caution in patients with renal impairment.

Drug Interactions. The effects of gallamine may be enhanced or prolonged by beta-adrenergic blocking agents. The central respiratory depressant effects of opioid analgesics especially those commonly used as adjuncts to anesthesia may be additive to the respiratory depressant effects of neuromuscular blocking agents. Gallamine may decrease the risk of opioid analgesic–induced bradycardia or hypotension because of its vagolytic activity. Neuromuscular blocking activity of inhalation anesthetics, especially enflurane or isoflurane may be additive to that of non depolarizing neuromuscular blocking agents. Dosage reduction should be considered. Calcium salts usually reverse the effects of non depolarizing neuromuscular blocking agents. Prior administration of depolarizing neuromuscular blocking agents may enhance the blockade of non depolarizing neuromuscular blocking agents. If a depolarizing n-m blocker (e.g. succinylcholine) is used before a non depolarizing agent, administration of the non depolarizing agent should be delayed until the effects of the depolarizing agent have decreased. Potassium-depleting drugs such as amphotericin B, corticosteroids, mineralocorticoids, ethacrynic acid, furosemide, and thiazide diuretics may enhance the action of no depolarizing neuromuscular blocking agents.

Pharmaceutical Formulations. The drug is available as gallamine triethiodide in 20 mg per mL solution for injection.

GENTAMICIN

Synonyms—Gentamycin.

Proprietary Names—Genticin˙; Gentasol˙.

Chemical Class—Aminoglycoside aminocyclitol.

Pharmacological Class—Antibiotic; Antimicrobial drug.

Source. Natural; produced by *Micromonospora purpurea* or *M. echinospora*.

Solubility, Stability and Storage—Gentamicin is soluble in water and insoluble in alcohol. Topical gentamicin sulfate preparations should be stored at 2-30°C. Gentamicin sulfate injection should be stored at a temperature less than 40°C, preferably between 15-30°C; freezing should be avoided. Gentamicin sulfate injection for IM or IV administration should not be mixed with other drugs.

Pharmacological Actions—Gentamicin is rapidly bactericidal to many gram-positive and gram-negative bacteria including Staphylococci, coliform organisms, *Pseudomonas aeruginosa*, Proteus and Serratia. The drug is inactive against fungi, viruses, and most anaerobic bacteria but minimally active against streptococci.

Mechanism of Action—Gentamicin binds to the 30S and also 50S ribosomal subunit to interfere with the initiation of protein synthesis leading to accumulation of abnormal initiation complexes. It may also induce misreading of the RNA template resulting in incorrect amino acid incorporation into the growing polypeptide chains.

Indications—Treatment of acute urinary tract infections, pneumonia, eye and ear infections caused by susceptible bacteria such as *Pseudomonas aeruginosa*, *Enterobacter*, *Klebsiella*, *Serratia* and other species resistant to less toxic antibiotics. Concurrent use of Gentamicin with ticarcillin gives synergistic effect against *Pseudomonas* infections.

Dosages—

Dog, cat	5 mg/kg IM or SC, q12h for 1 day, then once daily.
Pig	Colibacillosis in neonate; 5 mg PO or IM.
	Colibacillosis in other pigs; 1.1 mg/kg/day in drinking water for 3 days.
	Pig dysentery; 2.2 mg/kg/day in drinking water for 3 days.
Cattle	5 mg/kg IM every 8 hours.
Horse	2-4 mg/kg IM every 8-12 hours.
Rabbit	2-5 mg/kg IM, SC three times a day for 5 days.
NHP	2 mg/kg IM three times a day for 7-10 days.
Guinea pig	5-8 mg/kg SC once a day.

Route(s) of Administration—Per os; intramuscular; subcutaneous.

Absorption. Gentamicin is not absorbed from the GIT but readily absorbed from IM sites. Peak plasma concentration is attained within 0.5-1.5 hours. It is not usually absorbed following topical application to intact skin but it is absorbed systemically following topical application to wounds. Greater absorption may occur with topical application of gentamicin cream than with topical application of gentamicin ointment.

Distribution—Vd = 0.31 ± 0.10 L/kg (human). Vd is increased in edema and fluid overload but decreased in dehydration. Penetration into eye, CNS, bronchial secretions, peritoneal fluid, bone and prostate are poor. Gentamicin penetrates well into pleural and synovial fluids as well as pulmonary and renal tissues. It crosses the placenta.

Plasma Protein Binding—Less than 30%.

Plasma Half-life—2 to 4 hours; increased in renal failure; t½ for tissue-bound drug = 53 ± 25 hours. A very long terminal elimination phase of several days has also been reported.

Clearance—Plasma clearance, about 1 mL/min/kg.

Route(s) of Excretion—Rapidly excreted in the urine with 90% or more of the dose as unchanged drug.

Dialysis Status—Dialyzable.

Toxicity and Adverse Effects—Gentamicin has low safety margin. Nephrotoxicity and irreversible ototoxicity are serious adverse effects at therapeutic doses. Neurotoxicity may appear as curare-like effects producing neuromuscular blockade and respiratory paralysis at high doses.

Management of Overdose/Toxicity—Maintain good urine output.

Contraindications—Hypersensitivity to gentamicin and other aminoglycoside antibiotics.

Precautions—Reduce the dose in cases of renal impairment. Do not use for long term treatment. Use cautiously in cases with pre-existing renal impairment.

Drug Interactions—Penicillins, cephalosporins, amphotericin B and loop diuretics increase the nephrotoxic potential of gentamicin. Neuromuscular blocking agents increase its neuromuscular blocking action. Carbenicillin and ticarcillin synergize its action against *Pseudomonas aeruginosa*. There is partial cross-resistance between gentamicin and other aminoglycosides.

Pharmaceutical Formulations—Available as a mixture of the sulfate salts of gentamicin C_1, C_2, and C_{1A} in 2-, 10—and 40—mg/ml solutions for injection; oral solutions; and soluble powder.

Also available in 0.1% cream, 0.3% ophthalmic ointment, 0.1% topical ointment, 0.3% ophthalmic solution and in ophthalmic and otic drops.

GLIPIZIDE

Synonyms—Glydiazinamide.

Proprietary Names—Glucotrol®; Glibenese®.

Chemical Class—Sulfonylurea.

Pharmacological Class—Antidiabetic agent.

Source—Synthetic.

Solubility, Stability and Storage—Glipizide is practically insoluble in water and ethanol. Glipizide tablets should be stored in tight, light-resistant containers at room temperature.

Glipizide

Pharmacological Actions—Glipizide lowers blood glucose concentration in diabetic and non diabetic subjects.

Mechanism of Action—Not clearly established; but the drug initially appear to lower blood glucose concentration principally by stimulating secretion of endogenous insulin from the beta cells of the pancreas. Glipizide also increases tissue sensitivity so that smaller doses of insulin may have greater effect. Like other sulfonylureas, glipizide alone is ineffective in the absence of functioning beta cells.

Indications—Glipizide is used as a last resort in cats when insulin administration cannot be given or for a select few cats that are sensitive to insulin.

Dosages—0.25 to 0.5 mg/kg twice daily.

Route(s) of Administration—Per os.

Absorption—Glipizide is readily absorbed after oral administration.

Bioavailability—Oral bioavailability is almost 100%.

Distribution—Vd = about 0.2 L/kg (human).

Plasma Protein Binding—About 98% (human).

Metabolism—Almost completely metabolized mainly in the liver by hydroxylation to inactive metabolites.

Plasma Half-life—2 to 4 hours (human).

Clearance—Plasma clearance is about 0.6 ml/min/kg.

Route(s) of Excretion—About 65 to 85% of a dose is excreted in urine in 24 hours, with about 3 to 10% as unchanged drug. About 11% of a dose is eliminated in the faeces.

Toxicity and Adverse Effects—Hypoglycemia is reported to occur in approximately 15% of cats on glipizide. Nausea and appetite loss can occur in some individuals. Acute glipizide overdosage is manifested principally as hypoglycemia.

Management of Overdose/Toxicity—Undertake measures that could empty the stomach in case of acute overdose. Administer glucose and give supportive therapy.

Contraindications—Hypersensitivity to glipizide or other sulfonylureas.

Precautions—Monitor the patient for the first month or so since it will not be known if a cat will respond. Use glipizide cautiously with thiazide diuretics as these may aggravate diabetes mellitus.

Drug Interactions—Chloramphenicol, monoamine oxidase inhibitors, and probenecid may enhance the hypoglycemic effect of sulfonylurea antidiabetic agents including glipizide. The use of miconazole, fluconazole and some other antifungal antibiotics concomitantly with oral antidiabetic agents has resulted in increased plasma concentrations of glipizide. Cimetidine may potentiate the hypoglycemic effects of glipizide through inhibition of sulfonylurea hepatic metabolism.

Pharmaceutical Formulations—Glipizide is available in 5 mg tablets.

GLYCERIN

HO ⎯ OH

OH

Glycerin

Synonyms—Glycerol; Glycerine.

Proprietary Names—Osmogynl®; Ophthalgan®; Sani-supp®; Fleet®; Babylax®.

Chemical Class—Trihydric alcohol.

Pharmacological Class—Osmotic diuretic; Laxative; Demulcent; Emollient.

Source—synthetic.

Pharmacological Actions—Glycerin increases the osmotic pressure of plasma thereby causing the movement of water from the extracellular space to the blood. It causes diuresis, dehydration and reduced intraocular and intracranial pressures. It also increases osmotic pressure of the colon, draws fluid into the colon and stimulates evacuation. Glycerin has emollient properties on the skin and a soothing effect on mucous membranes.

Mechanism of Action—Glycerin acts mainly by its osmotic effect to increase the osmotic pressures of plasma and glomerular filtrate.

Indications—To relieve constipation, reduce intraocular and intracranial pressures, and manage corneal edema. As osmotic diuretic, it is useful prior to ophthalmological procedures.

Dosages—1-2 g/kg orally.

Route(s) of Administration—Per os.

Absorption—Glycerin is rapidly absorbed from the intestine. Peak plasma concentration is attained within 90 minutes. It is poorly absorbed from the rectum.

Onset of Action—10 to 30 minutes [reduction of intraocular pressure (IOP) in humans]; 10-60 minutes (reduction of intracranial pressure in humans); 15-30 minutes (to relieve constipation in humans).

Peak Action—IOP reduction: within 1 hour (dogs), 1-1.5 hours (humans). Reduction of intracranial pressure: 60-90 minutes (humans).

Duration of Action—IOP reduction: 4-8 hours (humans); 8-10 hours (dogs). Reduction of intracranial pressure: 2-3 hours (humans).

Distribution—Glycerine is widely distributed.

Metabolism—It is metabolized in the liver into glucose. About 20% is metabolized in the kidneys.

Plasma Half-Life—30 to 45 minutes (human).

Route(s) of Excretion—Glycerin is eliminated via urine with 10% as unchanged drug.

Toxicity and Adverse Effects—Vomition is the most common adverse effect. Nausea, diarrhea, polydipsia have been reported. Hyperglycemia and glucosuria are potential adverse effects due to its degradation to glucose.

Contraindications—Hypersensitivity to glycerin; anuria; severe dehydration; pulmonary edema; severely decompensated heart.

Precautions—Use glycerin cautiously in cases of hypovolemia, cardiac disease, or diabetes.

Pharmaceutical Formulations—Glycerin is available in solutions for ophthalmic (with 0.55% chlorobutanol), oral (50%) and rectal applications. Also available as suppository in combination with sodium stearate.

GLYCOPYRROLATE

Synonyms—Glycopyrronium bromide.

Proprietary Names—Robinul˚.

Chemical Class—Quaternary ammonium compound.

Pharmacological Class—Parasympatholytic drug; Antimuscarinic drug.

Source. Synthetic.

Solubility, Stability and Storage—Glycopyrrolate is soluble in water and alcohol. It is unstable in media of pH > 6 and incompatible with most alkaline drugs. Store glycopyrrolate products at room temperature. Tablets should be kept in tight containers.

Glycopyrrolate bromide

Pharmacological Actions—Glycopyrrolate has actions similar to those of atropine, but glycopyrrolate has restricted access to the CNS, being a quaternary ammonium compound. Glycopyrrolate causes tachycardia which is less of a problem than that produced by atropine. It relaxes the gastrointestinal smooth muscle and reduces gastric secretions. Glycopyrrolate reduces exocrine secretions especially from salivary glands. It dilates the bronchioles and reduces bronchial secretions. It also dilates the pupil and relaxes the urinary smooth muscle.

Mechanism of Action—Glycopyrrolate competitively inhibits the actions of acetylcholine and other cholinomimetic agents at muscarinic receptor sites.

Indications—Preanesthetic medication; treatment of anticholinesterase and cholinomimetic agent overdose.

Dosages—10 mcg/kg.

Route(s) of Administration—Parenteral routes are mostly used in animals. The oral route is also used in human beings

Absorption—Glycopyrrolate is poorly absorbed from the GIT.

Bioavailability—Oral bioavailability is less than 10%.

Onset of Action—1 minute (IV); within 50 minutes (oral); 20-40 minutes (IM).

Peak Action—30 to 45 minutes (IM or SC); Within 1 hour (oral).

Duration of Action—2 to 3 hours (vagolytic action); 7 hours (antisialoqogue action); 8-12 hours following oral administration.

Distribution—Glycopyrrolate is highly ionized; hence it does not cross the blood-brain-barrier and placenta appreciably.

Plasma Protein Binding—Unknown.

Metabolism—Small amount of glycopyrrolate is metabolized.

Plasma Half-life—Vary with route of administration.

Clearance—Glycopyrrolate is rapidly cleared from plasma.

Route(s) of Excretion—Excreted mainly in urine as unchanged drug. Unabsorbed portion of orally administered drug is eliminated in feces.

Dialysis Status—Nondialyzable.

Toxicity and Adverse Effects—The CNS related side effects of glycopyrrolate are less than those of atropine because glycopyrrolate poorly penetrates the CNS. Adverse effects include dry mouth, constipation, decreased sweating, mydriasis, tachycardia, hyperpnoea, restlessness, and respiratory failure. Glycopyrrolate causes irritation at injection site.

Management of Overdose/Toxicity—Give general antidotal therapy. Anticholinesterase agents (e.g. physostigmine) are antidotes.

Contraindications—Acute angle glaucoma; tachycardia; obstruction of the GIT and/or urinary tract; cardiac ischemia; acute hemorrhage; paralytic ileus; myasthenia gravis; hypersensitivity to glycopyrrolate.

Precautions—Use glycopyrrolate cautiously in hepatic, renal and cardiac diseases It should also use with caution in hyperthyroidism and in old animals.

Drug Interactions—Procainamide, quinidine, phenothiazines, pethidine, benzodiazepines, and antihistamines may enhance the effect of glycopyrrolate because they possess some anticholinergic actions. Primidone, disopyramide, prolonged use of corticosteroids may enhance the toxic potential of glycopyrrolate. Glycopyrrolate may enhance the actions of nitrofurantoin, thiazide diuretics, and sympathomimetic agents.

Pharmaceutical Formulations—Available in 0.2 mg/ml solution for injection. Glycopyrrolate is also available in 1 mg and 2 mg tablets. Other pharmaceutical formulations for human use are available.

GRISEOFULVIN

Griseofulvin

Synonym—Curling factor.

Proprietary Names—Fulcin®; Fulvicin®; Griseovin®.

Pharmacological Class—Antimycotic agent; Antibiotic.

Source. Natural; produced by *Penicillium griseofulvin dierckx.*

Solubility, Stability and Storage—Griseofulvin is slightly soluble in water and sparingly soluble in alcohol. Store griseofulvin products at room temperature in tight, light-resistant containers.

Pharmacological Actions—Griseofulvin has fungistatic action against Dermatophytes such as *Microsporum, Trichophyton*, and *Epidermophyton*. Other pathogenic fungi are resistant.

Mechanism of Action—Griseofulvin arrests cell division in metaphase by disrupting the cell's mitotic spindle. It may also interfere with cytoplasmic tubule formation.

Mechanism of Selective Toxicity—Griseofulvin attains high concentration in susceptible fungi because of active uptake mechanism.

Indications—Treatment of ringworm and mycoses of hair and claws caused by susceptible fungi in most animal species.

Dosages—

For micronized preparations.

Dog and Cat	65 mg/kg/day for at least 6 days
Guinea pig	75 mg/kg PO once a day for 2 weeks or 1.5% in dimethyl sulfoxide applied topically bid for 14 days.
Mouse	25 mg/100 g PO every 10 days.
NHP	20 mg/kg PO once a day.
	200 mg/kg PO once every 10 days.
Rat	25 mg/100 g PO every 10 days.
Rabbit	12.5-25 mg/kg PO bid for 30 days.

Ultra micronized preparations. 2.5-5 mg/kg every 12-24 hours in most animal species.

Route(s) of Administration—Per os.

Absorption—Absorption is enhanced when given with a fatty meal. Micronized form is absorbed to a variable (25-70%) extent. The ultra micronised form is almost completely absorbed.

Distribution—Griseofulvin accumulates in the stratum cornea of the skin. It attains high concentration also in hair, nails, fat, skeletal muscle liver and binds strongly to keratinocytes where it remains and eliminates the causative organism until keratin is shed. Griseofulvin crosses the placenta.

Metabolism—Griseofulvin undergoes demethylation and glucuronidation into inactive products. Cats may be more susceptible to its adverse effects because of poor glucuronidation in the species.

Plasma Half-life—9 to 12 hours (human); 47 minutes (dog).

Route(s) of Excretion—It is eliminated mainly via urine with less than 1% as unchanged drug.

Toxicity and Adverse Effects—Griseofulvin causes low incidence of adverse effects in animals. Nausea is the most common adverse effect. Vomiting and diarrhea may be observed. Cats are more susceptible and kittens are more sensitive than adult cats. Griseofulvin may cause blood dyscrasia characterized by neutropenia and lymphopenia in cats especially those infected with feline immunodeficiency virus. It causes birth defects in cats. Griseofulvin may inhibit spermatogenesis and may also cause photosensitization.

Management of Overdose/Toxicity—General antidotal therapy.

Contraindications—Feline immunodeficiency virus infection; hepatic dysfunction; hypersensitivity to griseofulvin; pregnancy.

Precautions—Continue treatment until the patient's fungal culture is negative.

Drug Interactions—Phenobarbitone reduces the rate of absorption of griseofulvin. Griseofulvin may inhibit fenthion metabolism; it may also reduce the anticoagulant action of coumarin anticoagulants.

Pharmaceutical Formulations—Available in micronized (4 μm diameter particle size) and ultra-micronized (< 1 μm diameter particle size). Micronized forms are available in 2.5 g powder (suitable for horses); 250 mg and 500 mg tablets (suitable for dogs and cats). Also available in 125 mg and 250 mg capsules; 125 mg/5 ml oral suspension with 0.2% alcohol for human use. Ultra micronized form is available in 125 mg, 165 mg, 250 mg, and 330 mg tablets.

HALOTHANE

Proprietary Names—Flu thane˙.

Chemical Class—Halogenated compound.

Pharmacological Class—General anesthetic agent; Inhalational anesthetic agent; Volatile anesthetic agent.

Source—Synthetic.

Solubility, Stability and Storage—Halothane is soluble 1 in 400 of water. It is miscible with dehydrated alcohol, chloroform, and ether. Halothane is better stored below 40°C in a tight, light-resistant container. Halothane SUP contains thyme and ammonia. The thyme does not vaporize so it may accumulate in the vaporizer causing yellow discoloration.

F—C—C—H structure

Halothane

Pharmacological Actions—Halothane depresses the CNS causing reversible loss of consciousness accompanied by analgesia and muscle relaxation. It also causes respiratory depression (pronounced in ruminants), myocardial depression, hypotension, vasodilatation and depression of the body temperature regulating centers and increased cerebral blood flow.

Mechanism of Action—Uncertain.

Indications—To induce and maintain anesthesia in both large and small animals.

Dosages—

Horse	Induction: 4-5% in an oxygen-enriched semi-closed large animal circle system. Maintenance: 2.503%.
Other domestic animals	Induction: 2 to 3% of the vapor by inhalation. Maintenance: 0.5 to 1.5%.
Fish	40 mg/L of water. Place fish in the solution until it turns belly up. The fish recovers when placed in fresh water.

Route(s) of Administration—Administered by inhalation, commonly by closed—or semi-closed circuit anesthetic device vaporized by a flow of oxygen or nitrous oxide-oxygen mixture in terrestrial animals.

Absorption. Rapidly absorbed upon inhalation.

Blood/gas partition coefficient—About 2.4.

Effective Concentration—Minimal Alveolar Concentrations (MAC) in oxygen are 0.76% in dog; 0.82% in cat; 0.88% in horse and 0.76% in human.

Distribution—Halothane accumulates in adipose tissue. It is distributed into milk.

Metabolism—It is metabolized to variable extent by the liver to trifluoroacetic acid, chlorine and bromine radicals.

Route(s) of Excretion. About 60 to 80% of an absorbed dose is exhaled unchanged from the lungs in 24 hours and smaller amounts continue to be exhaled for several days or weeks. Its metabolites are excreted in urine.

Toxicity and Adverse Effects—Cardiovascular effects characterized by vasodilation and hypotension are common. Halothane sensitizes the heart to catecholamines leading to cardiac arrhythmias followed by shivering and tremor on recovery. A malignant hyperthermia-stress syndrome has been reported in pigs, horses, dogs and cats.

Contraindications—Hypersensitivity to halothane; impaired liver function.

Management of Toxicity/Overdose—Give volume expanders and dobutamine for halothane-induced hypotension. Cardiac dysrhythmias may be treated with lidocaine.

Precautions—Rubber and some plastics are soluble in halothane leading to their rapid deterioration. Do not use acetaminophen as postoperative analgesic after halothane anesthesia. Reduce the doses of catecholamines if needed with halothane anesthesia.

Drug Interactions—Halothane sensitizes the myocardium to the effects of sympathomimetics, especially catecholamines, including dopamine, epinephrine, norepinephrine, ephedrine, metaraminol, etc. The use of non-depolarizing (competitive) neuromuscular blocking agents (e.g. d-tubocurarine, gallamine etc.), and systemic aminoglycosides (e.g. streptomycin, gentamicin etc.) with halogenated anesthetic agents may give additive neuromuscular blocking effect. In addition, d-tubocurarine may cause significant hypotension if used with halothane. Concomitant administration of depolarizing neuromuscular blocker, e.g. succinylcholine with inhalation anesthetics such as halothane, cyclopropane, nitrous oxide, and diethyl ether may increase the incidence of cardiac dysrhythmias, sinus arrest, apnea, and in susceptible patients, malignant hyperthermia.

Pharmaceutical Formulations—Halothane is available as volatile liquid with thymol 0.01% and ammonia 0.00025%.

HEPARIN

Synonyms—Heparin sodium.

Proprietary Names—Calciparine*; Certoparin*; Clexane*; Clivarin*; Clivarine*; Dalteparin*; Depo-Heparin*.

Chemical Class—Sulfated glycosaminoglycan.

Pharmacological Class—Anticoagulant.

Source—Natural; commonly obtained from porcine intestine or bovine lung.

Solubility, Stability and Storage—Heparin sodium and calcium are soluble in water and practically insoluble in alcohol. Heparin solutions are better stored at room temperature without excessive exposure to heat.

Pharmacological Actions—Heparin inhibits reactions that lead to the clotting of blood and the formation of fibrin clots both *in vitro* and *in vivo*. Clotting time is prolonged by full therapeutic doses of heparin sodium. Heparin does not have fibrinolytic activity; therefore, it will not lyse existing clots but it allows the body's natural clot lysis mechanisms to work normally to break down clots that have already formed. The diprotonated form of histamine binds specifically to heparin. Heparin also enhances the release of lipoprotein lipase, thereby increasing the clearance of circulating lipids and increasing plasma levels of free fatty acids.

Mechanism of Action—Heparin binds to the enzyme inhibitor antithrombin III (AT-III; heparin cofactor) in small amounts and induces a conformational change which exposes AT-III active site for rapid (1000–fold increase) interaction with thrombin and other proteases involved in blood clotting, most notably factor Xa. At high doses, heparin inactivates thrombin and blocks the conversion of fibrinogen to fibrin. Heparin also prevents the formation of a stable fibrin clot by inhibiting the activation of the fibrin stabilizing factor (factor XIII).

Indications—Treatment of Disseminated Intravascular Coagulation (DIC) and thromboembolic disease in small animals and horses. Heparin gel (topical) may be used to treat sports injuries.

Dosages—

Adjunctive treatment of DIC:

Cat	200 units/kg SC, 3 times daily
Dog	40-80 units/kg SC, 3 times daily or10-20 units/kg IV initially, then 5 units/kg every 3hours.
Horse	80-100 units/kg IV, every 4-6hours.

Blood transfusion: 1 unit/mL blood

As anticoagulant: 10 units/mL blood.

Route(s) of Administration—Intravenous or subcutaneous routes are preferred.

Absorption—Heparin is not absorbed from oral route. It is absorbed well from subcutaneous site. Peak plasma concentration is attained within two to four hours following subcutaneous administration, although there are considerable individual variations.

Onset of Action—Anticoagulant activity begins immediately after direct intravenous bolus injection, but may take up to one hour after deep subcutaneous injection.

Distribution—Heparin does not appreciably cross the placenta or enter milk.

Plasma Protein Binding—Heparin is extensively metabolized primarily to fibrinogen, low-density lipoproteins and globulins.

Metabolism—It is metabolized in the liver and reticulo-endothelial system.

Plasma Half-life—Biphasic; a rapidly declining alpha phase ($t_{1/2}$=10 minutes) and a slower beta phase. Biologic half-life is approximately one hour.

Dialysis Status—Nondialyzable.

Toxicity and Adverse Effects—A serious side-effect of heparin is heparin-induced thrombocytopenia (HIT syndrome), an immunological reaction characterized by platelet aggregation within the blood vessels leading to reduced levels of coagulation factors. Formation of platelet clots can lead to thrombosis, while the loss of coagulation factors and platelets may result in bleeding. Other side effects include alopecia, osteoporosis, diminished renal function (following prolong use at high doses), rebound hyperlipidemia, hyperkalemia, alopecia, suppressed aldosterone synthesis, and priapism. Subcutaneous injection of heparin may result in hematoma, pain, and irritation. Overdose causes bleeding. Because of its source, heparin may stimulate hypersensitivity reactions.

Management of Overdose/Toxicity—Administer protamine sulfate.

Contraindications—Hypersensitivity to heparin; severe thrombocytopenia or uncontrollable bleeding (caused by something other than DIC).

Precautions—Avoid injecting heparin intramuscularly because of the potential for forming hematomas. Heparin should be used therapeutically only by professionals familiar with it. The drug should be used cautiously in pregnancy.

Drug Interactions—Antihistamines, intravenous nitroglycerin, propylene glycol, digoxin, and tetracyclines may partially counteract the actions of heparin. Drugs that can cause changes in coagulation status or platelet function (e.g., aspirin, phenylbutazone, dipyridamole, warfarin, etc.) may increase the toxicity of heparin. Heparin may antagonize the actions of corticosteroids, insulin or ACTH. It may increase plasma levels of diazepam.

Pharmaceutical Formulations—Available as heparin sodium and heparin calcium in various strength.

HOMIDIUM

Homidium

Synonyms—Ethidium (homidiun bromide); Novidium (homidium chloride).

Proprietary Names—Ethidium˚; Novidium˚.

Chemical Class. Phenathridium compound.

Pharmacological Class—Trypanocide.

Source. Synthetic.

Solubility, Stability and Storage—Soluble 1 in 20 of water and 1 in 750 of chloroform.

Pharmacological Actions—Homidium is active against *Trypanosoma congolense* and *T. vivax*, but less active against *T. brucei*. It confers prophylaxis for about one month. One hour exposure to Homidium may render trypanosome motile but non infective. Homidium is mutagenic.

Mechanism of Action—Uncertain, but it is thought to interfere with several functions such as glycosomal functions, the function of adenosine monophosphate (AMP)-binding protein, trypanathione metabolism and the replication of kinetoplast minicircles giving rise to dyskinetoplastic trypanosomes.

Indications—Treatment of trypanosomosis caused by *T. brucei, T. vivax* and *T. congolense* in cattle. Used in the research laboratory environment as a nucleic acid stain.

Dosages—0.25 to 1mg per kg body weight as a 1% aqueous solution.

Route(s) of Administration—Deep intramuscular injection.

Distribution—Low concentrations of between 0.1 and 0.3 ng/mL remain in circulation for up to 90 days post-treatment.

Dialysis Status—Unknown.

Toxicity and Adverse Effects—Undesirable side effects include transient liver damage especially at high dosage. Severe local reactions can result from subcutaneous injection.

Pharmaceutical Formulations—Available as homidium chloride (novidium˚) and homidium bromide (ethidium˚) in powder for reconstitution into injectable solution.

HYDROCHLOROTHIAZIDE

Hydrochlorothiazide

Synonyms—HCTZ.

Proprietary Names—Hydrodiuril*; Esidrix*; Oretic*; Hydrosaluric*; Hypothiazide*; Hydrozide*—

Chemical Class—Sulfonamide derivative.

Pharmacological Class—Thiazides (benzothiadiazine) diuretic.

Source—Synthetic.

Solubility, Stability and Storage—Hydrochlorothiazide is slightly soluble in water but soluble in alcohol. Store hydrochlorothiazide tablets, capsules and oral solutions in tightly closed containers at 15–30°C. The formulations must be protected from light, moisture, and freezing.

Pharmacological Actions—HCTZ causes increased urinary excretion of sodium and water by inhibiting the reabsorption of sodium in the early distal tubule. It may reduce glomerular filtration due to direct action on renal vasculature. It increases the excretion of potassium, magnesium, phosphate, iodide, and bromide.

Mechanism of Action—HCTZ blocks the electroneutral Na^+-Cl^- co transport mechanism primarily at the cortical diluting segment. It has low carbonic anhydrase inhibitory action.

Indications—HCTZ is used to mobilize edema fluid, treat systemic hypertension and nephrogenic diabetes insipidus, prevent calcium oxalate urolith in dogs, prevent lactation in pseudo pregnancy, hasten the excretion of toxic substances and supplement antibacterial treatment of urinary tract infections.

Dosages—

Dog, cat	1-2 mg/kg PO, daily or 12.5-25 mg IM, daily.
Pig	50-75 mg IM, daily.
Horse, cattle	Initial dose: 500 mg PO daily.
	Maintenance dose: 250 mg PO, IM or IV
Cow	Udder edema: 125-250 mg IV or IM, once or twice a day; may continue for several days if necessary.

Route(s) of Administration—Per os and intravenous (in cattle).

Absorption—Hydrochlorothiazide is well (65-75%) absorbed from the GIT of humans with plasma concentration reaching its peak within one hour.

Bioavailability—71 ± 15%.

Onset of Action—2 hours—

Peak Action—4 to 6 hours.

Duration of Action—8 to 12 hours.

Distribution—Vd = 0.83 ± 0.31 L/kg.

Plasma Protein Binding—58 ±17%.

Metabolism—Not metabolized.

Plasma Half-Life—2.5 ± 0.2 hours.

Clearance—4.9 ± 1 (ml/min/kg)

Withdrawal Period—72 hours before milking.

Route(s) of Excretion—Kidney (95% as unchanged drug).

Dialysis Status—Not known.

Toxicity and Adverse Effects—HCTZ causes weakness, hypokalemia, metabolic alkalosis, impaired carbohydrate tolerance, hyperuricemia, hyperlipidemia and hyponatremia. It may also cause allergic reactions and rashes which are sometimes photosensitive.

Management of Toxicity/Overdose—Give supportive therapy with IV fluids, and electrolytes.

Contraindications—Digitalis therapy; known hypersensitivity to HCTZ.

Precautions—Potassium supplement may be required during hydrochlorothiazide therapy. Concurrent digitalis glycoside and thiazides therapy requires electrolyte monitoring since loss of K may enhance the therapeutic and toxic actions of digitalis. Use HCTZ with caution in borderline renal and or hepatic insufficiency.

Drug Interactions—HCTZ potentiates other antihypertensive therapy; may be alternately administered with K⁺-sparing diuretics. Its antihypertensive action is decreased by NSAIDs. Cholestyramine resins may reduce its absorption. HCTZ causes decreased effect of oral hypoglycemic drugs.

Pharmaceutical Formulations—HCTZ is available in 25 mg, 50 mg, and 100 mg tablets; and also as oral solution containing 10 mg/ml for human and small animal use. A 25 mg/ml injection solution is available for use in cattle.

HYDROCORTISONE

Hydrocortisone

Synonyms—Compound F; Cortisol; 17-Hydroxycorticosterone.

Proprietary Names—Hydrocortisone˙ A-hydrocort˙; Cortate˙; Cortef˙; Cortoderm˙; Hycort˙; Hydrosone˙; Vioform˙.

Chemical Class—Corticosteroid.

Pharmacological Class—Anti-inflammatory agent; Glucocorticoid.

Source—A natural hormone secreted by the adrenal cortex.

Solubility, Stability and Storage—Hydrocortisone and its esters are insoluble in water. Hydrocortisone is sparingly soluble, hydrocortisone acetate is slightly soluble, and hydrocortisone cypionate is soluble in alcohol. Solutions and suspensions of hydrocortisone and its derivatives are heat labile. Hydrocortisone preparations should be stored preferably between 15-30°C. Freezing of the oral and sterile suspensions should be avoided. Hydrocortisone tablets should be stored in well-closed containers. Reconstituted solutions of hydrocortisone sodium succinate should be stored at 25°C or below. Reconstituted solutions of the drug should not be used unless they are clear, and unused solutions should be discarded after 3 days.

Pharmacological Actions—Hydrocortisone is short-acting with equal anti-inflammatory and sodium ion retaining potencies.

Mechanism of Action—The drug binds to specific glucocorticoid receptors at the cytosol and the hormone-receptor complex is then transported into the cell nucleus where it binds with glucocorticoid response elements (GRE) on various genes and alters their expression. Activated hormone receptors may also interact with specific transcription factors and prevents the transcription of targeted genes. Glucocorticoids are able to prevent the transcription of any of immune genes, including the IL-2 gene.

Indications—Replacement therapy in patients with adrenocortical insufficiency. Hydrocortisone or cortisone is usually the corticosteroid of choice in this condition because these drugs have both glucocorticoid and mineralocorticoid properties—Hydrocortisone is also used for the relief of shock; treatment of inflammatory conditions of the skin (such as eczematous conditions, allergic dermatosis, seborrheic dermatitis, and intractable pruritus); suppression of scar tissue formation in infections or lesions of the cornea or ear, or when injected into keloid. For anti-inflammatory or immunosuppressive uses, synthetic glucocorticoids which have minimal mineralocorticoid activity are preferred.

Dosages—

Horse	1-4 mg/kg.
Cattle	100-600 mg.
Dog, cat	5 mg/kg PO, twice daily or 5 mg/kg IM or IV daily.
Circulatory shock in all species.	50 mg/kg, repeat after 3-6 hours if required.

Route(s) of Administration—Chosen route would depend on the ester form. See table below.

Hydrocortisone	Per os
Hydrocortisone sodium succinate XE	IM or IV routes.
Hydrocortisone sodium phosphate	IM, SC, or IV routes.
Hydrocortisone cypionate XE	Per os.
Hydrocortisone acetate	intra-articular, intrabursal, intralesional, intrasynovial or soft tissue injection.

Absorption—Hydrocortisone is readily absorbed after oral administration and through the skin. Hydrocortisone acetate is less well absorbed.

Distribution—Vd = 0.3 L/kg.

Plasma Protein Binding—More than 90%.

Metabolism—Hydrocortisone is metabolized in the liver and other tissues by reduction, hydroxylation, side-chain cleavage, and conjugation with glucuronic acid.

Plasma Half-life—about 1.5 h.

Route(s) of Excretion—About 90% of a dose is excreted in the urine in 24 hours with less than 1% as unchanged drug

Toxicity and Adverse Effects—Hydrocortisone delays wound healing; causes gastrointestinal ulceration, increased susceptibility to infection, edema from increased sodium retention, and abortion in late pregnancy. It causes liver degeneration in dogs. Iatrogenic hypoadrenocorticism may follow abrupt withdrawal following log-term use.

Contraindications—Concurrent infection; corneal ulcers; cardiac disorders; diabetes mellitus; burns; pregnancy; hypersensitivity to hydrocortisone or other corticosteroids.

Precautions—Glucocorticoid hormones should not be used in combination with NSAID drugs. Any latent infections can be unmasked by hydrocortisone use. Following chronic use, it is important that the dose be tapered to an every third day schedule once the condition is controlled. Patients taking corticosteroids should generally not receive live attenuated-virus vaccines.

Drug Interactions—The effects of hydrocortisone, and possibly other glucocorticoids, may be potentiated by concomitant administration with estrogens. Concurrent use with NSAIDs could lead to gastric bleeding and ulceration. Hydrocortisone decreases the effects of salicylates, vaccines and toxoids.

Pharmaceutical Formulations—Formulations vary with its ester forms. See table below.

Hydrocortisone	5 mg, 10 mg, and 20 mg oral tablets.
Hydrocortisone acetate	25 mg/ml and 50 mg/ml solution for injection
Hydrocortisone cypionate	oral suspension containing 2 mg/ml hydrocortisone in 120 ml.
Hydrocortisone sodium phosphate	50 mg/ml solution for injection.
Hydrocortisone sodium succinate	Solution for injection containing 100 mg-, 250 mg-, 500 mg-, and 1000 mg—per vial.

HYDROFLUMETHIAZIDE

Hydroflumethiazide

Synonyms—Trifluoromethylhydrothiazide.

Chemical Class—Sulfonamide derivative.

Pharmacological Class—Thiazide (benzothiadiazine) diuretic.

Source—Synthetic.

Proprietary Names—Saluron*; Diucardin*; Hydrenox*; Naclex*.

Pharmacological Actions—Hydroflumethiazide causes increased urinary excretion of sodium and water by inhibiting the reabsorption of sodium in the early distal tubule. It may reduce glomerular filtration due to direct action on renal vasculature. It increases the excretion of potassium, magnesium, phosphate, iodide, and bromide.

Mechanism of Action—Hydroflumethiazide blocks the electroneutral Na+-Cl⁻co transport mechanism primarily at the early distal tubule. It has low carbonic anhydrase inhibitory action.

Indications—Mobilization of edema fluid; adjunctive treatment of congestive heart failure. Hydroflumethiazide is used in combination with spironolactone (a potassium-sparing diuretic) to minimize the excessive loss of potassium in hypokalemic patients that require diuretic therapy or those refractory to loop diuretics.

Dosages—1 mg/kg orally every 24 hours.

Route(s) of Administration—Per os.

Absorption—Hydroflumethiazide is well absorbed from the GIT of humans; peak plasma concentration is attained within 1 hour.

Onset of Action—Within 2 hours—

Peak Action—Within 4 hours.

Duration of Action—12 to 24 hours.

Distribution—Hydroflumethiazide distributes more widely into body tissues than chlorothiazide because it is more lipid soluble.

Toxicity and Adverse Effects—Hydroflumethiazide may cause weakness, paresthesia, hypokalemia, metabolic alkalosis and hematologic signs characterized by aplastic anemia, hemolytic anemia, leukopenia, thrombocytopenia, and agranulocytosis. Photosensitivity, hyperglycemia, fluid and electrolyte imbalance characterized by hypomagnesaemia, hypocalcaemia, and hyponatremia associated with Hydroflumethiazide therapy have been reported. An overdose may cause hypermotility and weakness.

Management of Toxicity—Give supportive therapy with IV fluids and electrolytes.

Contraindications—Digitalis therapy; known hypersensitivity to hydroflumethiazide.

Precautions—Potassium supplement may be required. Concurrent digitalis glycoside and thiazides therapy requires electrolyte monitoring since loss of potassium may enhance the therapeutic and toxic actions of digitalis. Use hydroflumethiazide with caution in border line renal and or hepatic insufficiency.

Drug Interactions—Hydroflumethiazide potentiates other antihypertensive therapy. It may be alternately administered with K⁺ sparing diuretics. Its antihypertensive action is decreased by NSAIDs. Cholestyramine resins may reduce its absorption. It decreases the effects of oral hypoglycemic drugs.

Pharmaceutical Formulations—Available in 50 mg tablets.

HYDROMORPHONE

Hydromorphone

Synonyms—Dihydromorphinone.

Proprietary Names—Dilaudid˚; Dilaudid-HP˚.

Chemical Class—Opioid; Morphine derivative; Phenanthrene alkaloid derivative.

Pharmacological Class—Narcotic analgesic; Opioid analgesic.

Source—Semisynthetic.

Solubility, Stability and Storage—Hydromorphone is freely soluble in water and sparingly soluble in alcohol. Store hydromorphone products at room temperature; protect them from light.

Pharmacological Actions—The actions of hydromorphone are qualitatively similar to those of morphine. Hydromorphone produces CNS and respiratory depression. It causes analgesia and depression of cough center at lower doses. Hydromorphone is five times more potent an analgesic as morphine and it has low oral:parenteral potency ratio, high efficacy and addiction potential. Hydromorphone causes miosis, decreased motility and secretion of the GIT. It alters endocrine and autonomic system functions.

Mechanism of Action—Hydromorphone has strong agonist activity at opioid receptors. It binds to opioid receptors to cause inhibition of ascending pain pathways, altering the perception of and response to pain. Antitussive effect is due to depression of cough center at the medulla.

Indications—Control of cough and pain of moderate to severe intensity—

Dosages—Dog: 1.1-2.2 mg/kg.

Route(s) of Administration—Oral, intramuscular or subcutaneous routes are used.

Absorption—Like most opioids, hydomorphone is readily absorbed from the oral route. It is also well absorbed from the rectal, subcutaneous and intramuscular sites.

Bioavailability—Oral bioavailability is 62%.

Onset of Action—15 to 30 minutes.

Peak Action—30 to 60 minutes.

Duration of Action—4 to 5 hours.

Metabolism—Undergoes glucuronidation primarily in the liver.

Plasma Half-life—2 to 3 hours.

Route(s) of Excretion—Urine.

Toxicity and Adverse Effects—Respiratory depression and bradycardia are common adverse effects. Hydromorphone causes ADH release and lowers urine output. It produces less nausea, vomiting and GI upset than morphine in the dog. Decreased GI motility may result in constipation. Overdose may heighten respiratory depression and cause cardiovascular collapse, hypothermia and convulsions.

Management of Overdose/Toxicity—Initiate general antidotal therapy in conjunction with administration of naloxone.

Contraindications—Hypersensitivity to hydromorphone or other morphine derivatives.

Precautions—Use cautiously in animals with respiratory impairment, or severe liver and/or hepatic disease.

Drug Interactions—CNS depressants produce additive CNS depression when used with hydromorphone.

Pharmaceutical Formulations—Available as hydromorphone hydrochloride in 1 mg, 2 mg, 3 mg and 4 mg per ml solution for injection; 3 mg rectal suppository and also in 2 mg and 4 mg tablets. No specific veterinary formulations are available.

HYDROXYUREA

hydroxyurea

Synonyms—Hydroxycarbamide.

Proprietary Names—Hydrea®.

Chemical Class—Urea derivative.

Pharmacological Class—Antineoplastic drug; Anticancer agent; Cytotoxic drug.

Source—Synthetic.

Solubility, Stability and Storage—Hydroxyurea is freely soluble in water and slightly soluble in alcohol. Store products in tight containers at room temperature.

Pharmacological Actions—Hydroxyurea has cytotoxic action. It is cell-cycle specific, being active at the S phase of the cell cycle and causing cells to arrest at the G_1—S interface, a point at which cells are sensitive to irradiation. Hydroxyurea is teratogenic.

Mechanism of Action—Hydroxyurea inhibits ribonucleotide diphosphate reductase, an enzyme that converts ribonucleotides to deoxyribonucleotides. It inhibits the enzyme by destroying a tyrosyl free radical at the catalytic center. This limits the availability of deoxyribonucleotides needed for DNA synthesis by the cells.

Indications—Treatment of polycythemia vera, mastocytomas, and leukemia in dogs and cats.

Dosages—

25 mg/kg (for cats) or 50 mg/kg (for dogs) thrice a week or 30 mg/kg daily for one week followed by 15 mg/kg daily until remission.

Route(s) of Administration—Per os.

Absorption—Hydroxyurea is readily and significantly (>80%) absorbed from the oral route. Peak plasma concentration is attained within 2 hours.

Bioavailability (oral)—High.

Distribution—Distributes readily to tissues including brain, intestine, lungs and kidneys. Hydroxyurea is passed into milk.

Metabolism—50% of Hydroxyurea is degraded in the liver to urea and CO_2.

Plasma Half-life—2 to 4 hours.

Route(s) of Excretion—Urine (50% as unchanged drug); Urea, one of the metabolites is also excreted in urine. The CO_2 metabolite is excreted through the lungs.

Toxicity and Adverse Effects—Bone marrow depression characterized by anemia, leukopenia and thrombocytopenia is prominent. Others are gastrointestinal effects characterized by nausea, vomiting, diarrhea and stomatitis.

Management of Overdose—Set up general antidotal therapy.

Contraindications—Severe anemia; severe bone marrow depression; pregnancy; active infection; hypersensitivity to hydroxyurea.

Precautions—Use cautiously in patients with impaired renal function and those that have received previous cancer chemotherapy or irradiation. Use milk replacers in treated nursing bitches and queens.

Drug Interactions—Concomitant use of hydroxyurea with fluorouracil may increase the potential for neurotoxicity. Hydroxyurea may produce additive bone marrow depression with other antineoplastic drugs and bone marrow depressants (e.g. chloramphenicol, flucytosine, amphotericin B, and colchicine).

Pharmaceutical Formulations—Available in 500 mg capsules.

IBUPROFEN

Ibuprofen

Proprietary Names—Brufen˙; Motrin˙; Rufen˙; Advil˙; Nuprin˙; Profen˙; Tabalon˙ 400; Ibugesic˙; Ibu-slo ˙.

Chemical Class—Propionic acid derivative.

Pharmacological Class—Nonsteroidal anti-inflammatory drug (NSAID); Analgesic-antipyretic; Non opioid analgesic.

Source—Synthetic.

Solubility, Stability and Storage—Ibuprofen is practically insoluble in water but very soluble in alcohol. Preparations containing ibuprofen should be stored in well-closed, light-resistant containers at 15–30°C.

Pharmacological Actions—Ibuprofen possesses analgesic, antipyretic and anti-inflammatory actions. It inhibits platelet aggregation and prolongs bleeding time.

Mechanism of Action—Ibuprofen inhibits cyclooxygenase-1 (COX-1) and—2 (COX-2) in the biosynthesis of prostaglandins.

Indications—Symptomatic treatment of musculo-skeletal disorders such as rheumatoid arthritis, osteoarthritis, tendonitis, and bursitis; relief of mild to moderate pain.

Dosage—12 to 15 mg/kg. Higher doses usually are required for anti-inflammatory effects than for analgesia.

Route(s) of Administration—Per os.

Absorption—Ibuprofen is rapidly absorbed from the GIT. Peak plasma concentration is attained within 1-2 hours (human) and 0.5-3 hours (dog).

Bioavailability—> 80% (human); 77% (dog).

Distribution—Vd = 0.15 ± 0.02 L/kg (human); 0.164 L/kg (dog). Ibuprofen gets into synovial fluid and crosses the placenta barrier.

Plasma Protein Binding—99%.

Metabolism—Ibuprofen is metabolized in the liver to hydroxylated and carboxylated products.

Plasma Half-Life—2 ± 0.5 hours (human); 4.6 ± 0.8 hours (dog).

Clearance—0.7 ± 0.20 ml/min/kg (human); 0.49 ml/min/kg (dog).

Onset of Action—0.1 to 1 hour (analgesia); 7 days (anti-inflammatory action).

Duration of Action—4 to 6 hours (analgesia). Peak Action. 1-2 weeks (anti-inflammatory action).

Route(s) of Excretion—Urine (< 1% as unchanged drug) and bile.

Toxicity and Adverse Effects—Gastrointestinal irritation resulting in gastric ulceration and/or bleeding; thrombocytopenia; CNS effects (characterized by dizziness and blurred vision), renal damage and prolonged bleeding time have all been reported. Prolonged use may cause increase in liver enzymes values, jaundice, increased serum K^+ value, and hematopoietic disorders (e.g. anemia, impaired formation of WBC). Ibuprofen consistently causes GI erosion in dogs following therapeutic doses for 2-6 weeks. Overdose may cause apnea, metabolic acidosis, renal failure, nystagmus and coma.

Management of Overdose—Give symptomatic and supportive treatment.

Contraindications—Pregnancy; active peptic ulcer; abnormal bleeding tendency; hypersensitivity to ibuprofen.

Precautions—Administer ibuprofen with food or milk. Use the drug cautiously in patients with history of allergic conditions, liver or kidney damage, and cardiac insufficiency. Monitor lithium or K levels when used concurrently with lithium preparations or potassium containing or potassium sparing drugs.

Drug Interactions—Ibuprofen may reduce the diuretic effects of furosemide and the antihypertensive effects of thiazides, β—adrenergic antagonists and inhibitors of angiotensin converting enzyme. It may increase the serum concentration of digoxin and phenytoin if used concurrently with the drugs. It reduces the uricosuric effects of probenecid and sulfinpyrazone while both drugs reduce its excretion. Ibuprofen increases methotrexate concentration. The effects of warfarin and ibuprofen on GI bleeding are synergistic.

Pharmaceutical Formulations—Available as the acid and as the potassium salt in 200, 300, 400, 600, 800 mg tablets and 100 mg/5 ml oral suspension. Sustained—release capsules (300 mg) (Ibu-slo *) are also available.

IDOXURIDINE

Idoxuridine

Proprietary Names—Herpid*; Herplex*; Iduridin*; Idustatin*; Iduviran*; Ophthalmadine*.

Chemical Class—Pyrimidine derivative.

Pharmacological Class—Antiviral drug; Nucleic Acid Synthesis Inhibitor.

Source—Synthetic.

Solubility, Stability and Storage—Idoxuridine is soluble 1 in 500 of water and 1 in 400 of ethanol. Store idoxuridine preparations in a cool place or in the refrigerator; do not freeze.

Pharmacological Actions—Idoxuridine is virustatic against herpes simplex virus.

Mechanism of Action—Idoxuridine resembles thymidine, one of the four building blocks of DNA (the genetic material of the herpes virus). As a result, idoxuridine is able to replace thymidine in the enzymatic step of viral replication or "growth" catalyzed by thymidylate phosphorylase and specific DNA polymerases. The consequent production of faulty DNA results in the inability of the virus to infect tissue or reproduce.

Indications—Treatment of keratoconjunctivitis and keratitis caused by herpes simplex virus in cats.

Dosages—Apply the ophthalmic preparation to affected eyes at interval of 2-3 hours.

Route(s) of Administration—Topical.

Absorption—Idoxuridine penetrates the conjunctiva and cornea poorly except where there is ulceration. It is poorly absorbed even when swallowed because of rapid deamination in the gastrointestinal tract.

Metabolism—Idoxuridine is rapidly inactivated by deaminases or nucleotidases.

Toxicity and Adverse Effects—Idoxuridine is generally well tolerated. It may cause some local irritation and increased sensitivity of the eyes to light. $LD_{50} = 3080$ mg/kg (orally in mice).

Contraindications—Documented hypersensitivity to idoxuridine.

Precautions—Idoxuridine should not be used with topical ophthalmic corticosteroids in the treatment of corneal ulceration. Effective cure takes weeks and treatment should continue for an additional week past the resolution of all clinical signs.

Drug Interactions—Boric acid contained in any ophthalmic preparation may interact with idoxuridine preparation to cause the formation of a gritty substance or toxic effect in the eye.

Pharmaceutical Formulations—Idoxuridine is available in ophthalmic solution with dimethyl sulfoxide as well as in ointment.

IMIDOCARB

Proprietary Names—Imizol'.

Chemical Class—Carbanilide derivative.

Pharmacological Class—Antiprotozoan drug.

Source—Synthetic.

Solubility, Stability and Storage—Store at room temperature.

Pharmacological Actions—Imidocarb is active against certain protozoan organisms such as *Babesia, Anaplasma,* and *Erlichia* spp. It possesses anticholinesterase properties.

Imidocarb

Mechanism of Action—Uncertain; two mechanisms have been proposed. Firstly by interfering with polyamine synthesis and function and secondly by combining with nucleic acids of DNA in susceptible organisms, causing partial uncoiling and denaturation of the DNA double helix.

Indications—Treatment of babesiosis and anaplasmosis in cattle, horses, sheep, and dogs; treatment of canine ehrlichiosis and hepatozoonosis.

Dosages—The recommended dose is 6.6 mg/kg; repeat the dose in two weeks for a total of two treatments. A dose single subcutaneous injection of 1.5 mg/kg of imidocarb dihydrochloride or 3.0 mg/kg of imidocarb dipropionate is highly effective against *A. marginale*. Elimination of the carrier state requires the use of higher repeated doses (e.g., two injections of imidocarb dihydrochloride 5 mg/kg IM or SC two weeks apart).

Route(s) of Administration—Intramuscular, subcutaneous.

Absorption—Poor oral absorption.

Distribution—Detectable only in the liver, kidney, and gut. Imidocarb is unusually persistent in body tissues.

Plasma Protein Binding—72 to 91%.

Metabolism—Not metabolized.

Plasma Half-life—3.45 hours.

Residue Limit—The highest concentrations of residues are found in the liver and kidney. Residues could still be detected in these organs for 55 days. Maximum residue limits for bovine and ovine tissues are 300 mcg/kg (muscle), 50 mcg/kg (fat and milk), 2000 mcg/kg (liver) and 1500 mcg/kg (kidney).

Withholding Period—Imidocarb has long withholding periods; 90 days before slaughter of cattle and 21 days before milking.

Route(s) of Excretion—Imidocarb is slowly excreted; two-thirds of the dose in urine and one-third in faeces.

Toxicity and Adverse Effects—Signs of toxicity are generally consistent with the anticholinesterase activity of imidocarb and include lethargy, salivation, lachrymation, muscle fasciculation, ataxia, tremors, and convulsions. These may be accompanied by signs of gastrointestinal, liver, kidney and lung dysfunction. Post-treatment vomition has also been observed in dogs. Imidocarb is reported safe in dogs up to 9.9 mg/kg. It causes pain upon injection; ulceration of injection site occurs at high doses. Imidocarb is a suspected carcinogen. Overdose causes salivation, diarrhea, anorexia, dyspnea, tachycardia, listlessness and weakness.

Management of Overdose/Toxicity—Atropine may be beneficial.

Contraindications—Intravenous injection; pregnancy; nursing animals; known hypersensitivity to imidocarb.

Precautions—Use anticholinesterase insecticides with caution during treatment with imidocarb.

Drug Interactions—Concurrent use with anticholinesterase agents may enhance imidocarb toxicity.

Formulations—Available as imidocarb dipropionate in 12% solution for injection. Also available as imidocarb dihydrochloride.

IPECAC

Synonyms—Ipecacuanha.

Proprietary Names—Ipecac® syrup.

Chemical Class—Alkaloid.

Pharmacological Class—Emetic.

Source—Natural; contains the major alkaloids emetine and cephaeline

Solubility, Stability and Storage—Store away from heat and direct light; keep the syrup from freezing.

Pharmacological Actions—Ipecac syrup effectively produces emesis which is intended to remove ingested poisons from the stomach. Emesis is noninvasive, and utilizes a physiological mechanism.

Mechanism of Action—Unknown.

Indications—To induce vomition in the early management of acute oral drug overdosage and in certain cases of oral poisoning. The current first-line treatment for most ingested poisons is now activated charcoal, which operates much more quickly and effectively than ipecac treatments.

Onset of Action—Vomiting typically happens within 15 to 20 minutes.

Toxicity and Adverse Effects—Diarrhea, dyspnea, lethargy, nausea or vomiting (continuing more than 30 minutes), fast or irregular heartbeat, stomach cramps or pain, are common adverse effects. There is an increased risk of heart problems, such as unusually fast heartbeat, if the ipecac is not vomited.

Contraindications—Poisoning caused by strychnine, corrosives such as alkalies (lye) and strong acids, petroleum distillates such as kerosene, gasoline, coal oil, fuel oil, paint thinner, or cleaning fluid; unconscious patient; convulsion; known hypersensitivity to ipecac.

Precautions—Emesis may not evacuate more than 78% of gastric content; patients should be observed carefully for signs of increasing intoxication. Use ipecac within 60 minutes of ingestion of a poison. Ipecac's potential side effects, such as lethargy, can be confused with the poison's effects, thus, causing complication in diagnosis.

Drug Interactions—Milk or milk products may reduce the effect of ipecac.

Pharmaceutical Formulations. Available as syrup. Fluidextract or Ipecac tincture should not be used. These pharmaceutical formulations are too strong and may cause serious side effects or death.

IRON DEXTRAN

Synonyms—Iron-Dextran Complex.

Proprietary Names—INFeD'; Iron Dextran Injection-200'.

Chemical Class—Elemental iron complexed with polyglucose.

Pharmacological Class. Hematinic.

Source—Synthetic.

Solubility, Stability and Storage—Iron-Dextran is miscible with water and 0.9% sodium chloride. Store iron-dextran product at room temperature between 59 and 86°F (15 to 30°C) away from heat and light.

Pharmacological Actions—Iron-Dextran corrects the erythropoietic abnormalities that are due to a deficiency of iron. Iron deficiency causes anemia with unusual tiredness or weakness, decreased physical endurance, shortness of breath, decreased resistance to infections, and slow growth. Iron does not stimulate erythropoiesis nor does it correct hemoglobin disturbances that are not caused by iron deficiency.

Mechanism of Action. It replaces iron that is essential to the production of healthy red blood cells.

Indications—Treatment and prevention of iron deficiency anemia in suckling piglets where it is normally administered in the first week of life. It is also used in other animals when oral iron preparations are ineffective or cannot be used.

Dosages—The dosage of iron dextran is expressed in terms of milligram of elemental iron.

Piglet	Prevention: 100-200 mg at 1-3 days of age; repeated after 10-14 days in severe cases.
	Treatment: 200 mg elemental iron at the first sign of iron deficiency.
Horse	0.5-1g per week; inject calculated dose into two sites.
Dog	10-20 mg/kg once, followed by oral iron preparation such as ferrous sulfate.

| Cat | 50 mg at 18 days of age. |
| Poultry | 10 mg/kg; repeat in 7-10 days if PCV remains below normal. |

Route(s) of Administration—Intramuscular.

Absorption—Iron-dextran is absorbed from the site of injection in two stages principally through the lymphatic system. In stage one which lasts about 3 days, a local inflammatory reaction facilitates passage of the drug from the site of IM injection into the lymphatic system. In the second slower phase, iron dextran is ingested by macrophages, which then enter the lymphatic system and eventually the blood. About 60% of IM dose is absorbed after 3 days and up to 90% is absorbed after 1-3 weeks; the remainder is gradually absorbed over a period of several months or longer.

Distribution—Iron-dextran is gradually cleared from the plasma by the reticuloendothelial cells of the liver, spleen, and bone marrow. These cells separate iron from the iron dextran complex and the iron becomes a part of the body's total iron stores. Ferric iron is gradually released into the plasma where it rapidly combines with transferrin and is carried to the bone marrow and incorporated into hemoglobin. Small amounts may reach the fetus. Traces of unmetabolized iron dextran are distributed into milk.

Plasma Half-life—About 6 hours (higher in patients with renal disease).

Route(s) of Excretion—Traces of unmetabolized iron dextran are excreted in urine, bile or feces.

Dialysis Status—Negligible.

Toxicity and Adverse Effects—Iron dextran may cause muscular weakness and prostration in piglets. It may stain muscle if injected after 4 weeks of birth of piglets. Overdose may lead to hemosiderosis. Anaphylactic reactions to iron dextran, including fatal anaphylaxis, have been reported in humans. Iron dextran may cause local reactions characterized by soreness or pain, inflammation, sterile abscesses, necrosis, and swelling at IM injection site.

Contraindications—Known hypersensitivity to iron dextran; anemia not due to iron deficiency; acute renal infections; concurrent use with oral iron supplements.

Precautions—Use iron-dextran with caution in patients with serious renal and hepatic impairment.

Drug Interactions—Iron-dextran is physically incompatible with oxytetracycline and sulfadiazine sodium.

Pharmaceutical Formulations—Available in liquid containing 200 mg/ml of iron as iron-dextran complex.

ISOMETAMEDIUM

Proprietary Names—Samorin®.

Chemical Class—Phenanthridium compound.

Pharmacological Class—Trypanocide.

Source—Synthetic.

Solubility, Stability and Storage—Isometamedium is slightly soluble in water. Isometamedium solutions should neither be heated above 40°C nor kept at elevated temperatures for more than brief periods. Solutions should be used as soon as possible the same day.

Pharmacological Actions—Isometamedium eliminates existing trypanosomal infection and confers protection against *T. vivax*, *T. congolense* and *T. brucei* infection for a period of two to six months depending on the dosage and the intensity of fly challenge.

Mechanism of Action—It binds to trypanosome kinetoplast and cleaves the kDNA-topoisomerase complex.

Indications—Treatment and prevention of *T. congolense* and *T. vivax* infections of cattle and other species. It has also been shown to be effective against *T. brucei* infection in dogs. Isometamedium is effective in *T. evansi* infections in camels, donkeys, buffaloes and dogs.

Dosages—For curative purposes, 0.25-0.5 mg/kg; for prophylaxis, 0.5-1 mg/kg. It is administered as 1 to 4% solution; 0.25 mg/kg gives a 1% solution while 0.5 mg/kg and 1 mg/kg give 2% and 4% solutions respectively when 1 g of samorin is dissolved in 100, 50 or 25 ml. When field conditions necessitate a standard dose for cattle, 5.0 ml 2% samorin solution (100 mg of active ingredients) may be employed. This provides a dosage of 0.25 mg to 0.5 mg per kg over a weight range of 200 kg to 400 kg. In cattle maintained continuously under challenge conditions two to six treatments per year may be required, depending on the level of fly challenge.

Route(s) of Administration—Preferably by deep intramuscular injection at the middle third of the side of the neck. Injection may be made into the muscle of the rump or thigh.

Absorption—Isometamedium is incompletely absorbed from IM site; peak plasma concentration is attained within 20-60 minutes.

Bioavailability—65.7%.

Distribution—Vd=18.5-39.3 L/kg. Following administration, the drug can be detected in the liver, kidney and site of injection weeks after.

Plasma Protein Binding—Isometamedium binds extensively to tissue at the intramuscular injection site to form a primary depot responsible for most of the prolonged chemoprophylactic effect of the drug.

Plasma Half-life—Approximately 13.8 days in sheep and 17.4 days in goat.

Residue Limit—Acceptable residue values in cattle tissues are 100 mcg/kg in muscle; 500 mcg/kg in liver; 1000 mcg/kg in kidney; 100 mcg/kg in fat and 100 mcg/kg in milk.

Toxicity and Adverse Effects—At low dosage, isometamedium is well tolerated. Muscular swellings which may lead to induration have been observed at dosages above 0.5 mg/kg. IM injection of concentrated solution of isometamedium results in local necrosis followed by encapsulation. The incidence of systemic toxicity is low at dosages up to 1mg/kg. Toxicity signs at higher doses include depression, ataxia and dyspnea. Others are loss of weight, diminished spermatogenesis, abnormal genital epithelial cells in the testis and abnormal mast cell degranulation.

Contraindications—Known hypersensitivity to isometamedium.

Precautions—For optimum response, isometamedium doses should be computed according to weight. Avoid leakage into the subcutaneous tissues.

Pharmaceutical Formulations. Available as isometamedium chloride in powder for reconstitution with injection water.

ISOPROTERENOL

Synonyms—Isopropylnorepinephrine; Isopropylnoradrenaline; Isopropylarterenol; Isoprenaline.

Proprietary Names—Isuprel®; Isopro®; Norisodrine®.

Chemical Class—Catecholamine.

Pharmacological Class—Direct-acting sympathomimetic drug; β-adrenergic agonist.

Source—Synthetic.

Solubility, Stability and Storage—Isoproterenol hydrochloride is freely soluble in water but sparingly soluble in alcohol. Isoproterenol hydrochloride preparations gradually darken on exposure to air, light, and heat and must be stored in tight, light-resistant containers at 8–15°C.

Isoproterenol

Pharmacological Actions—Isoproterenol causes vasodilatation and thus lowers peripheral vascular resistance in skeletal muscle, renal and mesenteric vascular beds resulting in a fall in diastolic blood pressure. It has positive inotropic and chronotropic actions on the heart thus causing increased cardiac output. It relaxes bronchial and gastrointestinal smooth muscles when the muscular tones are high. Isoproterenol inhibits antigen-induced release of histamine and other mediators of allergic reactions. It stimulates the release of free fatty acids. Isoproterenol stimulates some insulin secretion and thus causes less hyperglycemia than epinephrine.

Mechanism of Action—Isoproterenol activates β-adrenergic receptors.

Indications—Treatment of bronchospasm and cardiac disorders such as bradycardia, cardiac arrest and A-V block.

Dosages—

  Heart disorders: 0.4 mg in 250 ml dextrose saline by slow IV infusion followed by 0.1-0.2 mg IM every 4 hours.

  Bronchospasm: 0.2 mg in 50 ml dextrose saline and infuse slowly.

Route(s) of Administration—Intravenous, intramuscular and subcutaneous.

Absorption—Absorption of isoproterenol from the GIT is erratic. Peak plasma concentration is attained within 1-2 hours. It is readily absorbed from muscular and subcutaneous sites.

Bioavailability—Oral bioavailability is low because it is rapidly inactivated in the GIT.

Onset of Action—Onset is immediate following intravenous administration.

Duration of Action—1 hour (oral); 2 hours (subcutaneous). Action is brief following intravenous administration.

Metabolism—Isoproterenol is inactivated in the liver and other tissues by catechol-o-methyl-transferase.

Plasma Half-Life—2.5 to 5 minutes.

Route(s) of Excretion—Urine.

Toxicity and Adverse Effects—These are transient due to the brief duration of action of the drug. However, isoproterenol commonly causes palpitations, tachycardia, and flushed skin. Overdose may cause hypertension and then hypotension in addition to cardiac arrhythmias.

Management of Toxicity/Overdose—Give supportive and symptomatic therapy following reduction in infusion rate. β-Adrenergic blockers may be used in patients without bronchospasm.

Contraindications—Acute or chronic heart failure.

Precautions—Isoproterenol should be used with caution and under the supervision of an expert. Use the drug cautiously in patients with coronary insufficiency, hyperthyroidism, diabetes, hypertension and renal disease. Isoproterenol should also be used cautiously in conjunction with potassium–depleting diuretics (e.g. furosemide).

Drug Interactions—Thiobarbiturates, digoxin, trichloroethylene, ethyl chloride, cyclopropane, halothane, chloroform, and methoxyflurane sensitize the heart to the actions of isoproterenol. Other sympathomimetic amines may produce additive effects and increase the likelihood of toxicity. β-Adrenergic blockers such as propranolol may antagonize its actions. Concurrent use with oxytocic agents may cause hypertension.

Pharmaceutical Formulations—Available as isoproterenol hydrochloride in 0.2 mg/ml (0.02%) aqueous solution for injection or as 10 mg and 15 mg tablets. Also available in aerosol and solution for oral inhalation in humans (Medihaler-Iso®).

ISOSORBIDE

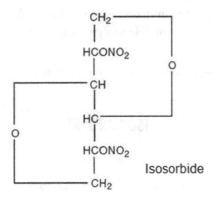

Isosorbide

Synonyms—Isosorbitol.

Proprietary Names—Ismotic®.

Chemical Class—Sugar alcohol; dihydric alcohol.

Pharmacological Class—Osmotic diuretic.

Source—Synthetic.

Pharmacological Actions—Isosorbide enhances the rate of urine flow that is accompanied by relatively smaller increment in the excretion of electrolytes. It also produces osmotic gradient that induces the diffusion of water from the intraocular fluid into plasma. These actions in the eye result in reduction of intraocular pressure.

Mechanism of Action—Isosorbide is osmotically active, therefore, it retains the fluid in the tubular lumen as well as extract some from the tissue.

Indications—Treatment of increased intraocular pressure.

Dosages—1.5 g/kg (dog).

Route(s) of Administration—Per os.

Absorption—Readily and almost completely absorbed after oral or sublingual administration.

Onset of Action—10 to 30 minutes in human.

Peak Action—1-1.5 hours in human.

Duration of Action—5-6 hours in human.

Distribution—Distributed in total body water.

Metabolism—Not metabolized.

Plasma Half-Life—5 to 9.5 hours.

Route(s) of Excretion—Urine.

Toxicity and Adverse Effects—Headache, disorientation, and vomiting have been reported in humans. Overdose may cause polyuria, dehydration, hypotension, cardiovascular collapse, and hyponatremia.

Management of Overdose/Toxicity—Discontinue the drug. Give supportive and symptomatic therapy—Pay attention to fluid and electrolyte balance.

Contraindications—Hypersensitivity to isosorbide; anuria; severe dehydration; pulmonary edema; severe renal disease; severely decompensated heart.

Precautions—Withdraw water from the subject for 4-6 hours following administration of isosorbide. Use the drug cautiously in patients with hypovolemia and impending pulmonary edema. Monitor and maintain fluid and electrolyte balance with multiple doses. Monitor urine output.

Pharmaceutical Formulations—Available in 45% oral solution.

ISOXSUPRINE

Proprietary Names—*Vasodilan®; Voxsuprine®. Navilox®.*

Pharmacological Class—Beta-adrenergic agonist; Vasodilator.

Source—Synthetic.

Solubility, Stability and Storage—Isoxsuprine is slightly soluble in water and sparingly soluble in alcohol. Store isoxsuprine products below 30°C in tight containers and in a dry place. Store Navilox® away from animal feeding stuffs. Reseal container after use.

Pharmacological Actions—Isoxsuprine causes direct relaxation of uterine and vascular smooth muscles. Its vasodilating actions are greater on the arteries supplying skeletal muscle than on those supplying skin. In horses with navicular disease, isoxsuprine raises distal limb temperatures. At high doses, isoxsuprine can decrease blood viscosity and reduce platelet aggregation.

Mechanism of Action—Isoxuprine stimulates beta-adrenergic receptors.

Indications—Treatment of navicular disease and laminitis. Isoxsuprine has been used to relax the uterus during the treatment of uterine infections in horses and to treat premature labor in other species.

Dosages—0.2 mg/kg to 0.6 mg/kg 2-4 times daily for 12 weeks. Administer Navilox® on empty stomach or approximately 30 minutes before feeding small quantity of feed.

Route(s) of Administration—Per os.

Absorption—In humans, isoxsuprine is almost completely absorbed from the GI tract.

Bioavailability (oral)—Low, probably due to a high first-pass effect.

Plasma Half-life—2.5 to 3.0 hours.

Route(s) of Excretion—Isoxsuprine may be detected in urine at low levels for long periods after administration.

Toxicity and Adverse Effects—The major side effects in horses are associated with the cardiovascular system and includes increased systolic and decreased diastolic pressures. Stimulation of the CNS characterized by uneasiness, hyperexcitability, and nose-rubbing have also been reported. Adverse effects in other species include nervousness, trembling, weakness, dizziness, palpitations, nausea, and vomiting. Overdose may cause sweating.

Management of Overdose/Toxicity—Stop the medication or reduce the dose. Give symptomatic and supportive therapy.

Contraindications—Pregnancy; within 14 days post-partum; arterial haemorrhage; horses intended for human consumption or competition; hypersensitivity to isuxsuprine.

Precautions—Avoid breathing the powder while mixing with feed. Do not eat, drink or smoke while using the product. Wash hands after use.

Drug Interactions—No clinically important interaction has been reported.

Pharmaceutical Formulations—Available as isoxsuprine hydrochloride in 10 mg and 20 mg tablets. Also available in white powder for addition to feeds (Navilox®) containing 3% isoxuprine hydrochloride with glucose as diluent. Each 10 g of powder contains 300 mg isoxsuprine hydrochloride.

ITRACONAZOLE

Synonyms—Oriconazole.

Proprietary Names—Sporonox®.

Chemical Class—Triazole compound.

Pharmacological Class—Antifungal agent.

Source—Synthetic.

Solubility, Stability and Storage—Itraconazole is practically insoluble in water but very slightly soluble in alcohol. Protect itraconazole products from light.

Pharmacological Actions—Itraconazole is effective against filamentous fungi, dimorphic fungi, and yeasts. It is particularly effective against *Aspergillus*. Itraconazole is fungistatic at the concentrations used systemically and fungicidal at the concentrations that may be achieved topically.

Mechanism of Action—Itraconazole inhibits cytochrome P450 oxidase mediated synthesis of ergosterol, an important component of the fungal cell wall. Without adequate ergosterol, the fungal cell becomes weak, leaky and ultimately dies.

Indications—Treatment of systemic fungal infections of dogs, cats and humans. It is also used topically in the treatment of ulcerative keratomycosis of horses.

Dosages—For aspergillosis in horses: 3 mg/kg twice a day; topical treatment every 2 hours for ulcerative keratomycosis.

Itraconazole

Route(s) of Administration—Per os and intravenous.

Absorption—Itraconazole is slowly but well absorbed after oral administration. A peak concentration is attained within 4 hours. Absorption is enhanced in the presence of food and in acidic intragastric environment.

Bioavailability (oral)—Highly variable; 50% or less with empty stomach; may approach 100% with food.

Distribution—Itraconazole is widely distributed throughout the body, particularly to tissues high in lipids. Itraconazole attains higher concentration in skin, female reproductive tract and pus greater than in serum. Only minimal concentrations are found in the CSF, aqueous humor and saliva.

Plasma Protein Binding—Highly protein bound (approximately. 99.8 % to albumin).

Metabolism—Metabolized by the liver to many different metabolites, including hydroxyitraconazole which is active.

Plasma Half-life—40 hours in horses and 21-64 hours in humans. Half-life increases following multiple dosing.

Clearance—Plasma, 18.7-22.9 L/h.

Route(s) of Excretion—Urine 40%, feces 8 to 18%.

Dialysis Status—Undialyzable.

Toxicity and Adverse Effects—Side effects of concern are anorexia, vomiting, and/or diarrhea. In dogs, hepatic toxicity appears to be the most significant adverse effect. At higher dose (10 mg/kg/day), some dogs may develop ulcerative skin lesions/vasculitis and limb edema. In cats, adverse effects such as anorexia, weight loss, vomiting, hepatotoxicity and depression have been noted. Uveitis may increase after the first day of therapy because of inflammation due to fungal death when used in the treatment of ulcerative keratomycosis.

Management of Overdose/Toxicity—Discontinue the medication. Oral antacids may help reduce absorption. If a large overdose occurs, consider gut emptying and give supportive therapy as required. After recovery, itraconazole can be restarted at a lower dose and/or reduced frequency.

Contraindications—Pregnancy; hepatic impairment; hypersensitivity to itraconazole or other azole antifungal agents.

Precautions. Itraconazole should be avoided in lactating animals.

Drug Interactions—Itraconazole may enhance the actions of amlodipine, digoxin, warfarin, quinidine and cyclosporine. Concurrent use with terfenadine and cisapride may cause serious heart abnormalities. Concurrent use of itraconazole and antacids reduces the absorption of itraconazole. It is recommended that at least 2 hours elapse between antacid administration and administration of itraconazole.

Pharmaceutical Formulations. Available in 100 mg capsules or as oral solution. The ophthalmic preparation of itraconazole contains 1% itraconazole, 30 % DMSO and artificial tears.

IVERMECTIN

Proprietary Names—Ivomec*; Iveen*; Ivojec*; Ivertin*; Lhivermectin*; Bimectin*; Mectizan*; Brema Mectin*.

Chemical Class—Macrocyclic lactone.

Pharmacological Class—Endectocide; Anthelmintic; Ectoparasiticide.

Source—Semisynthetic; obtained from a mixture of B_1 avermectins, products of *Streptomyces avermitilis*.

Solubility, Stability and Storage—Ivermectin is hydrophobic but soluble in organic solvents like propylene glycol, polyethylene glycol and vegetable oils. These and other solvents like glycerol, isopropyl alcohol have been used in ivermectin dosage forms. Ivermectin is rapidly degraded by UV light hence its products should be protected from light. Products may be stored at room temperature.

Pharmacological Actions—Ivermectin has nematocidal and ectoparasiticidal properties, hence it is also denoted as endectocide. It is extremely potent being active in microgram level. Its spectrum of activity includes major gastrointestinal nematodes, lung nematodes and ectoparasites of cattle, sheep, horses and pigs. Ear mites, sarcoptic mange, infective stage of *Dirofilaria immitis* in dogs and certain gastrointestinal nematodes and ectoparasites of chicken are susceptible to ivermectin. The drug is also effective against dung-breeding flies, *Onchocerca volvulus* and intestinal nematodes in humans. Ivermectin causes paralysis in parasites. It also reduces the reproductive potentials of nematodes, ticks, and dung-breeding flies. In *Onchocerca volvulus* infection, ivermectin causes marked decrease in microfilarial counts. It blocks the egress of microfilaria from the uterus of adult female worm and decreases the transmission of microfilariae to the *Simulium* vector.

Mechanism of Action—Ivermectin is known to increase neuronal chloride conductance by opening glutamate-gated chloride channels and also by potentiating the release and binding of GABA at certain synapses in invertebrates. This action results in hyperpolarization and reduced neuronal excitability thereby causing tonic paralysis of the peripheral musculature of susceptible parasites. It is not certain how ivermectin reduces reproductive potentials of parasites.

Mechanism of Selective Toxicity—High affinity avermectin receptors are absent in cestodes and trematodes. The sensitivity of avermectin receptors in nematodes and crustaceans is 100-fold higher than those in mammals.

Indications—Treatment of gastrointestinal nematode infections and control of ectoparasites in animals; control of onchocerciasis and treatment of scabies in human beings.

Dosages—

Horse, cattle, sheep, and goat. 0.2 mg/kg.

Pig. 0.3 mg/kg.

Dog. 0.006 mg/kg. (Higher doses (e.g. 0.05-0.5 mg/kg) expand the spectrum of activity).

Cat. 0.24 mg/kg (Higher doses may be required to eliminate hookworms).

Chickens. 0.2-0.3 mg/kg.

(See package insert for frequency and duration of treatment of different conditions).

Route(s) of Administration—Subcutaneous (SC); topical (pour-on); per os. Pharmacokinetic profile depends on route, species and formulation.

Absorption—Ivermectin is slowly absorbed from subcutaneous site. Up to 95% of oral dose is absorbed in simple stomachs; fewer amounts are absorbed in ruminants.

Bioavailability—Higher with SC injection than with per os; also higher with oral aqueous micelle formulation than with oral paste formulation. Ivermectin bioavailability is low in cats.

Peak Plasma Concentration—2 days (SC in cattle); 5.2 hours (per os in dogs); 0.5 days (per os in pigs); 2 days (SC in pigs); 4-5 hours (oral aqueous micelle formulation in horses); 15 hours (oral paste formulation in horses); 4 hours (per os in humans).

Duration of Action—> 2 weeks (SC injection).

Distribution—Vd = 1.9 L/kg in cattle; 4.61 L/kg in sheep. Ivermectin is well distributed into tissues. It accumulates in the liver, fat and bile. It crosses the blood-brain-barrier (BBB) poorly presumably because of a P-glycoprotein efflux pump operative at the BBB. Small amounts appear in milk.

Plasma Protein Binding—93% in human.

Metabolism. Ivermectin is degraded mainly in the liver. The products of metabolism vary with animal species. It is also partially inactivated in the rumen.

Plasma Half-life—2.8 days (IV in cattle); 1.6-1.8 days (IV in dogs); 2.7 days (IV in sheep); 8 days (SC in cattle); 3-5 days (per os in sheep); 27 hours (per os in humans).

Clearance—0.79 ml/min/kg in cattle.

Withdrawal Period—Varies with the formulation and species. withdrawal period before slaughter in cattle is 35 days (1% solution) or 24 days (oral paste) and 18 days in pigs.

Route(s) of Excretion—Excreted mainly in feces as unchanged drug; very little in urine; 5% may appear in milk of lactating animal.

Toxicity and Adverse Effects—Ivermectin has high safety margin apparently because the GABA-gated sites at which it acts is situated in the CNS in mammals to where it distributes poorly. However, high doses cause mydriasis and CNS toxicity with such signs as lethargy, ataxia, tremor, and eventually death in humans and animals, especially dogs. Collie dogs are particularly sensitive to ivermectin. It causes mild itching and swollen lymph nodes in humans with onchocerciasis. Hypersensitivity reactions to dying microfillariae have been reported in horses and dogs.

Management of Overdose/Toxicity—Give symptomatic and supportive therapy. Hypersensitivity reaction may be controlled with corticosteroids.

Contraindications—Hypersensitivity reaction to ivermectin or any component; milk producing animals; pregnant dairy cow within 28 days to calving; puppies less than 6 weeks.

Precautions—Reduce the dose of ivermectin in collie dogs. Avoid concurrent administration with drugs that cause CNS depression. Do not administer ivermectin in situations where the integrity of the blood-brain–barrier may be compromised as in meningitis.

Drug Interactions—Picrotoxin, a GABA antagonist can reverse 50% of ivermectin actions.

Pharmaceutical Formulations. Ivermectin is available in several formulations designed to suit every host species. These formulations include sterile solutions of 0.27% and 1% ivermectin (W/V) in 60% propylene glycol and 40% glycerol for SC injection; oral solutions of 0.08%, 0.4% and 1% ivermectin (W/V) in aqueous micelle (polysorbate 80); paste formulation containing 1.87% ivermectin (W/V) in 79% propylene glycol; pour-on formulation containing 0.5% ivermectin (W/V) in 80% isopropyl alcohol; extended release formulation containing 1.7g ivermectin in a wax vehicle designed to release ivermectin for up to 135 days; chewable cubes containing 68, 136, or 272 mcg ivermectin. Formulations of ivermectin in combination with other anthelmintics like 10% clorsulon (Ivomec Super˚) or pyrantel pamoate are also available. Availability of formulation depends on the market. Ivermectin is available in 6 mg tablets for use in human beings.

KAOLIN/PECTIN

Proprietary Names—Kaopec˚; Kaolin et morphine˚.

Chemical Class—Kaolin is an aluminum compound; pectin is a carbohydrate.

Pharmacological Class—Antidiarrheal agent; Adsorbent; Protectant.

Source—Natural; kaolin is a naturally occurring hydrated aluminum silicate. Pectin is obtained from the inner rind of citrus fruits, apple pomace and papaya.

Solubility, Stability and Storage—Kaolin is practically insoluble in water; pectin is sparingly soluble in water to form a viscous, colloidal solution. Kaolin/pectin should be stored in airtight containers; protect from freezing.

Pharmacological Actions—Kaolin/pectin possess both adsorbent and protective properties. They adsorb bacteria and toxins in the gut and the coating action of the suspension protects inflamed GI mucosa. The pectin component decreases intestinal pH by forming galacturonic acid.

Indications—Treatment of diarrhea and dysentery; it has also been used as an adsorbent following the ingestion of certain toxins.

Dosages—0.5-2 ml/kg every 2 to 6 hours.

Route(s) of Administration—Per os.

Absorption—Neither kaolin nor pectin are absorbed after oral administration.

Metabolism—Up to 90% of the pectin administered may disintegrate in the gut.

Toxicity and Adverse Effects—Kaolin/pectin may not cause adverse effects at usual doses. Constipation may occur at high doses. This effect is usually transient. In rats, kaolin/pectin has been demonstrated to increase fecal sodium loss in diarrhea. Overdose is unlikely to cause any serious effects, but constipation requiring treatment may occur.

Management of Overdose/Toxicity—Give symptomatic therapy.

Contraindications—Known hypersensitivity to kaolin/pectin.

Precautions—Kaolin/pectin should not replace adequate fluid/electrolyte monitoring or replacement therapy in severe or chronic diarrheas.

Drug Interactions—Kaolin/pectin may inhibit the oral absorption of lincomycin, tetracyclines, and anticholinergic drugs. If these drugs must be used, administer kaolin/pectin at least 2 hours before or 3-4 hours after the drugs. Kaolin/pectin is incompatible with alkalis, heavy metals, salicylic acid, tannic acid or strong alcohol.

Pharmaceutical Formulations—The drug is available as oral suspension containing one percent pectin and 20% kaolin. A mixture of kaolin and morphine is also available.

KETAMINE

Proprietary Names—Ketaset˙; Ketalar˙; Vetalar˙ (veterinary).

Chemical Class—Arylcycloalkylamine.

Pharmacological Class—General anesthetic; Dissociative anesthetic; Injectable anesthetic.

Source—Synthetic.

Solubility, Stability and Storage—Ketamine is soluble 1 in 4 of water, 1 in 14 of ethanol and 1 in 6 of methanol. It is sparingly soluble in chloroform but practically insoluble in ether.

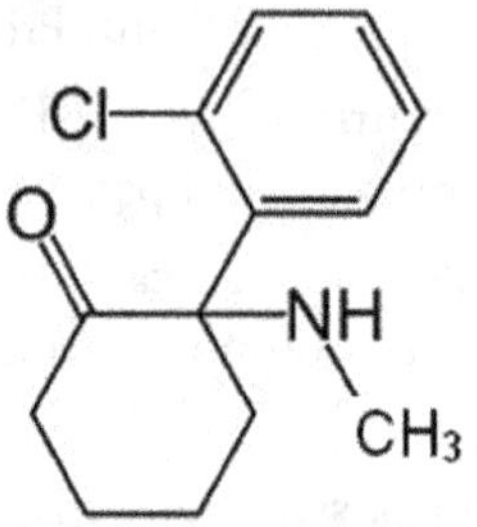

Ketamine

Pharmacological Actions—Ketamine depresses the CNS to cause sedation, rapid general anesthesia, amnesia, and marked analgesia. It creates a strong feeling of dissociation from the environment. Ketamine induces stages I and II anesthesia, not stage III. It causes slight hypothermia in cats. It also causes increased cardiac output and heart rate, variable peripheral resistance and increased intracranial pressure.

Mechanism of Action—Ketamine is an NMDA (N-methyl D-aspartate) receptor antagonist. NMDA receptor blockade is believed to mediate the analgesic effects of ketamine at low doses. At high doses, ketamine binds to opioid mu and sigma receptors. It has also been shown to act as a potent D_2 receptor partial agonist as well as a dopamine reuptake inhibitor.

Indications—Ketamine is used to induce general anesthesia in several animal species. It also used for chemical restraint in subhuman primates. Ketamine is suitable for in-patient use in small animals because of slow recovery. It is usually administered with sedatives such as acepromazine, xylazine or diazepam to provide muscle relaxation. It has also been used in combination with detomidine and medetomidine.

Dosages—

Ketamine alone:

Bird	10-50 mg/kg IM. Note: Rarely used alone.
Goat	22-44 mg/kg IM.
NHP	10-30 mg/kg IM
Sheep	22-44 mg/kg IM
Pig	15-25 mg/kg IM or 15-20 mg/kg IV.

Ketamine and acepromazine (respectively).

Bird	10-25 mg/kg IM and 0.5-1 mg/kg IM.
Cat	20 mg/kg IM and 0.11 mg/kg IM.
NHP	4 mg/kg IM and 0.4 mg/kg IM.

Ketamine and medetomidine (respectively) (not for major surgical procedures):

Cat	2-3 mg/kg IV and 30-50 µg/kg IV
	3-7 mg/kg IM and 40-80 µg/kg IM.
Dog	1-3 mg/kg IV and 10-20 µg/kg IV.
	3-5 mg/kg IM and 30-40 µg/kg IM.
Goat	1 mg/kg IM and 25 µg/kg IM.
Sheep	1 mg/kg IM and 25 µg/kg IM.
Pig	10 mg/kg IM and 0.08 mg/kg IM.

Ketamine and xylazine (respectively):

Bird	10-50 mg/kg IM and 1-10 mg/kg IM.
	2.5-5 mg/kg IV and 0.25-0.5 mg/kg IV.
NHP	10 mg/kg IM and 0.5 mg/kg IM.
Cat	22 mg/kg IM and 1.1 mg/kg IM and *atropine* (0.04 mg/kg IM).
Horse, donkey	2.2 mg/kg IV and1.1 mg/kg IM.
Pig	2-5 mg/kg IV (or 12-15 mg/kg IM) and 1.1 mg/kg IM.
Calf, sheep, goat	10 mg/kg IM and 0.2 mg/kg IM; with *atropine* 0.04 mg/kg IM.

Route(s) of Administration—Ketamine is administered parenterally but it may be effective orally.

Bioavailability—Oral bioavailability is 20.7%.

Effective Concentration—100 to 150 ng/ml.

Duration of Action—10 to 15 minutes to reach unconscious state; 30-40 minutes to induce analgesia; 1-2 hours for amnesia. Duration is dependent more on redistribution than metabolism.

Distribution—Vd = 1.8 ± 0.7 L/kg. Ketamine is rapidly distributed to all body tissues particularly adipose tissue, liver, lung and brain. Ketamine undergoes redistribution.

Plasma Protein Binding—50% (horse); 53% (dog); 37-53% (cat).

Metabolism—Occurs in the liver by N-demethylation and hydroxylation.

Plasma Half-Life—1 hour in animals; 2-3 hours ± 0.5 hours in human beings.

Clearance—15 ± 5 ml/min/kg.

Route(s) of Excretion—Excreted in urine (4 ± 3%) and bile.

Toxicity and Adverse Effects—Ketamine causes emergence phenomena characterized by disorientation, sensory and perceptual illusions and vivid dreams in humans, especially in adults above the age of 30 years. Seizures have been reported in 20% of cats. Hyper salivation and other autonomic signs have been observed. Tachycardia, muscle twitching and mild tonic convulsions have been reported in cats, horses and dogs following administration of ketamine alone.

Management of Overdose—Give supportive therapy. Administer atropine or glycopyrrolate to reduce autonomic signs.

Contraindications—Hypersensitivity to ketamine; elevated CSF pressure or head injury; hepatic or renal impairment; last trimester of pregnancy.

Precautions—Ketamine is potentially dangerous when intracranial pressure is elevated. Do not use ketamine as the lone anesthetic in horses, donkeys, or dogs.

Drug Interactions—The incidence of emergence phenomena can be reduced by prior administration of midazolam (a benzodiazepine). Recovery from ketamine-induced anesthesia may be prolonged by other CNS depressants. Ketamine is antagonized by physostigmine in humans. Chloramphenicol may prolong anesthesia induced by ketamine.

Pharmaceutical Formulations—The drug is available as ketamine hydrochloride supplied in solutions for injection in vials containing 10, 50, or 100 mg of ketamine base per milliliter.

KETOCONAZOLE

Ketoconazole

Proprietary Names—Nizoral®, Xolegel®, Extina®

Chemical Class—Imidazole derivative.

Pharmacological Class—Antimycotic agent; Antifungal drug.

Source—Synthetic.

Solubility, Stability and Storage—Ketoconazole is insoluble in water. Its formulations are better stored at room temperature in tightly closed containers.

Pharmacological Actions—Ketoconazole could be fungistatic or fungicidal depending on the dose and organism. Its spectrum of activity includes dermatophytes, yeasts and other fungi. Pathogenic fungi such as *Blatomyces, Coccidiodes, Cryptococcus, Histoplasma, Microsporum* and *Trichophyton* are susceptible. Ketoconazole inhibits the synthesis of cortisone and testosterone.

Mechanism of Action—Not certain; may be associated with cell membrane permeability arising from its interference with ergosterol synthesis.

Indications—Treatment of systemic and some cutaneous mycoses. Ketoconazole can be used in the treatment of Cushing's disease, where an excess amount of adrenal hormone is produced.

Dosages—

Bird	Psittacines. 30 mg/kg PO q12h.
Cat	10-20 mg/kg PO q8-12h.
Dog	10-20 mg/kg PO q8-12h.
Reptile	Tortoises. 30 mg/kg PO once a day for 2-4 weeks.

Route(s) of Administration—Per os.

Absorption—Ketoconazole is readily but incompletely absorbed; peak plasma concentration is attained within 1-4 hours in dogs. The drug is better absorbed from acid medium.

Bioavailability—Oral bioavailability is variable in dogs (ranges between 4-89%).

Distribution—Ketoconazole is widely distributed. It attains high concentration in body fluids such as bile, cerumen, saliva, synovial fluid, and tissues including liver, adrenals and pituitary glands. Ketoconazole level in the CSF increases when meninges are inflamed. Levels in kidney, lung, bladder, myocardium, bone marrow are moderate. It crosses the placenta and is distributed into milk.

Plasma Protein Binding—84-99%.

Metabolism—The drug is metabolized to inactive products.

Plasma Half-life—1 to 6 hours in dog and 6-10 hours in human.

Route(s) of Excretion—Ketoconazole is excreted mainly in feces via bile; 13% of dose is excreted in urine with 2-4% as unchanged drug.

Toxicity and Adverse Effects—Ketoconazole has wide safety margin. However, nausea, vomiting, and diarrhea are usual. It may cause hepatotoxicity at higher doses in cats. Its effects on testosterone secretion produce feminization effect in male animals. Ketoconazole is teratogenic and embryotoxic, at least, in rats. It may cause male infertility.

Management of Overdose/Toxicity—Give general antidotal therapy in cases of overdose. Vomition and diarrhea may be reduced by giving ketoconazole with food or by dividing a dose into several smaller doses.

Contraindications—Breeding male animals; known hypersensitivity to ketoconazole.

Precautions—Use ketoconazole cautiously in hepatic impairment and thrombocytopenia. Administer the drug with meal to reduce GI upset. The benefit of its use in pregnancy must be weighed against the risk of teratogenic and embryotoxic effects.

Drug Interactions—Ketoconazole may increase the blood levels of cyclosporine, cisapride, aminophylline, and warfarin. H_2–blockers (e.g. cimetidine) and antacids reduce the absorption of ketoconazole.

Pharmaceutical Formulations—Ketoconazole is available in 20 mg tablets and cream.

KETOPROFEN

Ketoprofen

Proprietary Names—Orudis'; Oruvail®; Ketofen® (veterinary).

Chemical Class—Propionic acid derivative.

Pharmacological Class—Nonsteroidal Anti-inflammatory Drug.

Source—Synthetic.

Solubility, Stability and Storage—Ketoprofen is practically insoluble in water and freely soluble in alcohol at 20°C. Ketoprofen capsules are better stored at room temperature in tightly closed containers away from light. The solution for injection store well at room temperature.

Pharmacological Actions—Ketoprofen has potent analgesic, antipyretic and anti-inflammatory actions.

Mechanism of Action—It is an inhibitor of cyclooxygenase and thus of prostaglandin synthesis. It also stabilizes lysosomal membranes and may antagonize the actions of bradykinin.

Indications—Ketoprofen is used for short-term management of post-surgical pain in dogs and cats; management of musculoskeletal pain due to soft tissue injury, synovitis, and osteoarthritis in horses. On occasion it may be used for the longer-term management of chronic pain particularly due to osteoarthritis.

Dosages—

Dog and cat: 2 mg/kg as a loading dose followed in 24 hours with 1 mg/kg daily.

Horse: 2.2 mg/kg daily for 5 days by IV.

Route(s) of Administration—Oral and intravenous routes are suitable.

Absorption—Ketoprofen is rapidly and almost completely absorbed from simple stomachs. Peak plasma concentration is attained within 1-2 hours. The rate of absorption is reduced by food and milk products.

Bioavailability—~100% (humans).

Onset of Action—2 hours post dose in horses.

Peak Action—12 hours after dose in horses.

Distribution—Vd = 0.15 ± 0.03 l/kg in human beings. Ketoprofen is distributed into canine milk.

Plasma Protein Binding—99.2 ± 0.1% (human); 93% (horse).

Metabolism—The drug is conjugated in the liver to ketoprofen glucuronide.

Plasma Half-Life—1.8 ± 0.3 hours (human); 1.5 hours (horse).

Clearance (ml/min/kg)—1.2 ± 0.3 (lower in the aged and uremia).

Route(s) of Excretion—Eliminated via urine (with < 1% as unchanged drug).

Toxicity and Adverse Effects—The most common side effects of ketoprofen include ulceration of the GI tract and a drop in the erythrocyte count due to GI bleeding. Rare side effects include kidney damage, bleeding disorders, and protein loss. Injection site reactions can occur if blood or the drug leaks into the site. Overdose may cause GI ulcers, protein loss, kidney and liver damage. Early signs of toxicity include loss of appetite, and depression.

Management of Overdose/Toxicity—Initiate general antidotal therapy. Give supportive and symptomatic treatment.

Contraindications—Active gastrointestinal ulceration or bleeding; known hypersensitivity to ketoprofen.

Precautions—Oral administration may be given with food. Use the drug cautiously in patients with impaired hepatic or renal function. Reduce the dose in animals with hypoproteinemia. Ketoprofen effects on fertility in breeding animals are not known; therefore it should be used in breeding animals with caution, when the potential benefits outweigh the potential risks. NSAIDs cause premature closure of patent ductus, thus, use of ketoprofen in late pregnancy should be avoided.

Drug Interactions—Ketoprofen is highly protein bound and may displace or be displaced by other protein bound drugs (such as anticoagulants, sulfonamides, phenylbutazone, hydatoins etc.) from binding sites. This may increase the free portion of displaced drugs in plasma. Ketoprofen increases blood concentration, half-life and likelihood of toxicity of methotrexate. Probenecid increases the half-life and reduces the protein binding of ketoprofen. GI bleeding or ulceration may be severe if used with drugs that alter hemostasis (e.g. heparin, warfarin) or cause ulceration (e.g. aspirin, phenylbutazone, corticosteroids etc.).

Pharmaceutical Formulations—Ketoprofen is available in 25 mg, 50 mg, and 75 mg immediate release capsules as well as 200 mg extended release capsules. The drug is also available in 100 mg/ml solution for parenteral administration.

LEVAMISOLE

Levamisole Hydrochloride

Proprietary Names—Ketrax'; Levasol'; Nilverm'; Ripercol'; Alfamisol®; Levaverm®; Levamisol®; Levaject®; Wormsol®; Levamizole®; Levadex®; Levi-worm®; Wormsol Plus® (in combination with rafoxanide); Vermicanis®; (in combination with niclosamide); Vermofas Drench® (in combination with oxyclozanide).

Chemical Class—Imidazothiazole compound; the l-isomer of dl tetramisole.

Pharmacological Class—Anthelmintic; Immunostimulatory agent.

Source—Synthetic.

Solubility, Stability, and Storage—Levamisole is soluble in water. Levamisole hydrochloride products should be kept at room temperature not exceeding 40°C. Levamisole phosphate products for injection may be refrigerated but not frozen. Unused drench may be stable for 7-12 days. The powder formulation administered in drinking water may be stable for 3 months after mixing provided it is kept in well capped container.

Pharmacological Actions—As an anthelmintic, levamisole is active against adult and larvae states of *Haemonchus, Ostertagia, Trichostrongylus, Cooperia, Nematodirus, Bunostomum, Oesophagostomum, Metastrongylus, Ascaris, Hyostrongylus, Trichuris* and *Dictyocaulus* in livestock. It is also effective against *Capillaria, Ascaridia* and *Heterakis* in poultry. Levamisole has immunostimulatory, nicotinic and muscarinic activities.

Mechanism of Action—Low levels of the drug cause ganglion stimulation leading to paralysis of the worm followed by expulsion. High levels of levamisole blocks the metabolic pathway leading to ATP production at the fumarate reductase and succinate oxidation sites. Its immunostimulatory action is due to stimulation of phagocytosis and restoration of cell-mediated immune function in T-lymphocytes.

Indications—Treatment and strategic dosing against gastrointestinal worms and lungworms in livestock, poultry and dogs. To stimulate immunity in calves, dogs, cats and human patients with immunodeficiencies, chronic infection, inflammatory disease and some malignancies. It has been used in humans to treat colorectal carcinoma (in combination with fluorouracil).

Dosages—

Cattle, sheep, goat and pig: 4-11mg/kg body weight.

Poultry: 18-36 mg/kg body weight.

Dog, cat and NHP: 5-10 mg/kg body weight

Fish: 100 mg/25 g food.

Route(s) of Administration—Per os; subcutaneous; topically (as pour-on).

Absorption—Levamisole is rapidly absorbed from the GIT and skin.

Distribution—The drug is widely distributed.

Metabolism—It is significantly metabolized. Only 6% appear as unchanged drug in urine.

Plasma Half-Life—4-6 hours (cattle); 1.8-4 hours (dogs); 3.5-6.8 hours (pigs).

Residue Limit—0.1 ppm negligible residue in edible tissues of cattle, sheep, and pigs.

Withholding Period—A slaughter clearance period of 2-9 days is recommended, depending on the formulation.

Route(s) of Excretion—Feces (41% of dose), Urine (40% of dose), and expired gases.

Toxicity and Adverse Effects—Levamisole has low safety margin, especially in horses and dogs. Toxic signs include salivation, lacrimation, head shaking, muscle tremors, mild excitability, and vomiting. There is usually tissue reaction at the site of injection. Signs of overdose with levamisole resemble those of organophosphate poisoning and include hypersalivation, hyperesthesia, defecation, urination, CNS depression, and collapse. Acute overdose may cause death due to respiratory failure.

Management of Overdose/Toxicity—Give supportive therapy.

Contraindications—Dairy animals of breeding age; known hypersensitivity to levamisole.

Precautions—The margin of safety is low in equines. Do not crush or make suspension from tablets.

Drug Interactions—Levamisole can safely be combined with other anthelmintics but its toxicity may be enhanced by drugs with parasympathomimetic actions (e.g. pyrantel, morantel, diethylcarbamazine, organophosphates, and neostigmine). Concurrent administration of levamisole and chloramphenicol has been reported to cause fatalities.

Pharmaceutical Formulations—The drug is available as levamisole hydrochloride in 40 mg tablets and 40 mg/5 ml syrup for humans. It is available as boluses, pellets, soluble drench, wettable powder for addition to drinking water, and injectable solution for animal use. Levamisole phosphate solution is more suitable for subcutaneous injection as it causes less irritation. A 10% pour-on formulation is also available for application to the midline of the back in animals. Formulations of levamisole in combination with cestocides (e.g. niclosamide) and trematocides (e.g. rafoxanide) are also available.

LEVOTHYROXINE SODIUM

Synonyms—L-Thyroxine sodium; L-T_4; Sodium levothyroxine; T_4 thyroxine sodium.

Proprietary Names—**Veterinary**: Soloxine*; Pan thyroid liquid*; Thyro-Tab*; Thyro—Form*; Thyro-L powder*; Thyrosyn*; Thyroxine-L*; Thyrozine*. **Human**: Levothroid*; Levoxyl*; Synthroid*; Levo-T*; Eltroxin*; Thyrex*.

Chemical Class—Iodinated thyronine derivative.

Pharmacological Class—Thyroid hormone.

Source—Synthetic.

Pharmacological Actions—Levothyroxine stimulates normal growth and development; increases basal metabolic rate and cholesterol metabolism; stimulates protein synthesis; promotes gluconeogenesis and increases utilization of glycogen stores. Qualitatively, levothyroxine possesses the same activity as thyroid extracts but 0.1 mg of levothyroxine is approximately equal in activity to 60 mg of the dried thyroid extract.

Mechanism of Action—Levothyroxine is converted to triiodothyronine which acts by interacting with specific receptors on nuclei, mitochondria and plasma membranes of cells. For instance, it activates plasma membrane-bound Na^+, K^+-ATPase to increase oxygen consumption.

Indications—Replacement or supplemental therapy in thyroid hypofunction and treatment of myxedema coma in all animal species; treatment of bilateral alopecia, obesity and urinary incontinence in dogs.

Dosages—

Dog	20-22 mcg/ kg orally every 12 hours initially. This may be reduced to once a day. Dogs with cardiac problems require 5 mcg/kg twice daily. This dose is gradually increased over 3-4 weeks.
Cat	10-20 mcg/kg/ day.
Horse	10 mg orally once daily or divided every 12 hours.
Cattle	50-100 mg PO, daily; 5-8 mg SC, daily.
Bird	0.1 mg tablet in 30-120 ml of water and administer for 15 minutes (for water drinkers).
Tortoise	0.02 mg/kg orally every other day.

Route(s) of Administration—It may be administered per os. Intramuscular and intravenous routes are used in myxedema coma.

Absorption—Incomplete and variable from the oral route; 42-74% is rapidly absorbed in humans; 10-50% is absorbed in dogs and 10.4% in cats. Absorption is increased by fasting. Peak plasma concentration is attained within 4-12 hours (in dogs), 2-4 hours (in humans) following oral administration.

Levothyroxine

Onset of Action—Oral, 3-5 days; IV, 6-8 hours.

Peak Action—Up to 10 days (oral); 24 hours (IV).

Distribution—Plasma pool is 46% in dog, 13% in cat and 32% in human. The rapidly equilibrating pool (liver and kidney) is 23% in dog, 19% in cat and 26% in human. Slowly equilibrating pool (muscle, skin) is 31% in dog, 68% in cat and 42% in human.

Plasma Protein Binding—99.7%.

Metabolism—Levothyroxine is metabolized in the liver to triiodothyronine.

Plasma Half-Life—6-7 days in human (3-4 days in patients with hyperthyroidism), 7-16 hours in dog and 10.7 hours in cat.

Clearance—(ml/min/kg)—0.24 (dog); 0.38 (cat); 0.017 (human).

Route(s) of Excretion—Feces and urine.

Dialysis Status—Non dialyzable.

Toxicity and Adverse Effects—Increased and irregular heart rate, forceful heartbeat, prominent arterial pulses, increased appetite, loss of weight, flushed moist and warm skin, weak and tremulous muscles, insomnia, restlessness and increased bowel movement are early manifestations of overdose. Excessive doses result in iatrogenic thyrotoxicosis characterized by polyuria, polydipsia, nervousness, weight loss, increased appetite, panting and fever.

Management of Overdose/Toxicity—Withdraw the drug; reduce gastrointestinal absorption; give general supportive therapy; give digitalis to control congestive heart failure; use beta adrenergic blocker (e.g. propranolol) to control enhanced adrenergic activities.

Contraindications—Myocardial infarction, thyrotoxicosis, uncorrected adrenal insufficiency, hypersensitivity to levothyroxine sodium or any component such as tartrazine dye.

Precautions—Reduce the initial dose and use with caution in patients with cardiovascular disease, concurrent hypoadrenocorticism, diabetes and the elderly. Administer when stomach is empty.

Drug Interactions—Phenytoin reduces levothyroxine effect by reducing its level. Cholestyramine reduces its absorption. Amiodarone decreases the conversion of thyroxine to triiodothyronine. Desmethylamodarone, a major metabolite of amiodarone decreases triiodothyronine binding to its nuclear receptors. Levothyroxine increases the effects of oral coagulants, catecholamines and sympathomimetic drugs. Tricyclic antidepressants increase its toxic potential.

Pharmaceutical Formulations—

Veterinary: Available in tablets containing 0.1 mg, 0.2 mg, 0.3 mg, 0.4 mg, 0.5 mg, 0.6 mg, 0.7 mg, and 0.8 mg. Also available in 0.22% powder for use in horses.

Human: Available in powder for injection in 6 ml and 10 ml vials containing 0.2 mg or 0.5 mg/vial. Also available in tablets containing 0.025 mg, 0.05 mg, 0.075 mg, 0.088 mg, 0.1 mg, 0.112 mg, 0.125 mg, 0.137 mg, 0.15 mg, 0.175 mg, 0.2 mg and 0.3 mg.

LIDOCAINE

Lidocaine

Synonyms—Lignocaine.

Proprietary Names—Xylocaine®.

Chemical Class—Xylidide derivative.

Pharmacological Class—Amide type local anesthetic agent.

Source—Synthetic.

Solubility, Stability and Storage—Lidocaine is very soluble in water and alcohol. Lidocaine hydrochloride solutions are highly resistant to acid or alkaline hydrolysis and can be autoclaved repeatedly. Epinephrine-containing solutions are not stable to autoclaving. Lidocaine hydrochloride injections should be stored at room temperature; freezing should be avoided.

Pharmacological Actions—Lidocaine reversibly blocks the initiation and conduction of nerve impulses thereby causing loss of sensation. It provides relief from pain when applied locally. Lidocaine is effective when applied to mucosa and abraded skin making it suitable for ophthalmic purposes, membrane anesthesia and pruritus.

Mechanism of Action—Lidocaine blocks the permeability of nerve axon membrane to Na^+ thereby preventing the generation of action potential. This renders the nerve unexcitable.

Indications—For topical, infiltration, and regional anesthesia, with or without adrenaline. Lidocaine has been administered intraperitoneally for anesthesia of the peritoneum and pelvic viscera. It is also used without epinephrine to treat ventricular arrhythmias.

Dosages—Dosage varies with anesthetic procedure, desired level of anaesthesia and individual patient response. The table below is a guide with the 2% solution of lidocaine hydrochloride.

Horse	Epidural: 6-10 mL. Infiltration: 200 mL maximum.
Cattle	Epidural: 5-6 mL. Infiltration: 200 mL maximum.
	Nerve block: up to 10 mL. Corneal injection: 2-6 mL.
Sheep	Epidural: 3-4 mL. Infiltration: 60 mL maximum.

Pig	Infiltration: 60 mL maximum.
Dog	Epidural: 0.2 mL/kg. Infiltration: 25-50 mL.
	Nerve block: 2-4 mL/site.
	Ventricular arrhythmias: 1-2 mg/kg IV every 20-30 minutes.
Cat	Epidural: 0.2 mL/kg. Infiltration: 5-20 mL
Topical (surface) anaesthesia	2-4% concentration applied to mucous membranes.

Route(s) of Administration—Topical; infiltration; regional (spinal, epidural, paravertebral).

Absorption—Lidocaine is readily absorbed from the gastrointestinal tract, mucous membranes, damaged skin (poor absorption from intact skin), and after IM injection. However, lidocaine is not effective orally because of high first-pass effect but if very high oral doses are given, toxic symptoms may occur before therapeutic levels can be reached apparently due to active metabolites.

Bioavailability—Oral bioavailability is low (about 35%) due to first-pass metabolism.

Effective Concentration (Plasma)—2.0 to 5.0 mg/L.

Onset of Action—Within 2 minutes following IV bolus dose.

Duration of Action—Intermediate (increases with adrenaline addition).

Distribution—Vd=1.0 to 2.0 L/kg in humans and 4.5 L/kg in dogs. Lidocaine is rapidly redistributed from the plasma into highly perfused organs such as kidney, liver, lungs, and heart. It has high affinity for fat and adipose tissue. Lidocaine crosses the placenta and the blood-brain—barrier and is distributed into milk.

Plasma Protein Binding—About 70%; there is considerable intersubject variation and binding appears to be concentration-dependent. It is bound primarily to α1-acid glycoprotein.

Metabolism—Lidocaine is metabolized rapid in the liver. In humans, about 90% of a dose is dealkylated to monoethylglycinexylidide and glycinexylidide which are active.

Plasma Half-life—1.0 to 2.0 hours for lidocaine (higher in hepatic impairment); 1.0 to 2.0 hours for monoethylglycinexylidide; about 10 hours for glycinexylidide in humans. Half-life of lidocaine in dogs has been reported to be 0.9 hours.

Clearance—5 to 20 (ml/min/kg).

Route(s) of Excretion—Excreted via urine with less than 10% as unchanged drug.

Toxicity and Adverse Effects—Serious adverse reactions are rare at usual doses when serum level remains within (1-5 mcg/ml). In dogs, serum levels of >8 mcg/ml may cause toxicity. Symptoms may include ataxia, nystagmus, depression, seizures, bradycardia, hypotension and, at very high levels, circulatory collapse. If an IV bolus is given too rapidly, hypotension may occur. Cats tend to be more sensitive to the CNS effects of lidocaine.

Management of Overdose/Toxicity—Withdraw the drug. Seizures or excitement may be treated with diazepam or either a short or ultra-short—acting barbiturate.

Contraindications. Known hypersensitivity to lidocaine or the amide-class local anesthetics.

Precautions—Solutions containing precipitates should not be used. Excessive use of local anesthetics in animals with hepatic damage should be avoided. Be careful not to use the product which contains epinephrine intravenously.

Drug Interactions—Concomitant administration of cimetidine or propranolol may increase lidocaine levels. Other antiarrhythmic drugs such as procainamide, quinidine, propranolol, and phenytoin may cause additive or antagonistic cardiac effects and toxicity may be enhanced if administered with lidocaine. Large doses of lidocaine may prolong succinylcholine-induced apnea.

Pharmaceutical Formulations—The drug is available as lignocaine hydrochloride alone or in combination with vasoconstrictors (adrenaline, phenylephrine or noradrenaline) in 1 and 2 percent solutions for injection. Solutions containing epinephrine may contain sodium metabisulfite as an antioxidant. Solutions of other strengths are available for human use.

LIOTHYRONINE SODIUM

Liothyronine sodium

Synonyms—Sodium L-triiodothyronine; T_3 sodium.

Proprietary Names—Cytobin® (veterinary); Cytomel®; Tetroxin®; Triostat®.

Chemical Class—Iodinated thyronine derivative.

Pharmacological Class—Thyroid hormone.

Source—Synthetic.

Solubility, Stability and Storage—Liothyronine is practically insoluble in water and most organic solvents. It is soluble 1 in 500 of ethanol and soluble in solutions of alkali hydroxides.

Pharmacological Actions—Liothyronine stimulates normal growth and development; increases basal metabolic rate and cholesterol metabolism; stimulates protein synthesis; promotes gluconeogenesis and increases utilization of glycogen stores. It has a more rapid onset of action than preparations containing thyroxine. It also has a shorter duration of action and is less prone to accumulation. In comparison, 25 mcg of liothyronine may produce the same clinical response as 65 mcg of thyroid or 100 mg of levothyroxine sodium.

Mechanism of Action—T_3 sodium interacts with specific receptors on nuclei, mitochondria and plasma membrane of cells. For instance, it activates plasma membrane-bound Na^+, K^+-ATPase to increase oxygen consumption.

Indications—Liothyronine is used to treat hypothyroidism and for T_3 suppression test.

Dosages—

Dog: 4-6 mcg/kg every 8 hours.

T3 Suppression Test in cats: 25 mcg every 8 hours for 2 days and a 7th dose on the morning of the 3rd day.

Large Animals: 400 mcg/day. Adjust dose according to response.

Route(s) of Administration—Administered mostly per os. IV is used in humans in myxedema coma.

Absorption—Liothyronine is very well and almost completely (85-90%) absorbed from the oral route. Peak plasma level is attained within 2-5 hours in dog. Absorption is not seriously affected by stomach contents.

Onset of Action—Onset is more rapid than thyroxine-containing preparations.

Distribution—90-95% is located in intracellular compartment mainly in slowly equilibrating tissues (muscle, skin).

Plasma Protein Binding—99.5 to 99.8%.

Metabolism—Liothyronine is metabolized in the liver to inactive products. Degradation rates (mcg/kg/day) are as follows. Human, 0.43-0.46; dog, 0.84-0.89; cat 0.52-2.2. It is less prone to accumulation.

Plasma Half-Life—5-6 hours (dogs and cats); 24-36 hours (human).

Clearance—(ml/min/kg)—1.99 (dog); 1.77 (cat); 0.32 (human).

Route(s) of Excretion—Bile and feces.

Dialysis Status—Nondialyzable.

Toxicity and Adverse Effects—Increased and irregular heart rate, forceful heartbeat, prominent arterial pulse, increased appetite, weight loss, flushed moist and warm skin, weak and tremulous muscles, insomnia, restlessness and increased bowel movement are early manifestations of overdose. Excessive doses results in iatrogenic thyrotoxicosis.

Management of Overdose/Toxicity—Withdraw the drug; reduce gastrointestinal absorption; give general supportive therapy; give digitalis for congestive heart failure and β-adrenergic blockers to control enhanced adrenergic activities.

Contraindications—Cardiac disease; thyrotoxicosis; hypersensitivity to liothyronine sodium; adrenal insufficiency.

Precautions—Use liothyronine cautiously in patients with coronary heart disease or other cardiovascular diseases.

Drug Interactions—Estrogens increase liothyronine level of plasma protein binding while binding is inhibited by salicylates and dicoumarol. Cholestyramine resin decreases its absorption. Amiodarone decreases the conversion of thyroxine to triiodothyronine. Desmethyl amiodarone, a major metabolite of amiodarone decreases triiodothyronine binding to its nuclear receptors.

Pharmaceutical Formulations—Tablets containing 5-, 25-, and 50—mcg, and solution for injection containing 10 mcg/ml are available for human use. Tablets containing 60 mcg and 120 mcg are available for veterinary use. One 20 mcg tablet is equivalent to 40-60 mg of thyroid extract.

LUFENURON

Lufenuron

Proprietary Names—Program*; Program Plus* (combination of lifenuron and milbemycin oxime).

Chemical Class—Benzoyl-phenyl-urea (BPU).

Pharmacological Class—Insect development inhibitor (IDI).

Source—Synthetic.

Solubility, Stability and Storage—The injectable solution for cats should be stored at room temperature.

Pharmacological Actions—Lifenuron breaks flea life cycle. Female fleas feeding on treated animals produce eggs which do not hatch to produce larvae. This causes long term interruption of the flea life cycle. It is ineffective on adult fleas, hence noticeable control may not be observed until several weeks after dosing when a pre-existing infestation is present. Lifenuron is also effective against fungal infections such as ringworm and some internal parasites like heartworm.

Mechanism of Action—Lufenuron interferes with chitin synthesis, polymerization and deposition in flea larvae.

Indications—Prevention and control of flea infestations in cats (six weeks of age and older) and dogs. Each injection will protect cats for 6 months. Program plus® is indicated for the concurrent prevention of flea infestation and heartworm (*Dirofilaria immitis*) disease as well as the treatment of gastrointestinal nematodes such as hookworms (*Ancylostoma caninum*), roundworms (*Toxocara canis*) and whipworms (*Trichuris vulpis*) in dogs.

Dosages—

    Cat: Injection, 10 mg/kg once in 6 months. Oral suspension, 30 mg/kg given once a month with a meal or immediately after feeding.

    Dog: 10 mg/kg orally with a meal or immediately after feeding.

Route(s) of Administration—Subcutaneous (in cats); per os.

Onset of Action—Effective blood levels of lufenuron are achieved within 21 days.

Duration of Action—Lufenuron protect cats for six months.

Distribution. Lufenuron is stored in the animal's body fat.

Toxicity and Adverse Effects—Injection site reactions characterized by pain on injection, granulomatous inflammation and fibrosis as well as vomiting, listlessness/lethargy and anorexia have been reported in cats. Severe local reaction such as is not seen in cats may occur in dogs which have received the injectable product. The orally administered pills sometimes cause stomach upset.

Management of Overdose/Toxicity—Give activated charcoal.

Contraindications—Hypersensitivity to lufenuron.

Precautions—Shake syringe vigorously to reconstitute the suspension and then inject immediately. Concurrent use of insecticides may be necessary for adequate control of adult fleas. Do not administer the injectable product to dogs. Treat all cats and dogs within a household at the same time to prevent the buildup of developing fleas in the environment.

Drug Interactions—Lufenuron is safe when administered to animals receiving products such as vaccines, anthelmintics, antibiotics, steroids and insecticides.

Pharmaceutical Formulations—Injectable solution containing 10 mg of lufenuron per ml in 0.4 ml and 0.8 ml prefilled syringes are available. Oral suspension containing 70 mg of lufenuron per gram is also available. Both formulations are used in cats. Tablets containing different doses of lufenuron and milbemycin oxime are also available. The strengths of the different combinations are

- 2.3 mg of milbemycin oxime and 46 mg of lufenuron.
- 5.75 mg of milbemycin oxime and 115mg of lufenuron.
- 11.5 mg of milbemycin oxime and 230 mg of lufenuron.
- 23 mg of milbemycin oxime and 460 mg of lufenuron.

LOMUSTINE

Lomustine

Synonyms—CCNU.

Proprietary Names—CeeNU®.

Chemical Class—Nitrosourea derivative; Alkylating agent.

Pharmacological Class—Antineoplastic drug.

Source—Synthetic; Lomustine is an analog of carmustine.

Solubility, Stability and Storage—Lomustine is practically insoluble in water. It is soluble in alcohol and highly soluble in lipids. Store lomustine products at room temperature and in tightly closed containers.

Pharmacological Actions—Lomustine has cytotoxic, carcinogenic and mutagenic properties. It is cell-cycle nonspecific and functions as a bifunctional alkylating agent to inhibit DNA and RNA synthesis, alter RNA, proteins and enzymes.

Mechanism of Action—The mechanism is not thoroughly understood. In addition to alkylation of target molecules, lomustine inhibits DNA and RNA synthesis by carbamoylation of lysine residues of proteins.

Indications—Adjunctive treatment of brain and gastrointestinal tumors.

Dosages—60-80 mg/m^2 orally every 5-8 weeks.

Route(s) of Administration—Per os.

Absorption—Lomustine is rapidly and completely absorbed from the GIT. It appears in plasma within 3 minutes. It is also absorbed following topical application.

Distribution—Lomustine crosses the blood-brain-barrier because it is highly lipophilic. It attains equivalent concentration in CSF as in plasma. Lomustine undergoes enterohepatic circulation. It appears in milk.

Plasma Protein Binding—50%.

Metabolism—Lomustine is rapidly hydroxylated in the liver to active and inactive metabolites.

Plasma Half-life—15 minutes for the parent drug; 1.3-2 days for active metabolites (human).

Route(s) of Excretion—Urine, feces (<5%), and expired air (<10%).

Dialysis Status—Dialyzable.

Toxicity and Adverse Effects—Lomustine causes stomatitis and GI upset characterized by nausea, vomiting and diarrhea. It also causes severe myelosuppression with severe thrombocytopenia which peaks at 7-10 of onset of treatment. Lomustine has been reported to suppress gonadal function.

Management of Overdose—There is no specific antidote. Give symptomatic and supportive therapy.

Contraindications—Hypersensitivity to lomustine; preexisting severe bone marrow depression or infection.

Precautions—Use lomustine cautiously in patients that have received previous chemotherapy or radiation and in those with hepatic, renal or pulmonary impairment. Use during pregnancy should be undertaken if the benefit to the bitch or queen outweighs the risk of teratogenic effect. Use live virus vaccines cautiously during lomustine therapy.

Drug Interactions—Lomustine may produce additive bone marrow depression with other antineoplastic agents and bone marrow depressants (e.g. chloramphenicol, flucytosine, amphotericin B, and colchicine). Azathioprine, cyclophosphamide, corticosteroids and other immunodepressants may increase the risk of infection when used concurrently with lomustine. Cimetidine potentiates the bone marrow depression of lomustine while phenobarbital reduces it efficacy.

Pharmaceutical Formulations—Lomustine is available in 10 mg, 40 mg and 100 mg capsules.

LOPERAMIDE

Loperamide

H–Cl

Proprietary Names—Imodium*; Kaopectate II*.

Chemical Class—Phenylpiperidine opioid derivative; Butyramide derivative.

Pharmacological Class—Antidiarrheal agent.

Source—Synthetic.

Pharmacological Actions—Loperamide causes increase in general muscle tone of the small intestine; inhibits peristalsis with consequent increase in intestinal transit time. These actions cause more absorption of water and nutrients and fewer diarrheas. Loperamide also increases intestinal luminal capacity, reduces fecal volume and viscosity, and decreases fluid and electrolyte loss. Thus, it reduces the amount of fluid presented to the large intestine by the small intestine. Loperamide also has antisecretory action. It is 40 to 50 times as potent an antidiarrheal agent as morphine. It may have a tightening effect on the internal anal sphincter.

Mechanism of Action—Loperamide activates mu-opioid receptors in the gastrointestinal tract.

Indications—Symptomatic control of acute and chronic nonspecific diarrhea. Also useful in dogs with fecal incontinence.

Dosages—Dogs: 0.1-0.2 mg/kg orally every 8 hours.

Route(s) of Administration—Per os.

Absorption—Poorly (<40%) absorbed from the GIT. Peak plasma concentration is attained within 4 hours.

Bioavailability—Low.

Onset of Action—0.5 to 1 hour.

Distribution—Loperamide is poorly distributed. It is excluded from the CNS and perhaps milk. It undergoes enterohepatic circulation.

Plasma Protein Binding—97%

Metabolism—> 50% are metabolized in the liver to inactive products.

Plasma Half-Life—7 to 14 hours.

Route(s) of Excretion—Loperamide is eliminated mainly in feces; 1 % is excreted in urine.

Toxicity and Adverse Effects—Loperamide produces few systemic side effects which include abdominal cramp, nausea and vomiting. In dogs, constipation and bloat with potential occurrence of paralytic ileus are common. Overdose may cause CNS and respiratory depression. Since loperamide is an opiate, tranquilization is a possible side effect.

Management Of Overdose/Toxicity—Reduce the drug level in the stomach through gastric lavage and administration of activated charcoal. Administer naloxone if CNS depression becomes evident.

Contraindications—Diarrheas involving intestinal toxins such as in parvovirus enteritis; liver failure; known hypersensitivity to loperamide.

Precautions—Loperamide may enhance bacterial proliferation and delay the disappearance of microbes from the feces. Opiates should not be given to patients concurrently taking or within 14 days of receiving monoamine oxidase inhibitors. Use of loperamide may falsely elevate laboratory tests for pancreatitis (amylase and lipase levels). Loperamide should not be used in debilitated patients. The absorption enhancing effects of loperamide could enhance the absorption of intestinal toxins.

Drug Interactions—Other CNS depressants may potentiate the actions of loperamide.

Pharmaceutical Formulations—The drug is available as loperamide hydrochloride in 2 mg capsules and tablets. It is also available in oral liquid containing 1 mg/ 5 ml.

MAGNESIUM SULFATE

Synonyms—Epsom salts. Magnesium Sulfate tetrahydrate.

Proprietary Names—Empsom salt*.

Chemical Class—Inorganic salt.

Pharmacological Class—Saline cathartic; Hyperosmotic laxative; Antacid; Anticonvulsant.

Source—Synthetic.

Solubility, Stability and Storage—Magnesium sulfate is freely soluble in water and sparingly soluble in alcohol. Store magnesium sulfate formulations at room temperature (15-30°C); do not freeze. Refrigeration of the injection solution may result in precipitation or crystallization. Magnesium sulfate is incompatible with alkali hydroxides, alkali carbonates, salicylates, fat emulsion, many metals and drugs including calcium gluceptate, dobutamine HCl, polymyxin B sulfate, procaine HCl, and sodium bicarbonate.

Pharmacological Actions—Magnesium is essential for the activity of many enzyme systems and plays important roles in neurochemical transmission and muscular excitability. Magnesium sulfate reduces skeletal muscle contractions and blocks peripheral neuromuscular transmission. It depresses the CNS and acts peripherally to produce vasodilation.

Mechanism of Action—The relaxant action of magnesium on smooth muscle including the myometrium is due to direct inhibition of action potentials in muscle cells by inhibiting Ca^{++} influx through dihydropyridine-sensitive, voltage-dependent channels. Magnesium prevents or controls convulsions by blocking neuromuscular transmission and decreasing the amount of acetylcholine liberated at the end plate by the motor nerve impulse.

Indications—Magnesium sulfate is used orally as a laxative to relieve constipation, evacuate the bowel for diagnostic purposes such as radiography and endoscopy or to reduce the rate of absorption of ingested poison. It is also used as laxative to soften faeces after intestinal or anal surgery and to prevent excessive straining in advanced pregnancy or prolapse. Parenteral magnesium sulfate is used for the treatment of hypomagnesaemia in cattle and for adjunctive treatment of malignant hyperthermia in pigs. Parenteral magnesium sulfate is also used in uterine tetany as a myometrial relaxant. The combination of chloral hydrate, pentobarbital, and magnesium sulfate is used for general anesthesia and as a sedative-relaxant in cattle and horses. In humans, magnesium sulfate is gaining popularity as an initial treatment in the management of various dysrhythmias and also as an anticonvulsant for the prevention and control of seizures (convulsions) in severe toxemia of pregnancy.

Dosages—

For oral administration:

Horse	0.5-1.0g/kg in 4-6 liter of warm water.
Cattle	250-500 g; or 1-2 g/kg.
Pig	25-125 g; 1-2 g/kg
Sheep	0.25-1 g/kg
Dog	5-25 g
Cat	2-5 g
Bird	0.5-1 g/kg as a 5% solution in drinking water.

For parenteral administration against hypomagnesaemia:

Cattle	350-400 ml of 20% solution SC.
Calf	Magnesium sulfate 10% 100 ml; followed by oral magnesium oxide at daily doses of 1 gram PO (0-5 weeks old), 2 gram PO (5-10 weeks old), and 3 grams PO (10-15 weeks old).
Sheep and goat	50-100 ml of 20% solution.

Change the site of injection two or three times. Warm the solution to body temperature before use.

The combination of chloral hydrate, pentobarbital, and magnesium sulfate is administered intravenously at a dose of 20 to 50 milliliters of the preparation per 220 kg of body weight for general anesthesia until the desired effect is produced. Cattle usually require a lower dosage on the basis of body weight. When used as a sedative-relaxant, magnesium sulfate is administered at a level of one-fourth to one-half of the anesthetic dose level.

Route(s) of Administration—Per os, intravenous, intramuscular and subcutaneous.

Absorption—20% of magnesium may be absorbed systemically.

Effective Concentration—2.5 to 7.5 mEq/liter (for anticonvulsant action in humans).

Onset of Action—Immediate (IV); 1 hour (IM).

Duration of Action—30 minutes (IV); 3-4 hours (IM)

Plasma Protein Binding—25-30%.

Metabolism—None

Route(s) of Excretion—Excreted in urine.

Toxicity and Adverse Effects—Adverse effects caused by parenteral magnesium sulfate are generally the result of magnesium overdose and may include flushing, sweating, hypotension, depressed reflexes, flaccid paralysis, hypothermia, circulatory collapse, cardiac and central nervous system depression proceeding to respiratory paralysis. Very high magnesium levels may cause neuromuscular blocking activity and eventually cardiac arrest.

Management of Overdose/Toxicity—Intravenous calcium may counteract effects of hypomagnesaemia.

Contraindications—Parenteral magnesium is contraindicated in patients with myocardial damage or heart block.

Precautions—Magnesium should be given with caution to patients with renal impairment. Administer the drug with caution in digitalized patients to avoid overdose and the consequent necessity to administer calcium. Serious changes in cardiac conduction which can cause heart block may occur if administration of calcium is required to treat magnesium toxicity.

Drug Interactions. Concurrent administration of parenteral magnesium sulfate and CNS depressants (e.g. barbiturates, narcotics or other hypnotics) may cause additive effects. CNS depression and peripheral transmission defects produced by magnesium may be antagonized by calcium. Excessive neuromuscular blockade may occur if parenteral magnesium sulfate is administered concurrently with neuromuscular blockers.

Pharmaceutical Formulations—Magnesium sulfate is available in several formulations and in combinations with several drugs and minerals or nutrients. The combination with chloral hydrate and pentobarbital contains 42.5 mg of chloral hydrate, 8.86 mg of pentobarbital, and 21.2 mg of magnesium sulfate in each milliliter of sterile aqueous solution containing water, 33.8 percent propylene glycol, and 14.25 percent ethyl alcohol.

MANNITOL

```
          CH₂OH
           |
   HO —— CH
           |
   HO —— CH
           |
      HC —— OH
           |
      HC —— OH    Mannitol
           |
          CH₂OH
```

Synonyms—D-mannitol.

Proprietary Names—Osmitrol®; Resectisol®; Mannitol injection®.

Chemical Class—Complex sugar alcohol chemically related to mannose.

Pharmacological Class—Osmotic diuretic.

Source—Naturally occurring in plants (e.g. *Fraxinus ornus*).

Solubility, Stability and storage—Mannitol is very slightly soluble in alcohol. It has a solubility of approximately 182 mg/mL in water at 25°C. Solutions of mannitol are chemically stable but mannitol may crystallize when exposed to low temperatures if solution is higher than 15% concentration. Mannitol solutions should be stored at 15-30°C and protected from freezing. Crystals can be dissolved by warming and shaking the solution.

Pharmacological Actions—Mannitol enhances the rate of urine flow that is accompanied by relatively smaller increment in the excretion of electrolytes, uric acid and urea. It also causes increase in renal medullary blood flow partly through a prostaglandin-mediated mechanism. Mannitol has nephro-protective effect by preventing the accumulation of nephrotoxins. In the eye, mannitol causes reduced plasma ultrafiltration within the ciliary blood vessels thereby inhibiting aqueous humor formation. It also produces osmotic gradient that induces the diffusion of water from the intraocular fluid into plasma. These actions in the eye result in reduced intraocular pressure.

Mechanism of Action—Mannitol is freely filtered at the glomerulus but it undergoes limited reabsorption. Being osmotically active, it prevents the reabsorption of fluid from the tubular lumen. It also extracts some fluid from the tissue into the lumen. This intracellular extraction of water leads to expanded extracellular fluid volume, decreased blood viscosity, inhibition of renin release and increased renal blood flow.

Indications—Treatment of increased intracranial and intraocular pressures; ophthalmic surgery; prophylaxis and early treatment of acute renal failure; differential diagnosis of acute oliguria; induction of polyuria.

Dosages—1-2 ml/kg of 5-10% solution are administered to effect at the rate of 4 ml/minute.

Route(s) of Administration—IV infusion.

Onset of Action—1 to 3 hours (diuresis in humans); 15 minutes (intracranial pressure); 30 minutes (intraocular pressure in dogs).

Duration of Action—3 to 6 hours (intracranial pressure); 4–6 hours (intraocular pressure).

Distribution—Mannitol distributes into the extracellular compartments. It does not enter the eye or CSF (unless if there is loss of integrity of the blood-brain barrier).

Metabolism—7-10% is metabolized to glycogen.

Plasma Half-Life—100 minutes (human); 40-60 minutes (cattle and sheep). 6-36 hours in renal failure (human).

Route(s) of Excretion—Urine with 90% as unchanged drug.

Dialysis Status—Dialyzable.

Toxicity and Adverse Effects—Mannitol causes hypersensitivity reactions and acute expansion of extracellular fluid volume. Overdose may cause polyuria, hypotension, cardiovascular collapse, and hypernatremia.

Management of Overdose/Toxicity—Give supportive and symptomatic therapy—Undertake hemodialysis.

Contraindications—Hearing failure; anuria due to severe renal disease; marked pulmonary congestion or edema; marked dehydration; intracranial hemorrhage.

Precautions—Discontinue infusion of mannitol if signs of progressive renal dysfunction, heart failure or pulmonary congestion appear.

Drug Interactions—Mannitol increases urinary excretion of lithium.

Pharmaceutical Formulations—Mannitol is available in 5-25% solution in volumes ranging from 50-1000 ml for intravenous infusion.

MEBENDAZOLE

Proprietary Names—Vermox˙; Natoa˙; Telmin˙.

Chemical Class—Benzimidazole.

Pharmacological Class—Anthelmintic.

Source—Synthetic.

Pharmacological Actions—Mebendazole has actions against the larval and adult stages of *Ascaris, Necator, Ancylostoma, Trichuris, Enterobius* species in humans; large and small *Strongyles, Oxyuris, Ascaris* and *Probstmayria* species in horses; *Syngamus, Ascarid* and *Capillaria* species in birds. It is ovicidal to *Trichuris* and *Ascaris* species. Mebendazole is effective against *Taenia* tapeworms of dogs, cats, and ruminants, and adult *Echinococcus* in dogs. It is larvicidal to *Taenia ovis* and *Taenia hydatigena*.

Mechanism of Action—Mebendazole inhibits microtubule polymerization in susceptible helminthes by binding to β-tubulin.

Mebendazole

Indications—Treatment and prophylaxis of most GI nematodes of horses and birds; treatment of nematodes and cestodes in ruminants, dogs, cats, as well as laboratory, zoo, and game animals.

Dosages—

Dog, cat.	22 mg/kg daily for 3 days in nematodes, 5 days in cestodes infections; 200 mg twice daily for 5 days in Echinococcus infections.
Horse	9-15 mg/kg in nematode, 15-20 mg/kg/day for 5 days in lugworm; 20 mg/kg single dose in tapeworm infections.
Sheep	20 mg /kg in Monieza infections
Bird	50 mg/kg as a single dose in ascarids, Capillaria and tapeworm infections.
Equine, ruminant	620 ppm in feed for 14 days.
Primate	5-10 mg/kg for 5 days in cestodes and nematode infections; 25 mg/kg twice daily for 7 days, followed by 7 days' rest, and then 50 mg/kg twice daily for another 7 days, followed by another 7 days rest, then 25 mg/kg twice daily for a final 7 days in *Strongyloids fuelleborni* and *S. stercoralis* infections.
Carnivore, rodent.	15 mg/kg in nematode and cestode infections.
Zoo birds	60-120 ppm in feed for 7 days.

Route(s) of Administration—Per os.

Absorption—Mebendazole is poorly absorbed from oral route. Plasma level is about 1% of administered dose. Peak plasma concentration is reached within 2-4 hours.

Plasma Protein Binding—95%.

Metabolism—Mebendazole is extensively metabolized in the liver.

Plasma Half-Life—1 to 11.5 hours (human).

Route(s) of Excretion—Feces (major) and urine.

Withdrawal Period—14 days for sheep; 6 months for the horse.

Toxicity and Adverse Effects—Mebendazole is very well tolerated; 70-90 times the therapeutic dose did not produce any ill-effects in the horse. The LD_{50} in dogs and guinea pigs is 640 mg/kg. In humans, transient abdominal pain and diarrhea have been observed in cases of massive worm infestation. Overdose may cause altered mental status.

Management of Overdose/Toxicity—Give supportive therapy—

Contraindications—Food animals and lactating animals whose milk are meant for human consumption; first 4 months of pregnancy in donkeys infected with *Dictyocaulus*; pigeons and parrots.

Precautions—Fasting or purging is not necessary with mebendazole.

Drug Interactions—Mebendazole is compatible with most drugs administered simultaneously, though; its metabolism may be enhanced by anticonvulsants like phenytoin and carbamazepine.

Pharmaceutical Formulations—Mebendazole is available in oral granules, oral paste, and oral powder for addition to feed. It is also available in 100 mg/5 ml suspension and 100 mg chewable tablets for human use. Mebendazole is available in combination with closantel in oral suspension.

MECHLORETHAMINE

Synonyms—Mustin; Nitrogen mustard; HN_2.

Proprietary Names—Mustargen®.

Chemical Class—Alkylating agent; Nitrogen mustard derivative.

Pharmacological Class—Antineoplastic drug.

Source—Synthetic.

Solubility, Stability and Storage—Mechlorethamine is very soluble in water and soluble in alcohol. Mechlorethamine solutions are unstable in neutral and alkaline media. Solutions should be prepared just before injection. Discard unused solution after 15 minutes. The powder for injection should be stored in light-resistant containers at 15–30°C; it should be protected from humidity.

Mechlorethamine

Pharmacological Actions—Mechlorethamine interferes with cell proliferation by disrupting DNA replication and transcription of RNA ultimately resulting in the disruption of nucleic acid function and cell division particularly in rapidly proliferating tissues. It also has radiomimetic and vesicant properties. Its cytotoxic action is not specific to any cell-cycle or phase although cells appear more sensitive in late G_1 and S phases. It has high (>90%) emetogenic potential and is teratogenic in laboratory animals. Mechlorethamine also possesses weak immunosuppressive activity.

Mechanism of Action—Mechlorethamine acts by forming highly reactive carbonium ion intermediates which react with strongly neucleophilic substituents like phosphate, amino,—SH,—OH,—COOH and imidazole groups to form covalent bonds. The target molecule is thus alkylated. The N-7 position of guanine in DNA is highly susceptible. Alkylation of guanine in the DNA leads to cross linkage of DNA strands, linking of DNA to a closely associated protein, base pairing of guanine with thymine instead of cytosine, or breakage of the DNA strand.

Indications—Adjunctive treatment of lymphoreticular neoplasms in small animals; treatment of pleural and peritoneal effusions.

Dosages—5 mg/m².

Route(s) of Administration—Intravenous and intracavitary (for treatment of pleural and peritoneal effusion).

Absorption. Mechlorethamine is incompletely absorbed from intracavitary sites. It is absorbed after oral or parenteral administration but the drug is extremely irritating to tissues and, therefore, must be administered IV.

Metabolism—Mechlorethamine undergoes rapid chemical change following injection.

Plasma Half-life—< 1 minute.

Route(s) of Excretion—Extremely low levels (0.01%) is recovered in urine as unchanged drug.

Toxicity and Adverse Effects—Nausea, vomiting, GI upset, bone marrow depression, reproductive irregularities, fetal abnormalities, convulsions, and paralysis are prominent adverse effects. Extravasation into subcutaneous tissues during IV administration results in painful swelling and sloughing. Intracavitary administration of mechlorethamine produces a sclerosing effect, causing an inflammatory reaction on serous membranes and subsequent adherence of serosal surfaces.

Contraindications—Preexisting severe myelosuppression or infection; hypersensitivity to mechlorethamine; pregnancy.

Precautions—Give IV injection with care. Extravasation should be avoided because the drug is a potent tissue irritant. Give allopurinol 2-3 days prior to therapy to prevent renal complications arising from tumor lysis. Neutralize any unused solution or equipment used in the administration of mechlorethamine (e.g., rubber gloves, tubing, glassware, etc.) by soaking for 45 minutes in an aqueous solution containing equal volumes of 5% sodium thiosulfate and 5% sodium bicarbonate.

Drug Interactions—Concomitant use with myelosuppressive and immunosuppressive drugs produce additive effects and may increase the risk of infection.

Pharmaceutical Formulations—Available as mechlorethamine hydrochloride in 10 mg powder for injection.

MECLOFENAMIC ACID

Meclofenamic acid

Proprietary Names—Meclomen˙; Arquel® (veterinary formulation).

Chemical Class—N-phenylanthranilic acid derivative.

Pharmacological Class—Nonsteroidal Anti-inflammatory Drug; Simple analgesic; Non-narcotic analgesic; Analgesic-antipyretic.

Source—Synthetic.

Solubility, Stability and Storage—Meclofenamic acid is freely soluble in water and soluble in alcohol. Store meclofenamic capsules below 30°C; protect from light and moisture—

Pharmacological Actions—Meclofenamic acid has analgesic, antipyretic and anti-inflammatory actions. It protects the bovine species against experimental anaphylaxis. It also antagonizes certain effects of prostaglandin $PGF_2\alpha$. Meclofenamic acid antagonizes the actions of histamine and kinins at high doses.

Mechanism of Action—Like other NSAIDs, meclofenamate inhibits cyclooxygenase (COX-1 and COX-2) in the conversion of arachidonic acid to the endoperoxide intermediate, PGG_2 in the synthesis of prostaglandins, thromboxanes and prostacyclin. NSAIDs appear to exert anti-inflammatory, analgesic, and antipyretic activity principally through inhibition of the

COX-2 isoenzyme; COX-1 inhibition presumably is responsible for the drugs' unwanted effects on GI mucosa and platelet aggregation. Unlike most other NSAIDs, the fenamates, including meclofenamate sodium, also appear to compete with prostaglandins for binding at the prostaglandin receptor site and thus potentially affect prostaglandins that have already been formed.

Indications—Treatment of acute and chronic inflammatory conditions associated with musculoskeletal system.

Dosages—

Horse. 2.2 mg/kg orally daily for 5-7 days reducing progressively.

Dog. 1.1 mg/kg orally for 5-7 days.

Route(s) of Administration—Per os.

Absorption—Meclofenamic acid is rapidly absorbed orally. Peak plasma concentration is attained within 0.5-1 hour in human; 0.5 hours and then 4-6 hours (calf). Food decreases both the rate and extent of absorption resulting in delayed and decreased peak plasma concentrations and decreased bioavailability.

Onset of Action—Slow (36-96 hours in horses).

Duration of Action—2-4 hours.

Distribution—Attains high levels in liver and kidney. It crosses the placenta readily.

Plasma Protein Binding—99.8% (principally to albumin).

Metabolism—Oxidized in the liver to an active 3-hydroxymethyl metabolite with elimination half-life of 12-15 hours in humans.

Plasma Half-Life—1-8 hours (horse); 2-4 hours (human); 4 hours (calf).

Route(s) of Excretion—Urine and feces.

Toxicity and Adverse Effects—Buccal erosions and gastrointestinal irritation resulting in distress, diarrhea and bleeding may be observed in horses. Meclofenamic acid decreases PCV levels and causes hypoproteinemia with chronic use. These effects in addition to leukocytosis have been reported in dogs. Meclofenamic acid has been observed to delay parturition and produce teratogenic effects in rodents.

Management of Overdose/Toxicity—Give general antidotal therapy.

Contraindications—Active GI ulcer; preexisting renal or hepatic disease; concurrent administration of aspirin; hypersensitivity to meclofenamic acid or salicylates.

Precautions—Reduce meclofenamic acid dose in animals with hypoproteinemia—Withdraw the drug if diarrhea appears in horses. NSAIDs cause premature closure of patent ductus; hence use in late pregnancy should be avoided.

Drug Interactions—Meclofenamic acid is highly protein bound and may displace other protein bound drugs (such as anticoagulants, sulfonamides, phenylbutazone, hydatoins etc.) from binding sites. It increases blood concentration, half-life and likelihood of toxicity of methotrexate. The effects of diuretics may be decreased by meclofenamic acid. Aspirin reduces the blood levels and effect of meclofenamic acid. Meclofenamic acid enhances the effects of warfarin.

Pharmaceutical Formulations—Meclofenamic is available in 500 mg granules for horses. It is also available as meclofenamate sodium in capsules and tablets containing the equivalent of 50-100 mg of meclofenamic acid. Each 100 mg capsule of meclofenamate sodium contains 0.34 mEq of sodium.

MEGESTROL

Proprietary Names—Ovarid*; Megace*; Syntex suppress*; Ovaban*.

Chemical Class—Steroid.

Pharmacological Class—Progestin; Progestagen.

Source—Synthetic.

Solubility, Stability and Storage—Megestrol is insoluble in water but sparingly soluble in alcohol. Megestrol acetate tablets should be stored in well-closed containers between 15-30°C.

Pharmacological Actions—Megestrol is similar to the naturally occurring progesterone. Like progesterone, megestrol induces the development of secretory endometrium, suppresses uterine contractility to create a favourable environment for the implantation of the fertilized ovum and maintenance of pregnancy. It acts with estrogen to cause the development and filling of the acini of the mammary gland during pregnancy. Megestrol causes slight increase in body temperature and tends to delay the onset of parturition in animal species like the rabbit. It blocks the release of pituitary gonadotropin. Megestrol demonstrates anti-estrogen properties and has some steroidal effects through which it causes adrenal suppression.

Megestrol

Mechanism of Action—Megestrol binds to specific receptors which are distributed in the female reproductive tract and influence the transcription of a limited number of genes in the synthesis of functional proteins which express the drug action in the cells.

Indications—Megestrol is used to suppress or deferment estrus in bitches and queens. It is used to treat prostatic hyperplasia in dogs, false pregnancy and estrogen-dependent mammary tumors in bitches, miliary eczema in cats and also to control undesirable behaviour characterized by aggression [either dominant or submissive (fear-induced)], mounting, territory marking by urination, roaming, excitability, and destructiveness in dogs.

Dosages—

Dog	Postponement of estrus or treatment of false pregnancy.	0.5 mg/kg daily for a maximum period of forty days. Start treatment at least 7 days (preferably fourteen days) before the effect is required.
	Treatment of mammary tumor.	2 mg/kg/day PO for 10 days.
	False pregnancy	0.5 mg/kg per day for 8 days.
	Undesirable behavior	1-4 mg/kg for 7-14 days.

Cat	Suppression of estrus	2.5 mg per cat once weekly for up to 30 weeks. Dosage should commence in anoestrus (the non-breeding season).
	Prevention of estrus.	5.0 mg per cat daily for three days commencing as soon as the signs of calling are seen.
	Miliary eczema (miliary dermatitis) and eosinophilic granuloma (rodent ulcer).	2.5 to 5.0 mg per cat every two to three days until the lesions begin to regress then once weekly until a satisfactory response is obtained. In some cases it may be necessary to give a maintenance dosage of 2.5 mg per cat weekly or fortnightly to prevent recurrence of the condition.

Route(s) of Administration—Per os.

Absorption—Megestrol is well absorbed from the GIT.

Metabolism—The drug may be completely metabolized to free steroids and glucuronide conjugates.

Plasma Half-Life—8 days (dog).

Route(s) of Excretion—Urine and feces.

Toxicity and Adverse Effects—Adverse effects include lethargy, vomiting, and diarrhea. Occasionally, increased appetite with consequent weight gain may be observed. Prolonged administration may cause pyometra and endometritis. Megestrol may cause adrenal insufficiency (creating Addison's disease-like syndrome) after few weeks of administering the drug in cats. Transient diabetes mellitus and liver disease have also been reported in cats. Megestrol may cause occasional temperamental changes, mammary development and CNS depression with overdose. Progestagens may inhibit parturition.

Management of Overdose/Toxicity—Medication should be withdrawn if mammary hypertrophy develops.

Contraindications—First estrus; uterine disease; pregnancy; diabetes; mammary tumor; male dogs intended for breeding; hypersensitivity to megestrol.

Precautions—Do not medicate bitches more than twice in any 12 month period. Do not administer for more than two consecutive treatments. Confine bitches for 3 to 8 days or until cessation of bleeding once therapy has started since dogs in proestrus accept a male. Do not allow mating if estrus occurs within 30 days after cessation of treatment.

Pharmaceutical Formulations—The drug is available as megestrol acetate in tablets of 5 mg, 20 mg and 40 mg.

MELOXICAM

Proprietary Names—Flexicam˙; Meloxidyl˙; Metacam˙.

Chemical Class—Oxicam derivative.

Pharmacological Class—Non-steroidal Anti-inflammatory drug; Analgesic; Non-narcotic analgesic; Analgesic-antipyretic.

Source—Synthetic.

Pharmacological Actions—Meloxicam exhibits anti-inflammatory, analgesic, anti-exudative and antipyretic actions. It reduces leukocyte infiltration into inflamed tissues. To a minor extent it also inhibits collagen-induced thrombocyte aggregation. Meloxicam also has anti-endotoxic properties because it has been shown to inhibit production of thromboxane B2 induced by intravenous *E. coli* endotoxin administration in calves and pigs.

Meloxicam

Mechanism of Action—Meloxicam inhibits the synthesis of prostaglandins through inhibition of cyclooxygenase-2 (COX-2) isoform of prostaglandin endoperoxide synthase [prostaglandin G/H synthase (PGHS)] to a greater extent than the COX-1 isoform. Meloxicam's COX-2 selectivity is dose dependent and is diminished at higher dosages. Therefore meloxicam sometimes has been referred to as a "preferential" rather than "selective" COX-2 inhibitor. There are 2 forms of cyclooxygenase (COX), COX-1, which is the constitutive form of the enzyme, and COX-2, which is the form induced in the presence of inflammation. Inhibition of COX-2 is therefore thought to be responsible for at least some of the analgesic, anti-inflammatory, and antipyretic properties of NSAIDs whereas inhibition of COX-1 is thought to produce some of their toxic effects, particularly those on the gastrointestinal tract.

Indications—Alleviation of inflammation and pain in both acute and chronic musculo-skeletal disorders in dogs; control of postoperative pain and inflammation associated with orthopedic surgery, ovariohysterectomy, and castration when administered prior to surgery in cats.

Dosages—Cat: 0.3 mg/kg as a single, one-time subcutaneous injection. Dog: 0.2mg/kg on the first day followed by a maintenance dose of 0.1mg/kg once daily.

Route(s) of Administration—Oral, intravenous and subcutaneous routes are used.

Absorption—Meloxicam is completely absorbed following oral administration. Peak plasma concentration is attained within 2-3 hours.

Bioavailability—Oral bioavailability is 98%.

Distribution—Vd = 0.12-0.3l/kg.

Plasma Protein Binding—98%.

Metabolism. Extensively metabolized to inactive metabolites.

Plasma Half-life. 7.7 hours.

Route(s) of Excretion—Meloxicam and its metabolites are excreted in urine and feces. It undergoes substantial biliary secretion and enterohepatic circulation.

Toxicity and Adverse Effects—Loss of appetite, vomiting, diarrhoea, faecal occult blood and apathy have rarely been reported. These side effects are transient and occur generally within the first week of treatment.

Management of Overdose/Toxicity—Discontinue treatment if adverse effects are serious. In the case of overdose, symptomatic treatment should be initiated.

Contraindications—Concurrent use with aspirin or other NSAIDs; hypersensitivity to meloxicam; dogs less than 6 weeks of age; pregnancy; lactating animals; gastrointestinal disorders such as irritation and haemorrhage; impaired hepatic, cardiac or renal function and haemorrhagic disorders.

Precautions—Avoid using meloxicam in any dehydrated, hypovolaemic or hypotensive animal due to potential risk of increased renal toxicity.

Drug Interactions—Patients receiving diuretics may have an increased risk of developing renal failure secondary to decreased renal blood flow resulting from prostaglandin inhibition by meloxicam. Meloxicam may reduce the natriuretic effects of furosemide and thiazides.

Pharmaceutical Formulations—Meloxicam is available in oral suspension of 1.5-, 5-, 15- or 20—mg/ml; solution for injection containing 5 mg/ml and chewable tablets.

MEPERIDINE

Meperidine

Synonyms—Pethidine.

Proprietary Names—Demerol˚, Pethadol˚, Dembrol˚, Dolantin˚, Dolantol˚.

Chemical Class—Phenylpiperidine derivative.

Pharmacological Class—Narcotic analgesic, Opioid analgesic, Morphine-like opioid agonist.

Source—Synthetic.

Solubility, Stability and Storage—Meperidine is very soluble in water and soluble in alcohol. Meperidine hydrochloride preparations should be protected from light; tablets should be stored at 15-30°C and injection solutions should be stored at 15-25°C.

Pharmacological Actions—Meperidine causes sedation, analgesia and respiratory depression. It has one-tenth the analgesic potency of morphine. It causes smooth muscle relaxation, and depresses intestinal peristalsis but the contraction of cattle uterus is not inhibited. Meperidine causes little or no constipation and has antitussive activity only in analgesic doses. It has advantage over morphine in situations where the intestinal muscle need not be depressed as in post-operative pain. Unlike morphine, it does not cause excitement in cats and horses at therapeutic doses. Topical application of the drug produces considerable local anesthesia, but meperidine is not utilized for local anesthesia because it also produces local irritation.

Mechanism of Action—Meperidine combines with and activates μ (mu) opioid receptors.

Indications—Meperidine is used in preanesthetic medication and as a sedative-analgesic in dogs and cats. It is also as an analgesic for the symptomatic relief of pain in spasmodic colic in horses and to allay parturition pains and calm nervous heifers and ewes.

Dosages—

Dog	2.5-6.5 mg/kg for preanesthetic medication; 5-10 mg/kg for analgesia
Cat	2.2-4.4 mg/kg for preanesthetic medication; 2-10 mg/kg for analgesia.
Pig	1-2 mg/kg for preanesthetic medication. Give with promazine (2 mg/kg) and atropine (0.07-0.09 mg/kg) for maximum efficacy.
Horse	4 mg/kg up to a maximum of 1000 mg IM or 500 mg IV
Cattle	500 mg maximum
NHP	2-4 mg/kg
Rabbit	10 mg/kg
Guinea pig	2 mg/kg
Other laboratory rodents	20 mg/kg

Route(s) of Administration—Intramuscular.

Absorption—Meperidine is absorbed from all routes. Absorption from IM site is erratic. Following absorption from the GIT, meperidine undergoes extensive metabolism on first pass through the liver, with approximately 50–60% of a dose reaching systemic circulation unchanged.

Bioavailability—Oral bioavailability is 52 ± 3% (80-90% in patients with cirrhosis).

Onset of Action—Analgesic effect appears 15-25 minutes after IM administration in the horse.

Peak Analgesic Action—1 hour (oral); 40–60 minutes (subcutaneous); 30–50 minutes (IM).

Duration of Action—Analgesia lasts 3 to 5 hours.

Distribution—Vd = 4.4 ± 0.9 L/kg in human and 2.4 L/kg in dog. Meperidine is widely distributed. It crosses the placenta barrier in reasonable analgesic doses but does not appreciably depress fetal respiration. Meperidine is distributed into milk.

Plasma Protein Binding—50-80% (decreases in uremia).

Metabolism—Meperidine is converted to normeperidine and meperidine acid in humans and some primates. Normeperidine has t½ of 15-20 hours and causes excitatory side effects. Parahydroxymeperidine has been identified as a metabolite in rats.

Plasma Half-Life is 3.2 ± 0.8 hours (human); 0.7 hours (cat); 0.75 hours (dog); 66 ± 8.7 minutes (horse).

Clearance (ml/min/Kg) is 17.0 ± 5.0 in human and 42.5 in dog.

Route(s) of Excretion—Urine (1-25% as unchanged drug).

Toxicity and Adverse Effects—The adverse effects associated with meperidine therapy are the same with equianalgesic dose of morphine but constipation and urinary retention are less common. Subcutaneous or intramuscular injection causes local irritation and tissue induration. Large doses at short intervals may produce excitatory symptoms in animals tolerant to its depressant action. Meperidine causes defecation in some cats following IM administration. It also induces hyperthermia in cats and causes excitement at high doses. Reduced systemic arterial pressure and bronchoconstriction have been observed in dogs. Unlike morphine, meperidine is no more toxic to the newborn than adult. It causes transient incoordination, trembling and immobility in horses soon after intravenous administration.

Management of Overdose/Toxicity—Naloxone antagonizes the respiratory depressant and other toxic effects of meperidine but not the CNS excitatory effects. Excitement can be controlled by low doses of barbiturates.

Contraindications—Renal function impairment; pregnancy; horses intended for human consumption; horses with obstructive colic; hypersensitivity to meperidine.

Precautions—Meperidine crosses the placenta barrier in reasonable analgesic doses to depress respiration in neonates. Intravenous administration must be done slowly to avoid circulatory collapse. Care should be taken with concomitant use of sedatives, analgesics and depressants as the depressant effects may be potentiated.

Drug Interactions—Severe reaction may occur in patients receiving MAO inhibitors. Flouxetine, and other serotonin reuptake inhibitors potentiate meperidine effects. Tricyclic antidepressants and phenothiazines (e.g. chlorpromazine) increase the respiratory depressant effect of meperidine. Concurrent administration with chlorpromazine or promethazine enhances sedation. Phenobarbitone and phenytoin increases systemic clearance and decreases oral bioavailability of meperidine. Concurrent administration of amphetamine enhances its analgesic effect.

Pharmaceutical Formulations—The drug is available as meperidine hydrochloride in 25 mg, 50 mg and 100 mg tablets; 50 mg/5 ml syrup; and solution of various strength for injection. No specific veterinary formulations are available.

MERCAPTOPURINE

Mercaptopurine

Synonyms—6-Mercaptopurine; 6-MP.

Proprietary Names—Purinethol®.

Chemical Class—Purine analog.

Pharmacological Class—Antineoplastic drug; Anticancer agent; Antimetabolite; Immunosuppressant.

Source. Synthetic.

Solubility, Stability and Storage—Mercaptopurine is insoluble in water but soluble in hot alcohol. It is stable when stored at room temperature.

Pharmacological Actions—6-MP has anticancer and moderate myelosuppressive actions through the inhibition of DNA and RNA synthesis. Mercaptopurine is also a powerful immunosuppressant. It strongly inhibits the primary immune response, selectively suppressing humoral immunity. Some inhibition of the cellular immune response also occurs. There is usually complete cross-resistance between mercaptopurine and thioguanine.

Mechanism of Action—Mercaptopurine is converted to the active nucleotide form (6-thioinosine-5' phosphate) by hypoxanthine-guanine phosphoribosyl-transferase. 6-thioinosine-5' phosphate inhibits several vital metabolic reactions as well as DNA and RNA syntheses.

Indications—Mercaptopurine is used in adjunctive treatment of lymphoid tumors and acute leukemia in dogs. It has also been used in the treatment of severe rheumatoid arthritis.

Dosages—50 mg/m^2 once a day for induction and then 50 mg/m^2 every 48 hours for maintenance.

Route(s) of Administration—Per os.

Absorption—Absorption of mercaptopurine from the oral route is variable and incomplete (16-50%). Peak plasma concentration is attained within 2 hours.

Bioavailability—Oral bioavailability is $12 \pm 7\%$. This increases to 60% when first pass metabolism is inhibited with allopurinol.

Distribution—Vd = 0.56 ± 0.38 L/kg. Mercaptopurine is widely distributed. It crosses the blood-brain barrier but does not attain therapeutic levels in the brain.

Plasma Protein Binding—19%.

Metabolism—The drug undergoes extensively first pass metabolism in the gastrointestinal mucosa and liver by xanthine oxidase.

Plasma Half-life—0.9 ± 0.37 hours.

Clearance—11 ± 4 (ml/min/kg).

Route(s) of Excretion—Urine with $22 \pm 12\%$ as unchanged drug.

Toxicity and Adverse Effects—Bone marrow depression characterized by anemia, leukopenia, and less severe thrombocytopenia. Nausea, vomiting, anorexia, and reversible cholestatic jaundice have all been reported. Mercaptopurine is mutagenic and teratogenic and may cause permanent sterility.

Management of Overdose/Toxicity—There is no antidote. Withdraw the drug if adverse effects are severe.

Contraindications—Hypersensitivity to mercaptopurine; severe renal or hepatic impairment; severe preexisting bone marrow depression; pregnancy.

Precautions—Feed kittens and pups with milk replacers if mercaptopurine is administered to nursing bitches and queens. Reduce dose in patients with renal impairment. Use cautiously in animals with history of urolithiasis. Pregnant women must avoid handling antineoplastic agents. Concomitant use with other drugs that can cause hepatotoxicity or alteration in liver metabolic function must be with caution.

Drug Interactions—Allopurinol inhibits the metabolism of mercaptopurine, thus increasing the toxicity of the latter. Consequently, the dose of mercaptopurine must be reduced by as much as 75% if both drugs are administered concurrently. Mercaptopurine may produce additive bone marrow depression with other antineoplastic agents, and bone marrow depressants (e.g. chloramphenicol, flucytosine, amphotericin B, and colchicine). Azathioprine, cyclophosphamide, corticosteroids and other immunodepressants may increase the risk of infection when used concurrently with mercaptopurine. Mercaptopurine inhibits the anticoagulant action of warfarin. Doxorubicin enhances the hepatotoxic effect of mercaptopurine. Cross-resistance exists between mercaptopurine and thioguanine.

Pharmaceutical Formulations—Mercaptopurine is available in 50 mg tablets.

METHADONE

Proprietary Names—Dolophine˚; Amidone˚.

Chemical Class—Diphenylheptane derivative.

Pharmacological Class—Narcotic analgesic; Opioid analgesic; Opiate agonist.

Source—Semi synthetic.

Stability and Storage—Methadone is soluble in water and freely soluble in alcohol. Methadone products should be stored in tight, light-resistant containers at room temperature.

Pharmacological Actions—The actions of methadone are similar to those of morphine but they are longer-acting. Methadone has slight action on the cardiovascular system and its emetic effect is low. Its analgesic, respiratory depressant activities and addiction potential reside in the l-isomer. The d-isomer possesses antitussive activity. Tolerance and physical dependence develops more slowly to methadone than to morphine. Methadone causes mild withdrawal syndrome. It inhibits drug metabolism following acute single oral dose but induces drug metabolism following repeated oral administration.

Methadone

Mechanism of Action—Methadone combines with and activates μ (mu) opioid receptors.

Indications—Methadone is used in preanesthetic medication before barbiturate anesthesia in dogs. It is used singly to control of severe pain and in combination with acepromazine for analgesia, sedation and restraint for minor surgery in horses.

Dosages—

Dog. 1.1 mg/kg SC for preanesthetic medication; or 0.11-0.55 mg/kg SC or IM for analgesia.

Horse. 0.11 mg/kg IV (in combination with 0.11 mg/kg acepromazine) for sedation and minor surgery; 0.25 mg/kg IM or SC for analgesia; 0.12 mg/kg IV for preanesthetic medication.

Route(s) of Administration—Methadone may be administered orally in humans. The subcutaneous, intramuscular and intravenous are used in animals.

Absorption—Methadone is well absorbed from all routes.

Bioavailability—Oral bioavailability is 92 ± 21%.

Effective Concentration—>100 ng/ml.

Onset of Action—To induce analgesia, 0.5-1 hour (oral route); 10-20 minutes (parenterally route); 30 seconds (methadone/acepromazine combination in the horse).

Peak Action—15 minutes (methadone/acepromazine combination in the horse); 1-2 hours (parenteral).

Duration of Action—6 to 8 hours (oral); 1 hour (methadone/acepromazine combination in the horse). Duration of action increases following repeated doses.

Distribution—Vd = 3.8 ± 0.6 L/kg (human). Methadone is widely distributed; it accumulates in tissues and also crosses the placenta.

Plasma Protein Binding—89 ± 1.4%.

Metabolism—Undergoes hepatic N-demethylation.

Plasma Half-Life—35 ± 12 hours (human).

Clearance—1.4 ± 0.5 ml/min/kg.

Route(s) of Excretion—Urine (21 ± 10% as unchanged drug) and bile. There is increased urinary excretion with acidic urine.

Toxicity and Adverse Effects—Methadone is more toxic than morphine although its toxicity is qualitatively similar to those of morphine. It depresses respiration, stimulates the vagus causing bradycardia and salivation in anaesthetized dogs. It causes excitation and seizure in cats. Methadone increases the tone of intestinal smooth muscle and may cause constipation due to inhibition of peristalsis. Large doses (0.5–1.0 mg/kg) cause incoordination and restlessness in horses.

Management of Overdose/Toxicity—Administer naloxone.

Contraindications—Hypersensitivity to methadone; severe hepatic impairment; shock of diverse origin.

Precautions—Use lower doses or give the drug over longer intervals with repeated use. Reduce the dose in patients with hepatic and/or renal impairment. Always administer methadone singly because methadone is incompatible with many drugs.

Drug Interactions—Rifampin, pentazocine, and phenytoin accelerate the metabolism of methadone. Atropine and scopolamine reduce the analgesic potency and duration of action of methadone. The CNS depressant effects of methadone is enhanced and prolonged by other CNS depressants e.g. phenothiazines.

Pharmaceutical Formulations—The drug is available as methadone hydrochloride in 5 mg and 10 mg tablets; 10 mg/ml solutions for injection; 5 mg/5 ml, 10 mg/5ml, and 10 mg/ml oral solutions. Tablets containing 40 mg is available for opioid addicts. No specific veterinary formulation is available.

METHENAMINE

Methenamine

Synonyms—Hexamine; Urotropine; Hexamethylenamine.

Proprietary Names—Hiprex®; Mandelamine®; Urex®; Urised®.

Chemical Class—Amine.

Pharmacological Class—Urinary tract antiseptic; Antimicrobial agent.

Source—Synthetic.

Solubility, Stability and Storage—Methenamine is soluble 1 in 1.5 of water and 1 in 8 of ethanol. Methenamine hippurate, which contains 44% methenamine and 56% hippuric acid is freely soluble in water and alcohol. Methenamine mandelate, containing approximately 48% methenamine and 52% mandelic acid is very soluble in water and has a solubility of approximately 100 mg/mL in alcohol at 25°C. Methenamine and its salts should be stored at room temperature.

Pharmacological Actions—Methenamine has diuretic and urinary antiseptic actions. It may be bacteriostatic or bactericidal depending on the amount of formaldehyde produced. Methenamine is hydrolyzed to formaldehyde and ammonia in acid urine. It has activity against a variety of Gram-positive and Gram-negative bacteria. *Enterobacter aerogens* and *Proteus vulgaris* are usually resistant. *E. coli* is particularly sensitive. Resistance does not usually develop during prolonged therapy with methenamine or its salts because its antibacterial products (formaldehyde, hippuric acid, and mandelic acid) have nonspecific antibacterial activity.

Mechanism of Action—Methenamine decomposes slowly in acid urine of less than pH 5.5 to formaldehyde and ammonia. Formaldehyde has nonspecific bactericidal action. Formaldehyde action combines with the bacteriostatic action of the acid portions (hippuric acid and mandelic acid) of methenamine salts (methenamine mandelate and methenamine hippurate). In turn, hippuric acid and mandelic acid enhance the liberation of formaldehyde from methenamine in vivo by maintaining urinary acidity.

Indications—Prophylaxis or suppression of recurrent urinary tract infections, especially when long-term therapy is considered necessary.

Dosages—

Dog, Cat	0.1-2 g in 2-4 divided doses depending on size of animal.	
Pig	2-8g twice daily.	
Horse	8-15 g twice daily.	

Route(s) of Administration—Per os.

Absorption—Methenamine is readily absorbed from the GIT.

Distribution—The drug crosses the placenta and is distributed into milk.

Metabolism—Methenamine is partly hydrolyzed in the liver to formaldehyde and ammonia; 1030% is hydrolyzed in the gastric juice unless protected by enteric coating.

Plasma Half-Life—3-6 hours.

Route(s) of Excretion—Urine (70-90% as unchanged drug).

Toxicity and Adverse Effects—Methenamine and its salts irritate the gastrointestinal and urinary tracts and may produce vomition, diarrhea, and abdominal cramps. Skin rashes may also occur. Albuminuria, hematuria, crystalluria, painful and frequent micturition may occur at high doses. Systemic methenamine is nontoxic.

Management of Overdose/Toxicity—Initiate general antidotal therapy.

Contraindications—Hepatic and renal insufficiency; sulfonamide therapy; severe dehydration; hypersensitivity to methenamine.

Precautions—Use methenamine only after the urinary tract infection has been eradicated by other appropriate anti-infectives. Do not use for acute or systemic infections. Use cautiously in patients with hepatic disease, gout and the elderly. Administer methenamine with food to minimize GI irritation. Accompany methenamine with sufficient fluids to ensure adequate urine flow. Give urine acidifiers (e.g. ascorbic acid).

Drug Interactions—Urinary alkalinizers decrease methenamine action. Sulfonamides may form insoluble precipitates with formaldehyde. Acidification of urine enhances its activity. Combination with sulfamethizole causes mutual antagonism. Tests for catecholamines may be falsely elevated.

Pharmaceutical Formulations—Available as methenamine mandelate in 250 mg, 500 mg, and 1 gram tablets; 1 gram granules and 250 mg/5ml, 500 mg/5 ml oral suspensions. It is also available as methenamine hippurate in 1 g tablets. Combined tablets containing 0.3 g methenamine and 0.15 gram sodium acid phosphate are available for animal treatment.

METHIMAZOLE

Methimazole

Synonyms—Thiamazole.

Proprietary Names—Tapazole®.

Chemical Class—Thioureylene compound.

Pharmacological Class—Antithyroid drug.

Source—Synthetic.

Pharmacological Actions—Methimazole inhibits the synthesis of thyroid hormones and consequently increases thyroid stimulating hormone activity and development of goiter. Methimazole has no effect on pre-existing circulating or stored thyroid hormones and it has no effect on supplemented thyroid hormones. It reduces basal metabolic rate. In livestock, it improves fattening rate but produces poor carcass quality. Thiamazole has immunomodulatory properties.

Mechanism of Action—Methimazole inhibits thyroid peroxidase enzyme-catalyzed oxidation of iodine to iodide. This action blocks organification (the incorporation of iodide into the tyrosyl groups in thyroglobulin).

Indications—Stabilization of feline hyperthyroidism prior to surgical thyroidectomy and for the long-term treatment of feline hyperthyroidism.

Dosages—

Stabilization: 2.5 mg tablet morning and evening. This should ensure euthyroidism within 3 weeks.

Long-term treatment: starting dose should be 2.5 mg twice daily. After 3 weeks, the dose should be titrated to effect according to the serum total T4. Dose adjustments should be made by increments of 2.5 mg. For long-term treatment of hyperthyroidism the animal should be treated for life.

Route(s) of Administration—Per os.

Absorption—Methimazole is readily absorbed.

Bioavailability—Oral bioavailability is 80-95% in human and 45-98% in cat.

Onset of Action—30-40 minutes. A lag time of 1-3 weeks between first administration and significant reduction in serum T_4 is observed.

Duration of Action—2-4 hours.

Distribution—Vd = 0.12-0.84 L/kg in cat. Methimazole concentrates in the thyroid gland, enters milk, and crosses the placenta.

Plasma Protein Binding—None.

Plasma Half-Life—2.3 to 10.2 hours in cat and 4-13 hours in human. Intrathyroid residence time is approximately 20 hours in human beings.

Route(s) of Excretion—Urine.

Toxicity and Adverse Effects—Adverse effects are commonly associated with long term use. In many cases symptoms may be mild and transitory. The more serious effects are reversible when medication is stopped. Vomiting, anorexia, lethargy, severe pruritus and excoriations of the head and neck and bleeding diathesis are common within therapeutic doses. Icterus associated with hepatopathy and haematological abnormalities (eosinophilia, lymphocytosis, neutropenia, lymphopenia, slight leucopenia, agranulocytosis, thrombocytopenia or haemolytic anaemia) are also common. These side effects resolved within 7-45 days after cessation of therapy. Signs are aggravated with overdose. Goiter is produced following excessive doses. Within the first few weeks of treatment, a small percentage of cats self-mutilate their faces and necks through scratching. Acquired myasthenia gravis has also been reported.

Management of Overdose/Toxicity—Discontinue treatment if adverse effects are serious. Neutropenic animals should be treated with prophylactic bactericidal antibacterial drugs and supportive therapy.

Contraindications—Pregnancy; lactation; tracheal obstruction; hypersensitivity to methimazole; systemic disease such as primary liver disease or diabetes mellitus; autoimmune disease; disorders of white blood cells, such as neutropenia and lymphopenia; platelet disorders and coagulopathies (particularly thrombocytopenia).

Precautions—Undertake frequent leukocyte count. Reduce the dose during pregnancy to avoid fetal goiter. Kittens out of queens receiving this drug should go on milk replacement after receiving colostrum. Use methimazole cautiously in patients receiving other drugs capable of causing agranulocytosis.

Drug Interactions—The use of methimazole and other thionamides during the week before and after radioiodine therapy may hinder response to radiation. Concurrent treatment with phenobarbital may reduce the clinical efficacy of methimazole. Concurrent treatment with benzimidazole anthelmintics (thiabendazole) may reduce the hepatic oxidation of methimazole and lead to increases in its circulating levels.

Pharmaceutical Formulations is Methimazole is available in 5 mg and 10 mg tablets.

METHOTREXATE

Methotrexate

Synonyms—Amethopterin; MTX.

Proprietary Names—Methotrexate® Folex®; Rheumatrex®.

Chemical Class—Folic acid analog.

Pharmacological Class—Antineoplastic drug; Anticancer agent; Antimetabolite.

Source—Synthetic.

Solubility, Stability and Storage—Methotrexate is practically insoluble in water and alcohol but methotrexate sodium is soluble in water. Store all products at room temperature in light resistant containers. Reconstituted solutions remain stable for one month at room temperature and three months if refrigerated. Dilute the drug solution for intrathecal use.

Pharmacological Actions—An S-phase specific anticancer drug with cytotoxic effects on rapidly proliferating neoplastic and normal cells. Methotrexate inhibits DNA synthesis and cell reproduction. It also has immunosuppressive, teratogenic and embryotoxic actions. MTX may affect spermatogenesis in male rats. Cells may become resistant due to decreased intracellular uptake of the drug. MTX produced the first cure of cancer when used against human choriocarcinoma.

Mechanism of Action—Methotrexate inhibits dihydrofolate reductase causing depletion of tetrahydrofolate, an important component in the synthesis of purine and thymidylate which are nucleic acid precursors. Its derivative, polyglutamyl MTX may also inhibit thymidylate synthetase.

Indications—MTX is used as an adjunct in the treatment of lymphomas and some solid tumors in dogs and cats.

Dosages—2.5 mg/m^2 daily orally. For high dose therapy, give 5-10 mg/m^2 orally or parenterally followed in 2-4 hours by 3 mg/m^2 calcium leucovorin. This form of therapy is expensive.

Route(s) of Administration—The oral, intravenous, intramuscular and intrathecal routes are appropriate.

Absorption—MTX is rapidly and well absorbed from the GIT at doses lower than 30 mg/m^2. Peak plasma concentrations are attained within 1-2 hours. Oral absorption is incomplete at high doses. Absorption is complete from intramuscular site with plasma concentration reaching its peak within 30-60 minutes.

Bioavailability (oral). 70 ± 27%.

Distribution. Vd = 0.55 ± 0.19 MTX is widely distributed. It is taken into cells and across membranes by an active transport mechanism. It crosses the blood-brain-barrier poorly and penetrates or leaves third space fluids (pleural effusion, ascites) slowly but attains high and sustainable concentrations in the kidneys, spleen, gallbladder, liver and skin. MTX crosses the placenta and appears to a limited amount in milk.

Plasma Protein Binding—46 ± 11% (human).

Metabolism—Less than 10% is metabolized. Metabolism occurs in the intestine, liver and in cells.

Plasma Half-life—Dose-dependent; 8-12 hours (high doses) and 3-10 hours (low doses).

Clearance—2.1 ± 0.8 ml/min/kg.

Route(s) of Excretion—$81 \pm 9\%$ excreted in urine in human. Small amount appear in feces.

Dialysis Status—Not dialyzable.

Toxicity and Adverse Effects—GI effects characterized by nausea, vomiting, diarrhea are most common at low doses. Ulceration, mucositis and stomatitis may be observed at high doses. Alopecia, myelosuppression (characterized by leukopenia, anemia and thrombocytopenia), and abnormalities of kidney, liver and lungs have also been reported. Renal damage may be due to precipitation of MTX in kidney tubules. Intrathecal administration may induce CNS toxicity. MTX has been reported to cause photosensitization in humans.

Management of Overdose/Toxicity—Prevent absorption by adopting general antidotal therapy. Administer Ca folinate (Ca leucovorin) within 24 hours of a high dose or as soon as toxicity signs appear. This is called folinic acid rescue. It terminates the effects of the drug and allows normal cells to recover. Hydrate the animal or alkalinize urine to prevent precipitation of methotrexate and its metabolites.

Contraindications—Severe renal or hepatic impairment; severe preexisting bone marrow depression; hypersensitivity to MTX.

Precautions—Use methotrexate with caution in old animals or in patients with renal or hepatic impairment. Handle products with gloves or wash hands almost immediately. Pregnant women must avoid handling antineoplastic agents. Do not administer MTX with NSAIDs. Closely monitor blood cells, hepatic, and renal functions regularly during therapy.

Drug Interactions—Salicylate blocks methotrexate active tubular excretion as well as displacing it from protein binding; thus increasing the risk of MTX toxicity. Probenecid inhibits tubular secretion of MTX. Highly protein bound drugs such as sulfonamides, phenytoin, phenylbutazone, oral anticoagulants may displace MTX or be displaced from binding by MTX. Oral neomycin reduces oral absorption of MTX. Pyrimethamine may increase MTX toxicity.

Pharmaceutical Formulations—The drug is available as methotrexate sodium in 2.5 mg/ml and 25 mg/ml solutions for injection. It is also available in 2.5 mg tablets, and 20 mg, 25 mg, 50 mg, 250 mg and 1 g powder for reconstitution. A preservative free solution for injection containing 25 mg is also available. No specific veterinary formations are available.

METOCLOPRAMIDE

Metoclopramide

Proprietary Names—Maloxon®; Octamide®; Reglan®; Reclomide®; Clopra®; Metoclopramide HCl®.

Chemical Class—Benzamide; para-aminobenzoic acid derivative.

Pharmacological Class—Antiemetic; Prokinetic agent; Dopamine-receptor antagonist.

Source—Synthetic.

Solubility, Stability and Storage—Metoclopramide is practically insoluble in water, soluble 1 in 45 of ethanol and 1 in 15 of chloroform—Store metoclopramide formulations at room temperature and in light resistant containers. Metoclopramide injection is stable in normal saline.

Pharmacological Actions. Metoclopramide acts peripherally on the upper gastrointestinal smooth muscle to cause prokinetic effects characterized by increased gastric motility and tone, relaxed pyloric sphincter, and increased peristalsis. It reduces gastrointestinal reflux. Its actions on the GIT are not associated with stimulation of gastric, biliary or pancreatic secretions. Metoclopramide also act centrally to cause sedation, extrapyramidal effects, stimulation of prolactin and anti-emesis. It blocks the emetic effects induced by drugs such as apomorphine and ergotamine.

Mechanism of Action—The exact molecular mechanisms are not clearly understood. Metoclopramide is known to inhibit dopamine and dopamine agonists at their receptor sites. It is also known to enhance the response of the upper GI muscles to acetylcholine. This peripheral effect is inhibited by atropine.

Indications—Prevention and treatment of emesis; treatment of gastric stasis disorders and gastrointestinal reflux.

Dosages—

Dog and Cat: 0.2-0.5 mg/kg every 6 hours orally and parenterally or as a continuous IV infusion in cases of emesis. Severe emesis may require 1-2 mg/kg every 24 hours or by slow IV infusion. Give same dose 30 minutes before meals in cases with gastric motility disorders.

Horse: 0.02-0.1 mg/kg IM or IV every 6 hours in foals with gastrointestinal stasis.

Route(s) of Administration—Per os, intramuscular and subcutaneous routes are suitable.

Absorption—Metoclopramide is well absorbed from the GIT. Peak plasma concentration is attained within 2 hours.

Bioavailability—50-70% following oral administration or 74-96% following IM injection.

Onset of Action—0.5-1 hour (oral); 1-3 minutes (IV).

Duration of Action—1-2 hours.

Distribution—Vd = 3.4 ± 1.3 in human. Metoclopramide is rapidly and well distributed. It is lipid soluble and readily enters the CNS and milk. It crosses the placenta.

Plasma Protein Binding—40 ± 4% in humans and 13-22% in animals.

Metabolism—Metoclopramide is metabolized in the liver by glucuronide and sulfate conjugation processes.

Plasma Half-Life—90 minutes in dog and 5.0 ± 1.4 in human. Half-life is increased in subjects with impaired renal function.

Clearance—6.2 ± 1.3 ml/min/kg in human.

Route(s) of Excretion—Urine (20-25% as unchanged drug); 5% of dose is excreted in feces via the bile.

Dialysis Status—Not dialyzable.

Toxicity and Adverse Effects—In dogs and cats, gastrointestinal side effect is characterized by constipation. CNS side effects include nervousness, restlessness, and disorientation. Tremors have also been reported. Horses, particularly adults, have been reported to show alternating periods of sedation and excitement, behavioral changes and abdominal pain. Overdose causes sedation ataxia, restlessness, extrapyramidal effects, nausea, vomiting, and seizures.

Management of Overdose/Toxicity—Initiate general antidotal therapy. Anticholinergic agents such as diphenhydramine and beztropine that can penetrate the CNS may control extrapyramidal effects.

Contraindications—Gastrointestinal obstruction or perforation; seizure; hypersensitivity to metoclopramide.

Precautions—Adjustment of insulin dosage may be required due to alteration in the delivery of food to the intestine. Metoclopramide may induce hypertensive crisis in patients with pheochromocytoma. Reduce metoclopramide dose in cases of renal impairment.

Drug Interactions—Metoclopramide effects are enhanced by bethanechol. Metoclopramide reduces the bioavailability of digoxin (and other drugs that are absorbed from the stomach) due to reduced absorption resulting from increased gastro motility. Atropine and opioid analgesics antagonize the gastrointestinal actions of metoclopramide. Phenothiazines (e.g. cpz) and butyrophenones (droperidol) may potentiate its extrapyramidal effects while sedatives may enhance its CNS effects.

Pharmaceutical Formulations—It is available as metoclopramide hydrochloride in 5 mg, 10 mg tablets; 1 mg/ml, 10 mg/ml oral solution; and 5 mg/ml solution for injection. There are no specific veterinary formulations.

METOPROLOL

Metoprolol

Proprietary Names—Lopressor®; Toprol XL® (extended release tablet).

Pharmacological Class—$Beta_1$-adrenergic receptor antagonist. Cardioselective beta blocker.

Source—Synthetic.

Solubility, Stability and Storage—Store metoprolol products at room temperature in light resistant container.

Pharmacological Actions—Metoprolol antagonizes the cardiovascular effects of isoprenaline and consequently cause reduction in sinus heart rate, blood pressure, cardiac oxygen demand, cardiac output, tachycardia and slowed AV conduction. It inhibits chronotropic response to electrical sympathetic nerve stimulation at lower doses than is required to inhibit the response to isoprenaline. It has no intrinsic sympathomimetic actions of its own. Unlike propranolol, metoprolol has little or no membrane stabilizing action. Metoprolol has little effect on the beta-receptor mediated peripheral vasodilator effect of adrenaline being mainly a $beta_1$-adrenergic receptor antagonist.

Mechanism of Action—Metoprolol competitively antagonizes the actions of beta-adrenergic agonists principally at $beta_1$ receptor sites. The $beta_2$ sites are antagonized only at high doses.

Indications—Treatment of systemic hypertension, supraventricular tachycardia, premature ventricular contractions in dogs and cats. Metoprolol is also indicated in hypertrophic cardiomyopathy in cats. Because of its cardio-selective properties at therapeutic doses, metoprolol is often preferred to propranolol in patients with bronchospastic disease and conditions for which a beta-adrenergic blocker is indicated.

Dosages—

    Dog: 5-50 mg (total dose) every 8 hours.

    Cat: 2-15 mg (total dose) every 8 hours.

Route(s) of Administration—Per os.

Absorption—Metoprolol is almost completely absorbed from the GIT.

Bioavailability—Oral bioavailability is 20-40% in dog and 40-50% in human.

Peak Effect—1.5-4 hours.

Duration of Action—10-20 hours.

Distribution—Vd = 5.52 ± 0.64 L/kg in cat and 3.09-3.61 L/kg in dog. Metoprolol is well distributed into most tissues and organs including the brain, lungs, liver, kidneys and mammary gland. It crosses the placenta and attains high levels in milk.

Plasma Protein Binding—Low (5-15%).

Metabolism—The drug is metabolized in the liver largely to inactive products. Metoprolol undergoes extensive first-pass.

Plasma Half-Life (hours)—1.3-1.7 (dog); 1.3 (cat); 3-4 (human).

Clearance—109 (ml/min/kg) in healthy human subjects.

Route(s) of Excretion—Urine.

Dialysis Status—Nondialyzable.

Toxicity and Adverse Effects—Metoprolol is well tolerated at therapeutic doses. Bradycardia, lethargy and depression have been reported. Vomition and increased salivation has also been observed at therapeutic doses. High doses cause incoordination, ataxia, mydriasis, hyperemia and tremor in dogs. Doses of 100-120 mg may cause fatality.

Management of Overdose/Toxicity—Give general antidotal therapy.

Contraindications—Heart failure; sinus bradycardia; hypersensitivity to metoprolol.

Precautions—Use metoprolol cautiously in patients with hepatic impairment, sinus node dysfunction, diabetes mellitus, and in pregnancy. Concurrent use with negative inotropic drugs like calcium channel blockers should be done cautiously. Metoprolol or other adrenergic blockers either of the cardioselective or nonselective group should be used cautiously in patients with preexisting heart disease since compensatory dominance of sympathetic activity may be in place to maintain hemodynamics in such cases. Sudden blockade of sympathetic input to the cardiac $beta_1$-adrenoceptors in a compensated heart may precipitate heart failure.

Drug Interactions—Sympathomimetic drugs with actions at the beta-adrenergic receptors (especially $beta_1$ subtype) may have their actions reduced by metoprolol. These agents may also reduce the action of metoprolol. Myocardial depression will be enhanced with concurrent use of metoprolol and cardiac depressants like anesthetic agents. Phenothiazines, furosemide, and hydralazine may enhance the hypotensive action of metoprolol. Metoprolol may prolong the hypoglycemic action of insulin.

Pharmaceutical Formulations—This drug is available as metoprolol tartrate in 50 mg and 100 mg oral tablets and 1 mg/5 ml solution for injection. It is also available as metoprolol succinate in extended release tablets equivalent to 50 mg, 100 mg, and 200 mg. No specific veterinary formulations are available.

METRONIDAZOLE

Proprietary Names—Flagyl`; Metrogyl`.

Chemical Class—Nitroimidazole.

Pharmacological Class—Antiprotozoal drug; Antibacterial drug.

Source—Synthetic.

Solubility, Stability and Storage—Metronidazole base is sparingly soluble in water and alcohol. Metronidazole hydrochloride is very soluble in water and soluble in alcohol. Metronidazole and metronidazole hydrochloride are stable in air but darken following prolonged exposure to light. Products should be stored in well-closed, light-resistant containers at room temperature.

Pharmacological Actions—Metronidazole has actions against bacteria, amoeba and trichomonas organisms. It has bactericidal action against most obligate anaerobes including *Bacteroides, Fusobacterium, Veillonella,* and *Clostridium* species. It is active against *Trichomonas, Giardia, Balantidium coli* and trophozoite forms of *Entamoeba histolytica*. It is said to have anti-inflammatory properties in the large intestine. Metronidazole is able to modify cell mediated immunity so as to normalize excessive immune reactions, especially in the large intestine.

Mechanism of Action—Its mechanism of action is not fully understood. The drug is reduced to intermediates which are toxic to the microbial cell by disrupting DNA and nucleic acid synthesis.

Indications—Treatment of *Giardia, Entamoeba, Trichomonas,* and *Balantidium* infections in dogs and cats; treatment of genital trichomoniasis in cattle and dogs. It is used primarily with other antibiotics in horses to treat mixed bacterial infections in which anaerobic bacteria are present, for example, pleuropneumonia, peritonitis, and abdominal abscesses. Metronidazole is also used prophylactically after colic or other abdominal surgery when the risk of mixed bacterial infections is real. Metronidazole is also used in radiotherapy for cancer to sensitize anaerobic tumor tissues to radiation making a smaller dose of radiation more effective. It may be used with corticosteroids in the treatment of inflammatory bowel disease, or gum disease (gingivitis/stomatitis) in cats. Topical metronidazole gel is used in the treatment of skin infections such as feline chin acne.

Dosages—

Canine Giardia and Entamoeba infections	15-30 mg/kg orally twice daily for 5-7 days
Feline Giardia and Entamoeba infections	10-25 mg/kg orally twice daily for 5-7 days
Equine Giardia infections	5 mg/kg orally three times daily for 10 days
Bovine genital trichomoniasis	75 mg/kg intravenously for three consecutive days

Route(s) of Administration—Oral, intravenous and topical routes are used depending on the disease condition and dosage form.

Absorption—Metronidazole is well absorbed following oral administration. Peak plasma concentration is attained within 1 hour. Absorption is enhanced in dogs but delayed in humans if given with food.

Bioavailability—50-100% in dogs; 57-100% in horses.

Distribution—Metronidazole is rapidly and widely distributed. It reaches high concentration in tissues and fluids including bones, abscesses, CNS and seminal fluid. The drug readily crosses the placenta and is rapidly distributed into fetal circulation. It is distributed into milk following oral or IV administration.

Plasma Protein Binding—Less than 20% in human.

Metabolism—Metronidazole is metabolized in the liver by oxidation and glucuronide formation.

Plasma Half-Life—Human, 6-8 hours (higher in neonates and hepatic dysfunctions); dog, 4-5 hours; horses, 2.9-4.3 hours.

Route(s) of Excretion—Mainly urine (20% as unchanged drug) and feces. Small amounts appear in saliva and milk.

Dialysis Status—Dialyzable.

Toxicity and Adverse Effects—Side effects are not commonly seen with metronidazole unless the patient is taking especially high doses. Excessive salivation, gagging, regurgitation, pawing at the mouth, nausea, vomiting, and decreased appetite are the most frequent complaints in dogs and cats. Glossitis, stomatitis are other potential adverse effects at therapeutic doses. An overdose may cause neurological signs characterized by staggering, head tilt to one side, dilated pupils, and nystagmus. Metronidazole is carcinogenic in rodents.

Management of Overdose/Toxicity—The side effects resolve in a matter of days when medication is withdrawn. Give symptomatic and supportive treatment in acute overdose.

Contraindications—Hypersensitivity to metronidazole, its component, or related nitroimidazole derivatives. Do not use metronidazole in severely debilitated, pregnant, or nursing animals.

Precautions—Use metronidazole cautiously in patients with hepatic dysfunction, blood dyscrasia, history of seizure and congestive heart failure. Avoid or use metronidazole with caution, at reduced doses, in animals with kidney or liver disease.

Drug Interactions—Phenobarbital and phenytoin cause increases, while cimetidine decreases the metabolism of metronidazole. Prothrombin time is increased in patients receiving warfarin or other coumarin anticoagulants. Consumption of alcohol following administration of metronidazole may induce disulfiram-like reaction in humans.

Pharmaceutical Formulations—Metronidazole is available in 200 mg and 400 mg tablets; 373 mg capsules and 500 mg/ml ready to use injection. It is also available as metronidazole hydrochloride in 500 mg powder for injection and 0.75% topical gel.

MIDAZOLAM

Proprietary Names—Versed®.

Chemical Class—Benzodiazepine; Imidazobenzodiazepine.

Pharmacological Class—CNS depressant; Sedative-hypnotic; Anxiolytic.

Source—Synthetic.

Solubility, Stability and Storage—The aqueous solubility of midazolam hydrochloride is pH dependent. The drug has solubilities of approximately 0.24, 1.09, 3.67, 10.3, or greater than 22 mg (of midazolam) per mL in water at pH 6.2, 5.1, 3.8, 3.4, or 2.8, respectively, at 25°C. Store midazolam formulations at room temperature in light resistant container. Midazolam hydrochloride injection is chemically and physically compatible with 5% dextrose, 0.9% sodium chloride, or lactated Ringer's solutions. It is physically compatible for at least 30 minutes with atropine sulfate, meperidine hydrochloride, morphine sulfate, or scopolamine hydrobromide, and for at least 8 hours with fentanyl citrate, glycopyrrolate, hydroxyzine hydrochloride, ketamine hydrochloride, nalbuphine hydrochloride, promethazine hydrochloride, or sufentanil citrate when mixed in the same syringe.

Midazolam

Pharmacological Actions—Midazolam depresses the CNS at the subcortical level and produces sedation, hypnosis, and stupor with increasing dosage. It decreases anxiety without decreasing alertness or impairing perceptive or cognitive capacities. It has anticonvulsant and muscle relaxant properties. Midazolam does not cause a true general anesthesia because awareness usually persists following its use.

Mechanism of Action—Midazolam binds to $GABA_A$ receptor/ion channel complex in the presence of GABA and allosterically modulates the action of GABA to produce increase in neuronal chloride conductance resulting in hyperpolarization and reduced neuronal excitability.

Indications—Preanesthetic medication.

Dosages—

Dog, cat	0.066-0.22 mg/kg
Bird	6 mg/kg IM
Goat	0.5 mg/kg IV

Mouse	5 mg/kg IM, IP
Rat	2 mg/kg IV ; 4 mg/kg IM; 5 mg/kg IP
Rabbit	0.5-2 mg/kg IM, IP, IV.
Horse	0.011-0.44 mg/kg.

Route(s) of Administration—Intramuscular and intravenous routes are used.

Absorption—Midazolam is rapidly and almost completely absorbed from muscular sites. Although not administered orally, absorption from oral route is rapid.

Bioavailability—31-72% (oral); 91% (IM).

Effective Concentration—50 ± 20 ng/ml.

Onset of Action—15 minutes (IM); 1-5 minutes (IV).

Peak Effect—0.5-1 hour.

Duration of Action—2-6 hours.

Distribution—Vd = 0.8-2.5 L/kg (human; Vd is higher in obesity). Midazolam is widely distributed, highly lipophilic and crosses the blood-brain-barrier.

Plasma Protein Binding—94-97% (human).

Metabolism—Midazolam is rapidly metabolized to α-hydroxymidazolam, which is active but transient because it is rapidly conjugated with glucuronic acid.

Plasma Half-Life—1.9 ± 0.6 hours (human).

Clearance—6.6 ± 1.8 ml/min/kg in human.

Route(s) of Excretion—56 ± 26% in urine (human).

Dialysis Status—Not dialyzable.

Toxicity and Adverse Effects—These have been reported in humans and are few. It causes phlebitis and pain at the site of injection. This is less severe than with diazepam. Other minor effects are respiratory depression, cardiac arrest, ataxia, nausea, vomiting and hiccups.

Management of Overdose—Follow general antidotal therapy in addition to adequate supportive measures. Flumazenil will specifically antagonize midazolam CNS depressant effect.

Contraindications—Hypersensitivity to midazolam or other benzodiazepines; acute narrow-angle glaucoma.

Precautions—Use midazolam cautiously in debilitated patients and patients with respiratory depression. Reduce the dose of anesthetic agent if used in conjunction with midazolam.

Drug Interactions—Concurrent administration of midazolam with other CNS depressants will give additive effects. Cimetidine may increase the blood concentration of midazolam. Theophylline may antagonize its sedative effect.

Pharmaceutical Formulations—The drug is available as midazolam hydrochloride in the form of 1 mg/ml and 5 mg/ml injectable solutions. Only formulations for human use are available.

MILBEMYCIN OXIME

Proprietary Names—Interceptor˙; Safeheart˙; Sentinel˙ (in combination with Lufenuron); Program® (in combination with Lufenuron); Milbemax˙ (in combination with praziquantel).

Chemical Class—Macrocyclic lactone.

Pharmacological Class—Ectoparasiticide; Endectocide; Anthelmintic

Source—Natural; obtained from *Streptomyces hygroscopicus aureolacrimosus*.

Solubility, Stability and Storage—Milbemycin oxime is poorly soluble in water. Store products at room temperature.

Pharmacological Actions—Milbemycin oxime has activity against nematodes and ectoparasites, particularly *Demodex canis*. It is effective against *Toxocara canis*, *Trichuris* and *Ancylostoma* species. Milbemycin is also effective against the developmental larvae of *Dirofilaria immitis*. It is highly active against microfilaria. It also blocks embryogenesis.

R: CH₃ (30 %)
R: CH₂CH₃ (70 %)

Milbemycin oxime

Mechanism of Action—Milbemycin oxime increases neuronal chloride conductance by opening glutamate-gated chloride channels and also by potentiating the release and binding of GABA at certain synapses in invertebrates. This results in hyperpolarization and reduced neuronal excitability thereby causing paralysis of the peripheral musculature of susceptible parasites. Lufenuron (contained in a formulation of milbemycin oxime) inhibits the production of chitin in insects thus preventing the hatching of flea eggs and the development of exoskeleton in flea larvae.

Indications—Prevention of dirofilariasis in dogs and cats; control of hookworm (especially ancylostomiasis), whipworms, and roundworms in dogs; control of demodecosis in dogs. The combination of milbemycin and praziquantel is indicated for the treatment of mixed infections by gastrointestinal nematodes and cestodes. Milbemycin/lufenuron combination is indicated for the prevention and control of flea populations, the prevention of heartworm (*Dirofilaria immitis*) disease and the treatment and control of roundworms (*Toxocara canis*, *Toxascaris leonina*), hookworms (*Ancylostoma caninum*) and whipworms (*Trichuris vulpis*) in dogs.

Dosages—0.5-0.99 mg/kg every month for prophylaxis of dirofilariasis and control of hookworm, whipworms and roundworms in dogs and cats; 0.5-1 mg/kg /day for 60-90 days for demodecosis.

Route(s) of Administration—Per os.

Absorption—Only 5-10% of a given dose is absorbed.

Onset of Action—Rapid.

Duration of Action—Milbemycin prevents the establishment of infection up to 45 days post exposure to infective larvae of *D. immitis*.

Distribution—Milbemycin is distributed into milk.

Route(s) of Excretion—90-95% of dose is excreted unchanged in feces while 5-10% excreted in bile.

Toxicity and Adverse Effects. Milbemycin oxime is well tolerated. Collie dogs may be sensitive to milbemycin at 10 times the recommended dose. Overdose in collie dogs may cause ataxia and periodic recumbency. Dogs with heavy filarial burden may show mild reaction characterized by depression, salivation, coughing, emesis, or tachypnea.

Management of Overdose/Toxicity—Reactions arising from presence of microfilaria in blood may be controlled by corticosteroids and IV fluids.

Contraindications—Hypersensitivity to milbemycin oxime.

Precautions—Administer milbemycin with prednisolone (or other corticosteroid) in microfilaremic dogs. Administer milbemycin within 30 days if discontinuing diethylcarbamazine.

Drug Interactions—There are no known adverse interaction with other drugs.

Pharmaceutical Formulations—Milbemycin is available as chewable tablets containing 2.3, 5.75, 11.5 or 23.0 mg of mixture of not less than 80% A_4 milbemycin oxime and not more than 20% A_3 milbemycin oxime. The drug is also available in combinations with lufenuron and praziquantel in oral tablets of different colors and strength.

MISOPROSTOL

Misoprostol

Proprietary Names—Cytotec˚; Arthrotec˚ (with Diclofenac); Napratec˚ (with Naproxen).

Chemical Class—Prostaglandin.

Pharmacological Class—Antiulcer agent.

Source—A synthetic analog of prostaglandin E_1 (alprostadil).

Solubility, Stability and Storage—Store misoprostol tablets at room temperature in a dry place and in well-closed containers.

Pharmacological Actions—Misoprostol is a gastric antisecretory agent with protective effects on the gastroduodenal mucosa. It inhibits gastric acid secretion and protects the mucosa from the irritant and/or other (e.g., pharmacologic) effects of certain drugs. Secretion is inhibited under basal conditions and also when stimulated by food, histamine, pentagastrin, betazole, tetragastrin, and NSAIDs. The degree of inhibition of gastric acid secretion is directly related to misoprostol dose. It may have similar antisecretory and mucosal effects in patients with gastric or duodenal ulcer. Misoprostol also increases the amplitude and frequency of uterine contractions, stimulates uterine bleeding and total or partial expulsion of uterine contents during pregnancy.

Mechanism of Action—Misoprostol reduces gastric acid secretion via a direct action on the parietal cells.

Indications—Short-term treatment of active duodenal benign gastric ulcers; maintenance therapy following healing of gastric ulcer to reduce ulcer recurrence; to reduce the risk of nonsteroidal anti-inflammatory drug (NSAID)-induced gastric ulcer in patients at high risk of developing complications from these ulcers and in patients at high risk of developing gastric ulceration. Misoprostol is also used to induce labor and treat serious postpartum hemorrhage in the presence of uterine atony.

Dosages—Dog, 2-5 µg/kg three times daily. In animals, doses smaller than those necessary for inhibition of gastric acid secretion have provided protection of the gastric mucosa.

Route(s) of Administration—Per os.

Absorption—Misoprostol is rapidly and almost completely absorbed from the GIT. Food and antacids decrease the rate of absorption.

Onset of Action—30 minutes.

Peak Action—60-90 minutes.

Duration of Action—About 3 hours (dose related).

Distribution—Vd = 6.6 L/kg. Misoprostol is widely distributed. It achieves concentrations in stomach, intestines, liver, blood, and kidneys.

Plasma Protein Binding—A misoprostol metabolite, misoprostol acid is approximately 80–90% bound to serum proteins.

Metabolism—Misoprostol is rapidly metabolized to misoprostol acid which is active.

Plasma Half-life—20-40 minutes for metabolite; shorter for parent drug; higher in renal impairment.

Route(s) of Excretion—Mainly in urine (with negligible amounts of unchanged drug); smaller amounts of metabolites are excreted in feces, probably via biliary elimination.

Toxicity and Adverse Effects—Diarrhea which is dose related and generally self-limiting is the most common adverse effect of misoprostol. Other minor signs are abdominal pain, nausea, vomiting, and constipation. Overdose produces diarrhea, GI lesions, emesis, tremors, mydriasis, focal cardiac necrosis, hepatic necrosis, renal tubular necrosis, testicular atrophy, hypertrophy of mucous cells, deepening of gastric pits, respiratory difficulties, reduced motor activity, and CNS depression.

Management of Overdose/Toxicity. Give symptomatic and supportive therapy

Contraindications—Pregnancy; hypersensitivity to misoprostol.

Precautions—Use cautiously in patients with hepatic impairment.

Drug Interactions—Magnesium-containing antacids may increase the incidence of misoprostol-induced diarrhea. In animals, misoprostol has been effective in reversing cyclosporine-induced nephrotoxicity. In this situation, misoprostol increases glomerular filtration rate, urinary flow rate, renal blood flow, sodium excretion, and urinary osmolarity and decreases renal vascular resistance.

Pharmaceutical Formulations—Misoprostol is available in 100 mcg and 200 mcg tablets. It is also available in combination with diclofenac sodium in tablets containing 200 mcg misoprostol outer layer and 50 mg diclofenac sodium enteric-coated core.

MITOTANE

Synonyms—o,p'-DDD

Proprietary Names—Lysodren®.

Chemical Class—Organochlorine compound (chemically similar to DDT).

Pharmacological Class—Antineoplastic drug; Anticancer drug; Cytotoxic drug; Selective inhibitor of adrenocortical function.

Source—Synthetic.

Stability and Storage—Mitotane is practically insoluble in water but soluble in alcohol. Store products at room temperature in light resistant container.

Pharmacological Actions—Mitotane is selectively cytotoxic to normal and neoplastic adrenocortical cells. It affects the mitochondria in adrenal cortical cells and decreases the production of adrenocorticosteroids. Therefore, it causes rapid reduction in blood and urine levels of adrenocorticosteroids. It also reduces the peripheral metabolism of adrenocorticosteroids.

Mechanism of Action. The mechanism is uncertain.

Indications—Treatment of adrenal hyperplasia, and adrenal carcinoma in dogs and cats.

Dosages—50 mg/kg daily for 4-7 days followed by once weekly.

Route(s) of Administration—Per os.

Absorption—30-40% of oral dose is absorbed. Peak plasma concentration is attained within 3-5 hours (human).

Bioavailability—Oral bioavailability is poor

Distribution—Mitotane is stored mainly in fat tissues.

Metabolism—It is degraded primarily in the liver by hydroxylation and oxidation to inactive metabolites.

Plasma Half-life—18-159 days.

Route(s) of Excretion—Urine and bile (with 60% as unchanged drug).

Toxicity and Adverse Effects—Early common adverse effects include lethargy, ataxia, and anorexia. Dose limiting adverse effects are associated with the GIT and CNS. Nausea, vomiting, diarrhea, CNS depression and vertigo have been reported.

Management of Overdose/Toxicology—Initiate general antidotal therapy.

Contraindications—Hypersensitivity to mitotane.

Precautions—Adverse effects of mitotane are related to low plasma cortisol level. Therefore, it is expedient to halt mitotane treatment temporarily and give glucocorticoids if adverse effects are severe. Give supplementary corticosteroids in patients with evidence of stress, shock or adrenal insufficiency. Use mitotane cautiously in patients with renal and/or hepatic impairment. Monitor patients with concurrent diabetes mellitus as their insulin requirements may be reduced following initial treatment with mitotane. Use the drug cautiously during pregnancy and consider milk replacers for offspring of nursing bitches and queens.

Drug Interactions—Mitotane may induce microsomal enzymes and influence the metabolism of drugs normally degraded by the enzymes (e.g. barbiturates, warfarin etc.). Mitotane may enhance the action of CNS depressants. Spironolactone abolishes the action of mitotane.

Pharmaceutical Formulations—Mitotane is available in 500 mg oral scored tablets.

MITOXANTRONE

Synonyms—DHAD; Dihydroanthracenedione.

Proprietary Names—Novantrone®.

Chemical Class—Anthracycline.

Pharmacological Class—Antineoplastic drug; Anticancer drug; Cytotoxic drug; Anticancer antibiotic.

Source—Synthetic; doxorubicin analog.

Solubility, Stability and Storage—Store unopened vials of mitoxantrone at room temperature. Opened vials are stable for 7 days at room temperature or 14 days if refrigerated. Mitoxantrone is incompatible with heparin and hydrocortisone. Do not mix mitoxantrone with other drugs before administration.

Pharmacological Actions—Mitoxantrone has activity against a wide variety of tumors. It is cell-cycle nonspecific although it is most active in the S phase. It inhibits DNA and RNA synthesis.

Mitoxantrone

Mechanism of Action—Mitoxantrone intercalates with DNA to inhibit DNA-dependent RNA synthesis. It also causes breaks in DNA strands by activating topoisomerase II.

Indications—Adjunctive treatment of wide variety of carcinomas and sarcomas (including lymphosarcoma) in dogs and cats.

Dosages—5-6 mg/m^2 every 3 weeks up to 240 mg/m^2.

Route(s) of Administration—Intravenous infusion.

Absorption—Oral absorption is poor.

Bioavailability—Oral bioavailability is low (5%).

Distribution—Vd = 14L/kg. Mitoxantrone is cleared rapidly from plasma to the heart, lungs, kidney, liver, spleen and erythrocyte.

Plasma Protein Binding—78%. It binds avidly to tissue proteins.

Metabolism—It is metabolized in the liver.

Plasma Half-life—37 hours (human).

Clearance—Rapidly cleared from plasma.

Route(s) of Excretion—Excreted in urine and bile both as unchanged drug and metabolites.

Toxicity and Adverse Effects—Mitoxantrone causes less cardiotoxicity, nausea, vomiting, tissue irritation and alopecia than doxorubicin. Cardiotoxicity has not been reported in dogs but rare in humans. Mitoxantrone causes acute myelosuppression and mucositis. It stains urine blue-green.

Management of Overdose/Toxicity—Give symptomatic and supportive therapy.

Contraindications—Hypersensitivity to mitoxantrone; preexisting myelosuppression or infection.

Precautions—Use mitoxantrone with caution in cases of hepatic impairment or hyperuricemia. Administer IV bolus slowly over 10-15 minutes preferably diluted to a concentration of 0.02-0.5 mg/ml in normal saline. Use live vaccines with caution, if at all, during therapy.

Drug Interactions—Mitoxantrone may produce additive bone marrow depression with other antineoplastic agents and bone marrow depressants (e.g. chloramphenicol, flucytosine, amphotericin B, and colchicine). Azathioprine, cyclophosphamide, corticosteroids and other immunodepressants may increase the risk of infection when used concurrently with mitoxantrone. Prior anthracycline therapy or mediastinal irradiation may predispose to cardiotoxicity.

Pharmaceutical Formulations—The drug is available as mitoxantrone hydrochloride in 2 mg/ml solution for injection.

MORANTEL

Proprietary Names—Banminth II˚; Paratect˚.

Chemical Class—Tetrahydropyrimidine compound.

Pharmacological Class—Anthelmintic.

Source—Synthetic; a methyl ester analog of pyrantel.

Pharmacological Actions—Morantel paralyzes and consequently causes the expulsion of adult and immature forms of gastrointestinal worms such as *Haemonchus, Ostertagia, Trichostrongylus, Cooperia, Nematodirus, Chabertia* and *Oesophagostomum* in cattle, sheep and goats.

Mechanism of Action—Morantel acts as a neuromuscular blocking agent by inhibiting acetylcholinesterase thereby causing accumulation of acetylcholine which induces marked nicotinic activation at the neuromuscular junction and produce spastic paralysis of the worm. It also inhibits the fumarate reductase enzyme in *Haemonchus* species.

Indications—Morantel is used for treatment of both adult and immature stages of most gastrointestinal roundworm infections in ruminants. It is also used to treat *Thelazia* eye infections in cattle.

Dosages—

Morantel tartrate: sheep and goats, 10 mg/kg; cattle, 8.8 mg/kg. Morantel fumarate: sheep and goats, 12.5 mg/kg.

Route(s) of Administration—Per os.

Absorption—Morantel is absorbed. Peak plasma levels are attained within 4-6 hours.

Bioavailability—Plasma levels are low (0.05 mcg/ml).

Metabolism—Absorbed portions are rapidly metabolized in the liver and excreted in urine within 96 hours.

Route(s) of Excretion—Feces and urine.

Withdrawal Period—14 days before slaughter. There is no withdrawal period for milk because of low levels in milk.

Toxicity and Adverse Effects—Morantel has a wide safety margin. It is safer than pyrantel. Its LD_{50} in mice is 5 g/kg.

Contraindications—Hypersensitivity to morantel.

Precautions—Do not use the sustained release formulation of morantel in cattle weighing less than 90 kg. Do not use morantel concurrently with pyrantel or levamisole to avoid toxicity resulting from similar mechanisms of action. Watch for adverse effects if used concurrently with organophosphates and diethylcarbamazine.

Drug Interactions—Piperazine may antagonize the actions of morantel. Mineral bullets may reduce its anthelmintic activity.

Pharmaceutical Formulations—The drug is available commonly as morantel tartrate in 2.2 g oral bolus and oral aqueous solution. Sustained release formulation containing 22.7 g morantel tartrate per cartridge is also available. A 4% ointment of morantel tartrate is available for the treatment of *Thelazia* eye infections in cattle. Other available salts are citrate and fumarate.

MORPHINE

Morphine

Proprietary Names—Roxanol˚; Astramorph˚; Duramorph˚.

Chemical Class—Phenanthrene alkaloid.

Pharmacological Class—Narcotic analgesic; opioid analgesic.

Source—Natural; contained in opium, the dried and powdered milky exudate of the unripe seed capsule of the poppy plant (*Papaver somniferum*).

Solubility, Stability and Storage—Morphine has solubilities of approximately 62.5 mg/mL in water and 1.75 mg/mL in alcohol at 25°C. Morphine sulfate darkens on prolonged exposure to light. Morphine products should be stored in tight, light-resistant containers at 15-30°C. Morphine sulfate injection and oral solution should not be frozen.

Pharmacological Actions—Morphine actions are diverse and seem to vary with species and at times with individual subjects. The drug produces CNS depression in humans, dogs, and primates and cause analgesia, drowsiness, changes in mood and metal clouding. Morphine causes excitement in cats, cattle, horses, goat and sheep due to action on hippocampal pyramidal cells in which it appears to inhibit GABA release. It stimulates emesis and produces antitussive effect and hypothermia in dogs. Morphine also causes miosis in humans and dogs as well as depresses respiration in most species. It causes decreased motility and secretion of the GIT, alters endocrine and autonomic system functions. Morphine stimulates the secretion of ADH and reduces urine output. It causes unpleasant reaction in subjects that have no pain. Repeated use results in tolerance and physical dependence in humans. This is rarely noticed in animals because opioids are only used on short term basis in animals.

Mechanism of Action—Morphine combines with and activates mu opioid receptors. It also has appreciable affinity for delta and kappa opioid receptors. These opioid receptors are thought to mediate inhibition of release of neurotransmitters.

Indications—Morphine is used in preanesthetic medication and to control severe pain, cough, and diarrhea.

Dosages—

Horse, cattle	0.22 mg/kg IM for analgesia or 0.12 mg/kg IV for preanesthetic medication.
Sheep, goat	0.2 mg/kg up to 10 mg total dose IM.
Pig	0.2 mg/kg up to 20 mg total dose IM.
Dog	0.5-1.0 mg/kg SC or IM for analgesia; 0.1-2 mg/kg SC for preanesthetic medication.
Cat	0.1 mg/kg SC.

Route(s) of Administration—Intravenous, intramuscular, subcutaneous and oral routes are appropriate depending on the dosage form.

Absorption—Morphine is readily absorbed from all routes.

Bioavailability—24 ± 12% following oral administration.

Onset of Action—Few minutes.

Peak Action—30-45 minutes (dog).

Duration of Action—1 to 2 hours (dog).

Effective Concentration—65 ± 80 ng/ml.

Distribution—Vd = 3.3 ± 2 L/kg. Morphine is distributed to and concentrated in kidneys, lungs, skeletal muscle and liver. It crosses the placenta and is secreted in milk. Concentration in the CNS decreases with age as the blood-brain barrier develops. The major metabolite, morphine-6-glucuronide penetrates the blood-brain-barrier less than the parent compound.

Plasma Protein Binding—35 ± 2%.

Metabolism—Morphine is conjugated with glucuronic acid to both active and inactive products. Morphine-6-glucuronide is a major active metabolite.

Plasma Half-Life—1.9 ± 0.5 hours (human); 1.5 hours (horse); 3.05 hours in cats (due to deficiency of uridine diphosphate glucuronic acid and related glucuronyl transferase enzyme). Morphine-6-glucuronide has higher t½ than the parent compound and accumulates following chronic morphine administration.

Clearance—24 ± 10 (ml/min/kg).

Route(s) of Excretion—Morphine is excreted in urine (mainly as morphine-3-glucuronide and small unchanged morphine), and feces (due to enterohepatic circulation).

Toxicity and Adverse Effects—Respiratory depression, nausea, vomiting, dizziness, mental clouding, dysphoria, pruritus, constipation have been reported. Respiratory depression may be pronounced and is usually the cause of death in morphine overdose. Restlessness and convulsive seizure at high doses may be noticed in most animal species including dog. Bronchoconstriction apparently due to histamine release has been noticed in dogs. Overdose causes stupor or coma, shallow breathing, cyanosis, and pinpoint pupils. Death is usually due to respiratory collapse. Newborn animals are more sensitive to the actions of morphine than adults hence toxicity decreases with age.

Management of Overdose/Toxicity—Initiate general antidotal therapy in conjunction with administration of naloxone, the specific antidote for morphine and its congeners

Contraindications—Cat; traumatic shock; convulsive seizure; hypersensitivity to morphine or its congeners.

Precautions—Acquired tolerance to and dependence on morphine can be induced with repeated dosing. It should be used with caution in patients with hepatic disease, impaired renal function, decreased respiratory reserve, head injury and hypotension.

Drug Interactions—The CNS depressant effects of morphine is enhanced and prolonged by phenothiazines, MAO inhibitors and tricyclic antidepressants. Amphetamine enhances its analgesic and euphoriant effects.

Pharmaceutical Formulations—It is available as morphine sulfate in solutions, tablets, controlled-release tablets and rectal suppositories.

MOXIDECTIN

Proprietary Names—Cydectin˙; ProHeart˙; Quest˙; Vetdectin˙; Moxidec˙.

Chemical Class—Macrocyclic lactone.

Pharmacological Class—Ectoparasiticide; Endectocide; Anthelmintic

Source—Semi synthetic; modified from nemadectin, a fermentation product of *Streptomyces cyaneorgriseus monocyanogenus*.

Solubility, Stability and Storage—Moxidectin is highly lipophilic. Store products at room temperature or below. Protect from light.

Pharmacological Actions—Like other endectocides, moxidectin is active against nematodes and ectoparasites. It is effective against adults and larvae of major gastrointestinal nematodes such as *Ostertagia, Bunostomum, Oesophagostomum, Trichostrongylus, Trichuris* and *Haemonchus* species of ruminants. *Dictyocaulus* spp of cattle are susceptible, so also are major gastrointestinal nematodes of horses. Sarcoptic, Psoroptes and a lesser extent, Chorioptes mites are susceptible. Moxidectin is efficacious against ticks and sucking lice. It eliminates the developing larvae of *D. immitis*.

Mechanism of Action—Moxidectin increases neuronal chloride conductance by opening glutamate-gated chloride channels and also by potentiating the release and binding of GABA at certain synapses in invertebrates. This results in hyperpolarization and reduced neuronal excitability thereby causing paralysis of the peripheral musculature of susceptible parasites.

Indications—Control of internal and external parasites in ruminants and horses; prophylaxis of dirofilariasis in dogs.

Dosages—

Ruminant.	200 mcg/kg (drench and injection formulations); 500 mcg/kg (pour-on formulation).
Dog	3 mcg/kg every month for prophylaxis of dirofilariasis.
Horse	400 mcg/kg.

Route(s) of Administration—Per os, subcutaneous or topical.

Duration of Action—Moxidectin may prevent reinfection for 28 days.

Distribution—Tissue levels persist longer than those of ivermectin. Moxidectin is distributed into milk.

Plasma Half-life. Plasma drug levels may be high for 14-15 days.

Route(s) of Excretion. Mainly feces.

Toxicity and Adverse Effects. Moxidectin is well tolerated. No adverse effects have been reported even following administration of 10 times the recommended dose in adult cattle. Collies and microfilaremic dogs have tolerated 5 times the recommended dose.

Contraindications—Hypersensitivity to moxidectin.

Precautions—Use moxidectin cautiously in calves weighing less than 100 kg.

Pharmaceutical Formulations—Moxidectin is available as 0.1% and 0.2% oral drench (for small ruminants); 1% solution for injection (in cattle); 0.5% pour-on in oil vehicle. Oral drenches and injection solution are formulated in propylene glycol. It is also available in tablets containing 7.5, 15, 30, 68 or 136 mcg of moxidectin, and in oral gel of 20 mg/ml.

NAFCILLIN

Proprietary Names—Nafcil ®; Nallpen ®; Unipen ®.

Chemical Class—6—aminopenicillanic acid derivative.

Pharmacological Class—Penicillinase resistant penicillin; Beta-lactam antibiotic.

Source—Semisynthetic.

Solubility, Stability and Storage—Nafcillin is freely soluble in water and soluble in alcohol. The powder may be reconstituted with sterile water for injection, bacteriostatic water for injection, or 0.9% sodium chloride injection. Reconstituted solutions containing 250 mg of nafcillin per mL are stable for 3 days at room temperature, 7 days when refrigerated, or 90 days when frozen.

Nafcillin

Pharmacological Actions—Nafcillin is bactericidal to penicillin G resistant *Staphylococcus* and other Gram-positive organisms. It is slightly more active than oxacillin but less potent than penicillin G against penicillin G-sensitive microorganisms.

Mechanism of Action—Nafcillin inhibits bacteria cell wall synthesis by similar mechanism with penicillin G.

Indications—Treatment of infections of respiratory tract, soft tissues, skin and suppurative osteomyelitis caused by penicillin G-resistant *Staphylococcus* and *Streptococcus*.

Dosages—7-11 mg/kg IM 4-6 times/day.

Route(s) of Administration—Per os and intramuscular.

Absorption—Nafcillin is irregularly absorbed from the GIT but it is absorbed well from IM site. Peak plasma concentration is attained within 1 hour following IM injection.

Bioavailability—36% (oral).

Distribution—Vd = 0.57–1.55 L/kg (human adult). Nafcillin is distributed into tissues and body fluid such as synovial, pleural, pericardial, and ascitic fluids. It attains higher concentration in bile than serum. It attains therapeutic concentrations in the CSF especially when meninges are inflamed. Nafcillin crosses the placenta.

Plasma Protein Binding—70–90%.

Plasma Half-Life—0.5-1.5 hours. Values are higher in neonates. It undergoes enterohepatic circulation.

Clearance (ml/min/kg)—7.5 ± 1.9.

Route(s) of Excretion—Bile and urine (10-30% as unchanged drug).

Dialysis Status—Not dialyzable.

Toxicity and Adverse Effects—Nafcillin causes pain and irritation at IM site. It may cause hypersensitivity reactions, nausea, diarrhea, neutropenia and acute interstitial nephritis at therapeutic doses. Overdose may cause neuromuscular hypersensitivity, electrolyte imbalance and renal failure.

Management of Overdose/Toxicity—If overdosed, withdraw the drug and give symptomatic treatment.

Contraindications—Hypersensitivity to nafcillin, the penicillins or their products or components.

Precautions—Avoid extravasation during injection; reduce dose in renal and hepatic impairment.

Drug Interactions—Chloramphenicol reduces nafcillin plasma levels while probenecid increases its levels. Nafcillin may increase the risk of bleeding with oral coagulants and heparin.

Pharmaceutical Formulations—The drug is formulated as nafcillin sodium in 250 mg capsules; 500 mg, 1 g, 2 g, 4 g, and 10 g powder for injection. It is also available in 250 mg/5 ml solution and 500 mg tablets. Intra mammary preparations are available for veterinary use. Each mg of nafcillin sodium contains not less than 820 mcg of nafcillin.

NALOXONE

Synonyms—N-allylnoroxymorphone.

Proprietary Names—Nalone˚; Naxolan˚; Zynox˚; Narcan˚.

Chemical Class—Oxymorphone derivative.

Pharmacological Class—Opioid antagonist.

Source—Semi synthetic; Naloxone is derived from thebaine.

Stability and Storage—Naloxone is soluble in water, slightly soluble in alcohol and practically insoluble in ether and chloroform. Store naloxone formulations at room temperature in light resistant containers. Dilute naloxone solution with sterile water for injection. Naloxone can be mixed with normal saline. It is unstable in alkaline medium.

Naloxone

Pharmacological Actions—Naloxone is devoid of agonist actions at low doses if the endogenous opioid system is inactivated or if opioid agonist has not been administered previously. Otherwise, it decreases tolerance to pain. Naloxone reverses opiate effects within 1-2 minutes and precipitates withdrawal syndrome. It reverses or attenuates the hypotension associated with shock in animals. Naloxone produces slight sedation at very large doses. The drug increases energy expenditure, interrupt hibernation and induce weight loss. At high doses, naloxone affects dopaminergic mechanism, antagonizes GABA and releases catecholamines which may cause increased arterial pressure and myocardial contractility.

Mechanism of Action—Naloxone competes with opioids and morphinomimetic peptides (e.g. β-endorphin) for binding sites in those areas of the brain believed to be responsible for pain perception. It has high binding affinity for μ (mu) opioid receptors. It binds less to δ (delta) and κ (kappa) receptors. Its use in hypovolemic shock is associated with its antagonism of the hypotensive effects of β-endorphin which is one of the potent compounds released during stress.

Indications—Treatment of acute opioid overdose; reversal of hypovolemic and endotoxic shock in dogs and cats; reversal of immobilizing actions of fentanyl and etorphine in game animals. Naloxone is used with 4-aminopyrine (0.5 mg/kg) to reverse the effects of fentanyl/droperidol in game animals.

Dosages—0.04 mg/kg. Repeat at 2-3 minutes interval.

Route(s) of Administration—Intravenous and intramuscular (require high dose).

Absorption—Absorption from the oral route is 91% but most of the drug is subject to first-pass metabolism.

Bioavailability—2.0%

Onset of Action—Action is immediate following IV injection but 1-5 minutes with IM or SC injection.

Duration of Action—45 to 90 minutes.

Distribution—Vd = 2.1 L/kg. Distributes rapidly and attains high levels in several organs including heart, kidney, spleen, brain, lungs and skeletal muscle. It crosses the placenta.

Metabolism—Naloxone is conjugated with glucuronic acid in the liver.

Plasma Half-Life—1.1 ± 0.6 hours.

Clearance—22.0 (ml/min/kg).

Route(s) of Excretion—Urine.

Toxicity and Adverse Effects—Increased systolic blood pressure, cardiac arrhythmia, and slight drowsiness at high doses are common. In humans naloxone may cause decreased performance on tests of memory. Naloxone has high therapeutic index but excessive doses may precipitate seizures.

Contraindications—Hypersensitivity to naloxone.

Precautions—Do not administer naloxone orally. Use the drug cautiously in patients with cardiovascular disease. Avoid high doses in patients that have received opioid during surgery because naloxone may increase blood pressure and reverse anesthesia.

Drug Interactions—Naloxone decreases effects of opioid analgesics. It also reverses the actions of opioid with mixed actions.

Pharmaceutical Formulations—The drug is formulated as naloxone hydrochloride in 0.02, 0.04 and 1 mg/ml solutions for injection.

NALTREXONE

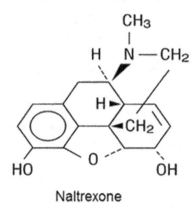

Naltrexone

Proprietary Names—Trexan*; ReVia*.

Chemical Class—Oxymorphone derivative.

Pharmacological Class—Pure Opioid Antagonist.

Source—Semi synthetic; Naltrexone is derived from thebaine.

Solubility, Stability and Storage—Naltrexone has a solubility of 100 mg/mL in water at 25°C. Naltrexone hydrochloride tablets should be stored in well-closed containers at 15-30°C.

Pharmacological Actions—Actions of naltrexone are similar to those of naloxone. Naltrexone has higher oral efficacy and longer duration of action than naloxone and it blocks the euphoric effects of opioids more effectively. Naltrexone increases the secretion of gonadotrophin releasing hormone and corticotropin-releasing factor and elevates plasma concentration of LH, FSH and ACTH.

Mechanism of Action—See naloxone.

Indications—Control of self-mutilating and tail-chasing behaviors in dogs and cats; control of pruritic dermatitis; prevention of crib biting in horses.

Dosages—

Horse, 0.4 mg/kg.

Dog, Cat, 1-2 mg/kg daily.

Route(s) of Administration—Per os, intravenous and subcutaneous.

Absorption—Naltrexone is rapidly and almost completely absorbed from the GIT of humans and simple stomach animals. Peak plasma concentration is attained within 1 hour.

Bioavailability—5 to 40%.

Duration of Action—Varies with the dose; lasts for 6 hours in horses at 0.4 mg/kg.

Distribution—Vd = 19 ± 5 L/kg. Naltrexone is widely distributed but individual variations exist. CSF levels may be as much as 30% of plasma levels.

Plasma Protein Binding—20%.

Metabolism—Naltrexone is converted mainly in the liver to 6-beta-naltrexol, a weak active metabolite with t½ of 8.8-13 hours.

Plasma Half-Life—2.7 ± 1.0 hours.

Clearance—48 ± 6 (ml/min/kg).

Route(s) of Excretion—Urine (<1%).

Toxicity and Adverse Effects—Naltrexone is a relatively safe drug even though nausea, vomiting, abdominal cramps, insomnia, nervousness and skin rashes have been reported in humans. Drowsiness and minor changes in behavior have been observed in dogs. Naltrexone has been shown to cause dose-dependent hepatotoxicity. Mild dysphoria has been observed in some cases at high doses. Overdose causes seizures and respiratory failure.

Management of Overdose/Toxicity—Initiate general antidotal therapy and give supportive and symptomatic treatment.

Contraindications—Hypersensitivity to naltrexone; severe hepatic impairment; opioid-dependent subjects.

Precautions—Use naltrexone cautiously in pregnant and nursing animals.

Drug Interactions—Naltrexone blocks the effects of pure and partial opioid agonists thus reducing the analgesic, antidiarrheal and antitussive effects of these drugs. Naltrexone causes withdrawal syndromes in opioid-dependent humans.

Pharmaceutical Formulations—It is available as naltrexone hydrochloride in 50 mg tablets.

NAPROXEN

Naproxen sodium

Proprietary Names—Naprosyn˙; Anaprox˙ (Naproxen sodium) Naprium˙; Naxen˙; Equiproxen®.

Chemical Class—Propionic acid derivative.

Pharmacological Class—Nonsteroidal Anti-inflammatory Drug; Non-narcotic analgesic; Analgesic-antipyretic.

Source—Synthetic.

Solubility, Stability and Storage—Naproxen is practically insoluble in water but soluble 1 in 25 of ethanol. Store naproxen products below 40° C; protect products from light.

Pharmacological Actions—Naproxen possesses analgesic, antipyretic and anti-inflammatory properties. It also inhibits the migration of leukocytes.

Mechanism of Action—Like other prototypical NSAIDs, naproxen inhibits cyclooxygenase-1 (COX-1) and—2 (COX-2) (also referred to as prostaglandin G/H synthase-1 (PGHS-1) and—2 (PGHS-2), respectively) in the conversion of arachidonic acid to endoperoxide intermediate, PGG_2 in the synthesis of prostaglandins. Anti-inflammatory, analgesic, and antipyretic activity are associated with inhibition of the COX-2 isoenzyme; COX-1 inhibition presumably is responsible for the unwanted effects of the drug on GI mucosa and platelet aggregation. Naproxen also appears to reduce intracellular concentrations of free arachidonate in leukocytes.

Indications—Treatment of lameness and myositis in horses and of inflammatory conditions of the musculoskeletal system in dogs.

Dosages—

Horse: 10 mg/kg orally twice daily for 14 days.

Dog: 5 mg/kg orally as loading dose followed in 24 hours with 1.5 mg/kg once a day.

Route(s) of Administration—Per os.

Absorption—Naproxen may be completely absorbed from the GIT depending on species and presence of food. Peak plasma concentration is attained within 2-3 hours in the horse or 0.5-3 hours in dog.

Bioavailability—99% (human); 50% (horse); 68-100% (dog).

Onset of Action. 1 hour to induce analgesia.

Peak Action—Anti-inflammatory: 5-7 days (horse).

Duration of Action—Analgesia lasts 7 hours in humans. The period is extended in dogs.

Distribution—Vd = 0.16 ± 0.02 L/kg (human); 0.13 l/kg (dog). Naproxen crosses the placenta; it appears in milk.

Plasma Protein Binding—99.7± 0.1% (human); 99% (dog)

Metabolism—Naproxen is demethylated, and conjugated with glucuronic acid.

Plasma Half-Life—14 ± 1 hours (human; value increases in the elderly); 4 hours (horse); 45-92 hours (dog; undergoes enterohepatic circulation).

Clearance (ml/min/kg)—0.13 ± 0.02 (human); 0.021 (dog).

Route(s) of Excretion—Urine (<1% as unchanged drug).

Toxicity and Adverse Effects—Naproxen is well tolerated in horses but gastrointestinal irritation resulting in distress, diarrhea and bleeding may be observed. Hypoproteinemia, reduced PCV and fluid retention may also be observed. GI ulcers and perforation have been reported in dogs. Renal and hepatic toxicities have also been observed in dogs.

Management of Overdose/Toxicity—Initiate general antidotal therapy. Give supportive and symptomatic treatment.

Contraindications—Active GI ulcer; hypersensitivity to naproxen; pre-existing hematologic, renal or hepatic disease; Concurrent administration of aspirin.

Precautions—Use naproxen cautiously in renal or hepatic dysfunction, heart failure, bronchoconstriction, history of GIT lesions, concurrent administration of protein-bound drugs, anticoagulants, lithium, beta-adrenergic blockers, furosemide, thiazide, and methotrexate. Avoid administration during pregnancy or lactation. Dogs are sensitive to naproxen; the use of naproxen in this species must be done cautiously. NSAIDs cause premature closure of patent ductus, therefore the use of naproxen in late pregnancy should be avoided.

Drug Interactions—The absorption of naproxen is enhanced by concurrent administration of sodium bicarbonate but reduced by magnesium oxide or aluminium hydroxide. Naproxen is significantly adsorbed by activated charcoal. It is highly protein bound and may displace other protein bound drugs from binding sites. It increases blood concentration and half-life of methotrexate. Probenecid increases the half-life of naproxen.

Pharmaceutical Formulations—Naproxen is available in 250 mg and 500 mg tablets; 125 mg/5 ml oral suspension; and 500 mg suppository for human use. It is also available as naproxen sodium containing 275 or 550 mg of salt (equivalent to 250 or 500 mg of naproxen). It is available in 10% solution for injection and in granules for addition to horse ration.

NEOMYCIN

Proprietary Name	Constituents Other Than Neomycin
Mycifradin*	None
Myciguent*	None
Biosol*	None
Neotreat*	Oxytetracycline and vitamins
Coryl SP*	Erythromycin thiocyanate, Colistin sulfate, Oxytetracycline, HCl and vitamins
Neoxytetramycin*	Oxytetracycline HCl and vitamins
Aseryl*	Oxytetracycline HCl, Colistin Sulfate, Erythromycin thiocyanate and vitamins
Neocloxin*	Oxytetracycline HCl and chloramphenicol
Neosan*	Oxytetracycline HCl
Teravite*	Oxytetracycline HCl, Furaldatoin HCl, Dihydrostreptomycin Sulfate, Chloramphenicol and vitamins
Poultaid C*	Oxytetracycline HCl, Streptomycin sulfate, Colistin Sulfate, Erythromycin thiocyanate, and vitamins
Ladseryl*	Erythromycin thiocyanate, Colistin Sulfate, Oxytetracycline HCl, Streptomycin sulfate, vitamins, inositol and calcium pantothenate
Neocillin*	Ampicillin trihydrate, Oxytetracycline HCl, and vitamins
Furacycline Plus*	Furazolidone, Oxytetracycline HCl, Streptomycin sulfate, Chloramphenicol

| Vetaseryl* | Colistin Sulfate, Oxytetracycline HCl, Erythromycin thiocyanate, Streptomycin sulfate, vitamins, and amino acids. |
| Bivacyn* Powder | Bacitracin |

Chemical Class—Aminoglycoside aminocyclitol.

Pharmacological Class—Aminoglycoside antibiotic; Broad spectrum antibiotic.

Source—Natural; obtained from *Streptomyces fradiae*.

Solubility, Stability and Storage—Neomycin is readily soluble in water but slightly soluble in alcohol. Store neomycin formulations in tight containers at room temperature. They should be protected from light.

Pharmacological Actions—Neomycin has bactericidal action against some Gram-positive and Gram-negative bacteria. Gram-negative species which are inhibited include *E. coli, Enterobacter aerogenes, Klebsiella pneumoniae* and *Proteus vulgaris*. Gram-positive organisms that are susceptible are *Staphylococcus aureus, E. fecalis. Mycobacterium tuberculosis* is also sensitive. Neomycin causes increase in plasma cholesterol.

Mechanism of Action—Neomycin binds to the 30S and 50S ribosomal subunit to interfere with the initiation of protein synthesis leading to accumulation of abnormal initiation complexes. It may also induce misreading of the RNA template resulting in incorrect amino acid incorporation into the growing polypeptide chains.

Indications—Treatment of colibacillosis (bacterial enteritis) caused by *Escherichia coli* susceptible to neomycin sulfate in cattle, pigs, sheep and goats; skin, eye, and ear infections; mastitis in dry cow (usually in combination with penicillin). It is also used in preoperative reduction of gut flora prior to colon surgery.

Dosages—

Horse, cattle	4-7.5 g/day
Calf, foal	2-3 g/day
Lamb, young pig	0.75-1 g/day
Dog	0.2-0.5 g/day

All doses should be divided into 2 or 3 equal parts and administered at regular intervals. On a mg/kg basis, a dose of 4.5 mg/kg is recommended for cattle, sheep, goats and pigs.

Route(s) of Administration—Per os and topical.

Absorption—Neomycin is poorly absorbed from the GIT and percutaneous sites. The amount absorbed may increase with reduced gut motility or ulceration of GIT mucosa.

Bioavailability—Oral bioavailability is poor.

Distribution—Vd = 0.36L/kg. Neomycin penetrates the blood brain barrier following intramuscular administration.

Plasma Half-Life—3 hours (following IM administration).

Route(s) of Excretion—Urine with 30-50% as unchanged drug; 97% of an oral dose is eliminated unchanged in feces.

Maximum Residue Limit. Kidney 5 mg/kg; muscle, liver and fat; 0.5 mg/kg for cattle, sheep, goats, pigs, turkeys, ducks, and chickens. The MRLs recommended for chicken eggs and cow's milk are 0.5 mg/kg and 0.5 mg/l respectively. MRL are expressed as parent drug.

Withdrawal Period—Cattle, 1 day; Sheep, 2 days; Pigs and goats, 3 days.

Toxicity and Adverse Effects—Skin rashes due to hypersensitivity reaction may occur. Neomycin causes renal damage, deafness, and neuromuscular blockade with respiratory paralysis. Ototoxicity is often delayed in onset; total or partial deafness may occur long after neomycin has been discontinued. Intestinal malabsorption syndrome for a variety of substances including fat, nitrogen, cholesterol, carotene, glucose, xylose, lactose, sodium, calcium, cyanocobalamin and iron as well as superinfection may accompany oral administration even at low doses. Diarrhea may develop following oral administration. Neomycin may also produce mild morphological changes of intestinal villi, precipitates bile salts within the lumen of the intestine thus increasing fecal bile excretion. Dehydration enhances toxicity.

Management of Overdose/Toxicity—Give symptomatic and supportive treatment; stop therapy.

Contraindications—Intestinal obstruction; hypersensitivity to neomycin, other aminoglycoside antibiotics or their components.

Precautions—Avoid prolong use of neomycin. Concurrent and/or sequential systemic, oral or topical use of other aminoglycosides, including paromomycin and other potentially nephrotoxic and/or neurotoxic drugs such as bacitracin, cisplatin, vancomycin, amphotericin B, polymyxin B, colistin and viomycin, should be avoided because the toxicity may be additive. The concurrent use of neomycin with potent diuretics such as ethacrynic acid or furosemide should be avoided, since certain diuretics by themselves may cause ototoxicity.

Drug Interactions—Neomycin may decrease GI absorption of digoxin and methotrexate. It has synergistic effects with penicillins. Neomycin potentiates the effects of oral anticoagulants and inactivated by compounds containing sulphonic acid. Oral neomycin inhibits the gastrointestinal absorption of penicillin V, and oral vitamin B_{12}. The possibility of the occurrence of neuromuscular blockage and respiratory paralysis should be considered if neomycin is administered to patients receiving anesthetics, neuromuscular blocking agents such as tubocurarine, succinylcholine, and decamethonium. Other aminoglycosides and potentially nephrotoxic and/or neurotoxic drugs may cause additive toxic effects with neomycin. Diuretics may enhance neomycin toxicity by altering the antibiotic concentration in serum and tissues.

Pharmaceutical Formulations—The drug is available as neomycin sulfate in 500 mg tablets, 125 mg/5 ml oral solution, and 5 mg/g of ointment and cream. Neomycin is also available in combination with other antibiotics like polymyxin B, bacitracin and with corticosteroids like hydrocortisone (Cortisporin˙) and dexamethasone in creams and ointments for use in humans. Neomycin is available in combination with several antibacterial agents and vitamins for animal treatment.

NEOSTIGMINE

Proprietary Names—Prostigmin˙.

Chemical Class—Quaternary ammonium compound.

Pharmacological Class—Reversible cholinesterase inhibitor; Indirect-acting cholinomimetic drug.

Source—Synthetic.

Stability and Storage—Neostigmine bromide and neostigmine methylsulfate are very soluble in water and soluble in alcohol. Store neostigmine formulations at room temperature in light resistant container. Injection solution is compatible with IV fluids.

Pharmacological Actions—Neostigmine produces generalized cholinergic responses including miosis, increased tonus of intestinal and skeletal musculature, constriction of bronchi and ureters, bradycardia, and stimulation of secretion by salivary and sweat glands. At low doses, neostigmine and other anticholinesterase agents augment the nervous stimulation of secretory glands including bronchial, lacrimal, sweat, salivary, gastric, and intestinal glands. Higher doses produce increased secretion of these glands. Neostigmine has a direct cholinomimetic effect on skeletal muscle. It may cause twitching of skeletal muscle at high doses as a result of direct nicotinic receptor activation. It causes persistent depolarization of the motor end plate if acetylcholinesterase is sufficiently inhibited resulting in neuromuscular blockade. The CNS is stimulated at low doses but depressed at high doses of neostigmine and other anticholinesterases. Anticholinesterase agents cause miosis, blockade of accommodation reflex and conjunctiva hyperemia if applied directly to the conjunctiva. They also reduce intraocular pressure.

Neostigmine bromide

Mechanism of Action—Neostigmine competes with acetylcholine for acetylcholinesterase enzyme. It is less rapidly hydrolyzed than acetylcholine. This allows acetylcholine to accumulate leading to prolongation and exaggeration of its effect. Neostigmine may directly stimulate nicotinic receptors of the motor end plate.

Indications—Treatment of ruminal atony, paralytic ileus, and urinary retention; diagnosis and treatment of myasthenia gravis; reversal of muscle relaxation caused by curare and other non-depolarizing neuromuscular blockers; treatment of curare overdose.

Dosages—

Dog: 1-2 mg IM; 0.05 mg/kg IM for diagnosis of myasthenia gravis; 0.022 mg/kg for reversal of curare muscle relaxation.

Large animals: 0.01 mg/kg

Route(s) of Administration—Intramuscular, subcutaneous and intravenous routes are suitable.

Absorption—Neostigmine is poorly and incompletely absorbed from the GIT. It is absorbed better from the nasal mucosa than from the GIT.

Onset of Action—1 to 20 minutes (IV); 20 to 30 minutes (IM)

Duration of Action. 1 to 2 hours (IV); 2 to 4 hours (IM).

Distribution—Vd = 0.7 ± 0.3 in human. Neostigmine crosses membranes poorly because of its quaternary ammonium constituent.

Plasma Protein Binding—15 to 25%.

Metabolism. Neostigmine is hydrolyzed by cholinesterase to weakly active metabolite.

Plasma Half-life—1.3 ± 0.8 hours in human. It is prolonged in patients with renal impairment.

Clearance—8.4 ± 2.7 ml/min/kg in human.

Route(s) of Excretion—Mainly urine with > 50% as unchanged drug.

Dialysis Status—Nondialyzable.

Toxicity and Adverse Effects—Severe muscle weakness, nausea, vomiting, diarrhea, miosis, and dyspnea are the most common adverse effects caused by neostigmine. It produces hypotension and bradycardia at high doses. Overdose causes signs characteristic of excessive cholinergic stimulation (cholinergic crisis). The signs include excessive salivation, sweating, miosis, lacrimation, bronchial secretion, bronchospasm, hypotension, and muscle weakness. Death may result from paralysis of respiratory muscles compounded with excessive bronchial secretion.

Management of Overdose/Toxicity—Atropine is an antidote.

Contraindications—Hypersensitivity to neostigmine; peritonitis; intestinal or urinary tract obstruction; late pregnancy; concurrent treatment with other anticholinesterase.

Precautions—Administer neostigmine with atropine when the former is used to reverse curare muscle relaxation.

Drug Interactions—Neostigmine reverses the actions of competitive neuromuscular blockers (e.g. tubocurarine) and augments those of depolarizing neuromuscular blockers (e.g. succinylcholine). Atropine obliterates the muscarinic effects of neostigmine because neostigmine effects are attributed to unhydrolyzed acetylcholine. The effect of neostigmine may be reduced by drugs that have neuromuscular blocking actions (e.g. aminoglycoside antibiotics and anesthetics).

Pharmaceutical Formulations—The drug is available as neostigmine bromide in 15 mg oral tablets and also as neostigmine methylsulfate in 0.25 mg/ml, 0.5 mg/ml, and 1 mg/ml solution for injection.

NITROXINIL

Synonyms—Nitroxynil.

Proprietary Names—Trodax*.

Chemical Class—Nitrobenzonitrile derivative.

Pharmacological Class—Anthelmintic; Trematocide.

Source—Synthetic.

Solubility, Stability, and Storage—Nitroxinil is insoluble in water but sparingly soluble in ether, and ethanol. Nitroxinil meglumine salt is readily soluble in water. The drug is stable under ordinary conditions. Store above 25°C in light resistant container.

Pharmacological Actions—Nitroxinil is active against Fasciola species. It also has some activity against gastrointestinal nematodes such as *Haemonchus contortus* in ruminants and *Syngamus trachea* in game birds. Nitroxynil is active against triclabendazole-resistant *Fasciola hepatica*.

Mechanism of Action—Nitroxinil act by uncoupling oxidative phosphorylation in liver flukes. It also reduces spermatogenesis in surviving flukes, resulting in fewer fertile eggs.

Indications—Treatment of fascioliasis in cattle and sheep. It is also used to treat adult and larval infections of *Haemonchus contortus* in cattle and sheep, *Haemonchus placei*, *Oesophagostomum radiatum* and *Bunostomum phlebotomum* in cattle as well as syngamiais in birds.

Nitroxinil

Dosages—

Cattle and sheep: 10 mg/kg.

Game birds: 24 mg/kg.

During outbreaks of acute fascioliasis infected and in-contact animals should be treated; repeat treatment as considered necessary, though not more frequently than once per 60 days in cattle and 49 days in sheep.

Route(s) of Administration—Per os (in game birds by addition to drinking water) and subcutaneous in cattle and sheep.

Absorption—Nitroxinil is slowly but well absorbed from the GIT. Peak plasma concentration is attained within 5 hours.

Distribution—Nitroxinil attains lower concentration in tissues than plasma.

Plasma Protein Binding—97-98% in cattle and sheep.

Metabolism. Nitroxinil is extensively metabolized in the liver.

Plasma Half-life—22 hours.

Maximum Residue Limit—400 mcg/kg (muscle, kidney); 200 mcg/kg (fat); 20 mcg/kg (liver).

Withdrawal Period—60 days (cattle); 49 days (sheep).

Route(s) of Excretion—Urine.

Toxicity and Adverse Effects—Nitroxinil is well tolerated at therapeutic doses. Hyperthermia and hyperpnoea may be observed at higher doses. It is safe for use in pregnant animals.

Contraindications—Lactating animals; hypersensitivity to Nitroxynil.

Drug Interactions—Concurrent administration of nitroxynil with nematocides (e.g. levamisole) or with clostridial vaccine produces no ill effects.

Pharmaceutical Formulations—Nitroxinil is available as the N-ethylglucamine salt in 20% and 34% injectable solution. It is also available as water soluble liquid containing 14 mg Nitroxynil.

NORFLOXACIN

Norfloxacin

Proprietary Names—Chibroxin™; Noroxin®; Quinabic'; Hipralona Nor-S'; Quintril'; Mycomas'; Norfloxacin 200'; Floxatril'; Agtril'.

Chemical Class—Fluorinated 4-quinolone (Fluoroquinolone).

Pharmacological Class—Antimicrobial agent.

Source—Synthetic.

Solubility, Stability and Storage—Norfloxacin is very slightly soluble in water and alcohol, having solubilities of approximately 0.28 mg/mL and 1.9 mg/mL respectively at 25°C. Solubility of norfloxacin in urine depends on pH and temperature. The drug is least soluble in urine at pH 7.5. Store norfloxacin tablets in tight containers at room temperature.

Pharmacological Actions—Norfloxacin has potent antimicrobial activity against aerobic bacteria including *E. coli, Pseudomonas aeruginosa* and *Staphylococcus* species. It has poor activity against anaerobic organisms. Norfloxacin is less potent than enrofloxacin and ciprofloxacin.

Mechanism of Action—Norfloxacin inhibits gyrase-mediated DNA negative super coiling leading to inability of the bacteria to maintain DNA super helical structure and effect DNA repair.

Indications—Treatment of infections caused by susceptible aerobic organisms.

Dosages—Dogs and Cats: 22 mg/kg twice daily.

Route(s) of Administration—Per os and topical.

Absorption—The drug is rapidly and very well absorbed after oral dose. Peak serum concentration is attained within 20 minutes in chickens and 1.5 hours in dogs. Food and antacids delay absorption.

Bioavailability—Oral bioavailability is 57% in chicken and 30-40% in human.

Distribution—Vd = 3.2 ± 1.4 L/kg. Norfloxacin penetrates tissues slowly. It crosses the placenta. Small amounts are distributed into milk.

Plasma Protein Binding—15-20% in human.

Metabolism—Norfloxacin is converted in the liver to desethylenenorfloxacin and oxonorfloxacin.

Plasma Half-Life (hours)—6.3-6.7 (dog); 8-12 (chicken); 2.4-2.82 (rhesus monkeys); 4.8 (human).

Clearance—7.2 ± 3.0 ml/min/kg in human.

Route(s) of Excretion—Urine and feces.

Dialysis Status—Non dialyzable.

Toxicity and Adverse Effects—Norfloxacin causes arthropathy at 50 mg/kg in dogs and 25 mg/kg in rabbits. Monkeys have shown reduced tolerance during pregnancy but no teratogenic effect has been demonstrated. Gastrointestinal effects characterized by vomiting and anorexia have been observed. Norfloxacin causes CNS effects characterized by headache, dizziness and fatigue in humans where overdose may cause renal failure and seizures.

Management of Overdose/Toxicity—Give supportive measures.

Contraindications—Hypersensitivity to enrofloxacin or any other quinolone.

Precautions—Avoid dehydration during norfloxacin therapy to prevent crystalluria. Administer norfloxacin two hours before or after the administration of antacids containing magnesium, calcium and aluminium.

Drug Interactions—Norfloxacin inhibits the metabolism of theophylline, caffeine, cyclosporine, and warfarin. Azlocillin and cimetidine increase the blood levels of quinolones. The absorption of norfloxacin is reduced if co-administered with antacids containing magnesium, calcium and aluminum. Probenecid blocks tubular secretion of norfloxacin and increases its half-life.

Pharmaceutical Formulations—Norfloxacin is available as 5% and 10% injectable solution; 50 g and 100 g water soluble powder. It is also available in 400 mg tablets and 0.3% ophthalmic solution.

NYSTATIN

Proprietary Names—Candistatin˚; Flagystatin˚; Mycostatin˚; Nyaderm˚; Theraderm˚; Viaderm˚.

Chemical Class—Amphoteric polyene macrolide.

Pharmacological Class—Antifungal antibiotic.

Source—Natural; produced by certain strains of *Streptomyces noursei*.

Solubility, Stability and Storage—Nystatin is slightly soluble in water but sparingly soluble in ethanol. It deteriorates on exposure to heat, light, moisture, or air. Nystatin preparations should not be frozen.

Pharmacological Actions—Nystatin has fungistatic or fungicidal activity against a variety of pathogenic and nonpathogenic yeasts and fungi. There is little difference between fungistatic and fungicidal concentrations for a particular organism. It is inactive against bacteria, protozoa, or viruses.

Nystatin A₁

Mechanism of Action—Nystatin binds to sterols, the predominant component of the fungal cell membrane and disrupts the selective barrier function of the membrane causing the loss of potassium and other cellular constituents.

Indications—Treatment of Candida infections.

Dosages—50,000-150,000 units PO every 6-8 hours.

Route(s) of Administration. Topical and per os.

Absorption—Nystatin is not absorbed from intact skin or mucous membranes.

Route(s) of Excretion—Feces, mainly as unchanged drug.

Toxicity and Adverse Effects—Adverse reactions to topically applied nystatin are very infrequent even during prolonged use. Although, irritation has occurred rarely. Hypersensitivity reactions to nystatin are also rare. High oral doses may cause gastrointestinal upset characterized by anorexia, vomition and diarrhea.

Contraindications—Hypersensitivity to nystatin.

Pharmaceutical Formulations—Nystatin is available as cream, ointment, powder or tablets. Topical formulations contain 100, 000 units per gram. Each mg of nystatin contains not less than 4400 units of activity. Nystatin creams and ointments are commercially available in combination with triamcinolone acetonide for the treatment of cutaneous candidiasis.

OMEPRAZOLE

Proprietary Names—Antra˙; Gastroguard˙; Gastroloc˙; Logastric˙; Losec˙; Mepral˙; Omepral˙; Omeprazen˙; Pepticum˙; Prilosec˙.

Chemical Class—Substituted benzimidazole.

Pharmacological Class—Antiulcer Agent; Gastric Antisecretory Agent; Acid-pump Inhibitor; Proton-pump inhibitor.

Source—Synthetic.

Solubility, Stability and Storage—Omeprazole is very slightly soluble in water, soluble in alcohol and very soluble in alkaline solutions. Omeprazole molecule is acid labile, hence it is administered orally as a delayed-release capsule, delayed-release tablet, or buffered oral suspension. Omeprazole tablets should be stored at room temperature in light-resistant, tight containers.

Omeprazole

Pharmacological Actions—Omeprazole inhibits basal and stimulated gastric acid secretion. The degree of inhibition is related to the dose and duration of therapy. Omeprazole is a more potent inhibitor of gastric acid secretion than are histamine H_2-receptor antagonists. Because of omeprazole's greater potency as an inhibitor of gastric acid secretion, the drug also causes secondary increases in plasma gastrin concentrations that exceed those produced by histamine H_2-receptor antagonists. Omeprazole does not appear to lower esophageal sphincter pressure or affect gastric emptying. It suppresses gastric *Helicobacter pylori* (formerly *Campylobacter pylori* or *C. pyloridis*) in humans with duodenal ulcer and/or reflux esophagitis infected with the organism.

Mechanism of Action—Omeprazole is activated in an acid medium to sulfenamide metabolite which inactivates hydrogen/potassium adenosine triphosphatase (H^+K^+-exchanging ATPase). This is also known as the proton, hydrogen, or acid pump in gastric parietal cells. The inhibition blocks the final step in the secretion of hydrochloric acid by these cells. Because the sulfenamide metabolite forms an irreversible covalent bond to H^+K^+-exchanging ATPase, acid secretion is inhibited until additional enzyme is synthesized, resulting in prolonged duration of action.

Indications—Treatment of gastroduodenal ulcers and prevention or treatment of gastric erosions caused by ulcerogenic drugs (e.g. aspirin). It is also used in combination with clarithromycin (dual therapy) or with amoxicillin and clarithromycin (triple therapy) in human adults for the treatment of *Helicobacter pylori* infection and duodenal ulcer disease.

Dosages—0.7-1.4 mg/kg PO once daily.

Route(s) of Administration—Per os.

Absorption—Omeprazole is rapidly absorbed from the intestine. Peak plasma concentration is attained within 30 minutes to 3.5 hours after administration of slow release formulation. Peak plasma concentrations of the drug occur at about 30 minutes (range 10-90 minutes) after oral administration of the suspension. Absorption is not affected by the presence of food.

Bioavailability—Oral bioavailability increases with duration of therapy (from about 35% after the first dose, to about 50% after several doses).

Onset of Action—1 hour.

Peak Action—Within 2 hours.

Duration of Action—Up to 72 hour.

Distribution—Vd = 0.27 to 0.45 L/kg. Omeprazole crosses the placenta in animals and in humans.

Plasma Protein Binding—Approximately 95%.

Metabolism—Omeprazole is almost completely metabolized in the liver.

Plasma Half-life—0.5 to 3 hours; the long duration of action may be due to prolonged binding of the drug to H^+K^+-exchanging ATPase.

Clearance—0.23 L/kg/h.

Route(s) of Excretion—About 80% of metabolites are excreted in urine, the rest in faeces.

Toxicity and Adverse Effects—Omeprazole is generally well tolerated. The most frequent adverse effects observed in humans include diarrhea, nausea, constipation, abdominal pain and vomiting. Limited veterinary experience indicates that omeprazole is well tolerated in animals at therapeutic doses. Potentially, GI distress which is common in humans could occur.

Management of Overdose/Toxicity—Give symptomatic and supportive treatment.

Contraindications—Nursing animal; hypersensitivity to omeprazole.

Precautions—Do not crush the pellets contained in the capsule. Mix the pellets carefully with fruit juices if needed to be administered as slurry. Use with caution in patients with hepatic impairment.

Drug Interactions—Omeprazole inhibits the metabolism of diazepam, warfarin, phenytoin and other drugs which are metabolized by cytochrome P-450. Omeprazole-induced increases in gastric pH may affect the bioavailability of drugs such as ketoconazole, ampicillin esters, iron salts and others where gastric acidity is an important determinant of oral absorption.

Pharmaceutical Formulations—Omeprazole is available in delayed-release capsules (containing enteric-coated granules) of 10 mg, 20 mg and 40 mg strengths. It is also available in suspension powder of 20 mg and 40 mg/packet.

OXACILLIN

Proprietary Names—Bactocill', Prostaphilin'.

Synonyms—Methylphenyl isoxazolyl penicillin.

Chemical Class—6-Aminopenicillinic acid derivative.

Pharmacological Class—An isoxazolyl penicillin; Beta-lactam antibiotic; Penicillinase resistant penicillin.

Source—Semisynthetic.

Solubility, Stability and Storage—Oxacillin is freely soluble in water. Oxacillin sodium powder for IM or IV injection should be stored at controlled room temperature. When oxacillin sodium powder for injection is reconstituted with sterile water for injection, solutions for IM injection containing 167 mg of oxacillin per mL (250 mg/1.5 mL) are stable for 3 days at room temperature or 7 days when refrigerated.

Oxacillin sodium

Pharmacological Actions—Oxacillin is bactericidal to penicillinase-producing *Staphyloccocus aureus* and penicillin G-sensitive *Staphyloccocus* and other Gram-positive bacteria. It is less active than penicillin G against penicillin G-sensitive microbes.

Mechanism of Action—Same as for other penicillins. See benzathine penicillin G.

Indications—Treatment and control of mastitis, soft tissue infections, wounds and burns, and septicemia due to infections by gram positive microbes especially penicillinase—producing staph.

Dosages—

Horse: 25-50 mg/kg IM or IV every 6-8 hours.

Other animals: 22-40 mg/kg orally every 8 hours or 5-12 mg/kg IV, IM every 8 hours.

Route(s) of Administration—Per os, intramuscular and intravenous route are appropriate.

Absorption—Oxacillin is rapidly but incompletely absorbed from the GIT. Peak plasma concentration is attained within 1-2 hours following oral administration or 30-60 minutes with IM. Food decreases the rate and extent of absorption.

Bioavailability—Oral bioavailability is 30-35% in human.

Distribution—Vd = 0.33 ± 0.09 L/kg in human and 0.3 L/kg in dog. Oxacillin is widely distributed. It is distributed into milk, crosses the placenta but penetrates CSF poorly.

Plasma Protein Binding—92.2 ± 0.6%.

Metabolism—Oxacillin is partly metabolized to active and inactive products.

Plasma Half—Life—Human: 0.4-0.7 hours (higher in neonates, children and renal insufficiency). Dog: 0.33-0.5 hours.

Clearance—6.1 ± 1.7 (ml/min/kg).

Route(s) of Excretion—Urine and Bile.

Dialysis Status—Dialyzable.

Toxicity and Adverse Effects—Hypersensitivity reaction ranging from skin rash to serum sickness-like reactions are common. Nausea, vomiting, diarrhea, hematologic disorders, hepatoxicity and hematuria have been observed at therapeutic doses. Overdose may cause neuromuscular hypersensitivity (characterized by agitation, hallucinations seizures and confusion), electrolyte imbalance and renal failure.

Management of Overdose/Toxicity—Set up hemodialysis and give supportive and symptomatic treatment.

Contraindications. Hypersensitivity to oxacillin or other penicillins, or their products and components.

Precautions—Administer oxacillin 1 hour before, or two hours after food. Use the drug cautiously in patients with history of cephalosporin use.

Drug Interactions—Efficacy of oral contraceptive in humans may be reduced by oxacillin. Effects of anticoagulants may be increased by oxacillin. Probenecid and disulfiram increase the plasma concentration of oxacillin. The drug is incompatible with oxytetracycline and tetracycline.

Pharmaceutical Formulations—Available as oxacillin sodium in 250 mg and 500 mg capsule and in powder for oral suspension containing 250 mg/5ml. Oxacillin is also available as powder for injection in vials containing 250, 500 mg, 1, 2, 4, and 10 g. Reconstituted powder for injection should contain 167 mg oxacillin per millilitre. Each mg of oxacillin sodium contains 815-950 mcg of oxacillin. Each gram of commercially available oxacillin sodium powder for injection contains approximately 2.5 mEq of sodium and is buffered with 20 mg of dibasic sodium phosphate.

OXAZEPAM

Oxazepam

Proprietary Names—Serax®; Zaxopam®.

Chemical Class—Benzodiazepine.

Pharmacological Class—CNS depressant; Sedative-hypnotic; Anxiolytic.

Source—Synthetic.

Solubility, Stability and Storage—Oxazepam is practically insoluble in water but slightly soluble in alcohol. Store oxazepam preparations at room temperature and in well closed containers.

Pharmacological Actions—Oxazepam depresses the CNS at subcortical levels and produces sedation and hypnosis. It decreases anxiety without decreasing alertness or impairing perceptive or cognitive capacities. It has anticonvulsant and muscle relaxant properties. Oxazepam stimulates appetite in cats.

Mechanism of Action—Same as for other benzodiazepines. See diazepam.

Indications—Treatment of anorexia in cats and dogs; adjunctive treatment of anxiety-related disorders.

Dosages—2 mg every 12 hours in cats.

Route(s) of Administration—Per os.

Absorption—Oxazepam is slowly but almost completely absorbed from the GIT. Peak plasma concentration is attained within 2-4 hours in humans.

Bioavailability—Oral bioavailability is 97 ± 11 in humans.

Distribution—Vd = 0.60 ± 0.20. Oxazepam crosses the placenta and is found in breast milk.

Plasma Protein Binding—98.8 ± 1.8% in humans.

Metabolism—Oxazepam is conjugated with glucuronic acid. The drug is an active metabolite of several benzodiazepines including chlordiazepoxide, clorazepate, demoxepam, desmethyldiazepam (nordazepam), diazepam, prazepam and temazepam.

Plasma Half-Life—8.0 ± 2.4 in humans.

Plasma Clearance—About 1 to 2 (ml/min/kg).

Route(s) of Excretion—Urine (< 1% as unchanged drug). Up to 10% of a dose is eliminated in the faeces mostly as unchanged drug.

Dialysis Status—Not dialyzable.

Toxicity and Adverse Effects—Oxazepam may cause transient sedation and ataxia. Overdose may cause confusion, coma, and decreased reflexes.

Management of Overdose/Toxicity—Follow general antidotal therapy in addition to adequate supportive measures. Flumazenil will specifically antagonize the CNS depressant effect of oxazepam.

Contraindications—Hypersensitivity to oxazepam or other benzodiazepines; acute narrow-angle glaucoma.

Precautions—Use with caution in seizure-prone patients since oxazepam has reportedly precipitated tonic-clonic seizures. Use cautiously during first trimester of pregnancy.

Drug Interactions—Concurrent administration with other CNS depressants will produce additive effects. Probenecid may interfere with glucuronide conjugation of oxazepam.

Pharmaceutical Formulations—Oxazepam is available in 10 mg, 15 mg, and 30 mg oral capsules and 15 mg oral tablets.

OXYMORPHONE

Proprietary Names—Numorphan*.

Chemical Class—Phenanthrene alkaloid derivative.

Pharmacological Class—Narcotic analgesic; opioid analgesic.

Source—Semi synthetic.

Solubility, Stability and Storage—Oxymorphone is freely soluble in water and sparingly soluble in alcohol. Store oxymorphone injection formulations at room temperature in light resistant container. Refrigerate suppository formulations. Do not mix oxymorphone with barbiturates and diazepam.

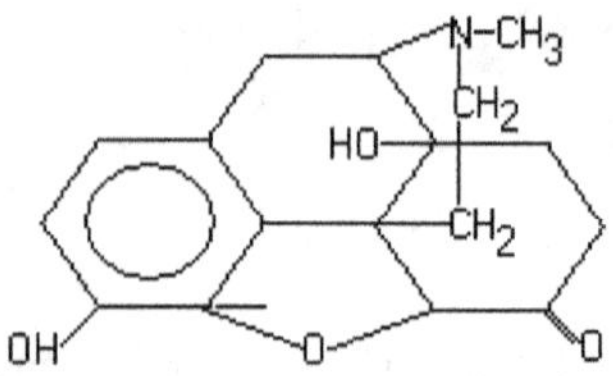

Oxymorphone

Pharmacological Actions. Oxymorphone has potent analgesic action. Its analgesic potency is ten times that of morphine. It causes mild CNS and respiratory depressions. It also decreases gut motility. Oxymorphone hydrochloride has little antitussive activity and may be less constipating than morphine.

Mechanism of Action. Oxymorphone combines with and activates opioid receptors.

Indications—Oxymorphone is used in preanesthetic medication and control of post-operative pain. It is also used in combination with tranquilizers (acepromazine, triflupromazine) and other sedatives like xylazine to induce neurolepsia.

Dosages—

Oxymorphone

Dog, Cat	0.2 mg/kg for preanesthetic medication or 0.1 mg/kg every 24 hours for postoperative pain.
NHP	0.075-0.15 mg/kg SC, IM, IV in monkeys.
Pig	0.15 mg/kg IM.
Horse	22 mcg/kg for colic or 30 mcg/kg for preanesthetic medication.

Oxymorphone and acepromazine (respectively).

Cat	0.05-0.15 mg/kg and 0.02-0.05 mg/kg
Dog	0.1-0.2 mg/kg and 0.02-0.1 mg/kg

Route(s) of Administration—Oxymorphone may be administered by intravenous, intramuscular and subcutaneous routes.

Absorption—Oxymorphone is readily absorbed from IM and SC sites.

Bioavailability—Oral bioavailability is low.

Onset of Action—5 to 10 minutes after IV administration and 10-15 minutes after subcutaneous or IM administration.

Duration of Action—3 to 6 hours.

Distribution—Oxymorphone is widely distributed and concentrates in kidneys, lungs, skeletal muscle and liver. It crosses the placenta.

Metabolism—Conjugated with glucuronic acid in the liver.

Route(s) of Excretion—Urine.

Toxicity and Adverse Effects—Respiratory depression and bradycardia are common adverse effects in most species. High doses in cats cause ataxia and behavioral changes. Oxymorphone decreases GI motility which may result in constipation. In equianalgesic doses, oxymorphone hydrochloride may cause more nausea, vomiting, and euphoria than does morphine sulfate. Overdose of oxymorphone may worsen respiratory depression and cause cardiovascular collapse, hypothermia and reduced muscle tone.

Management of Overdose/Toxicity—Initiate general antidotal therapy in conjunction with naloxone therapy.

Contraindications—Hypersensitivity to oxymorphone.

Precautions—Use oxymorphone with caution in patients with hepatic disease, impaired renal function, decreased respiratory reserve, head injury, hypothyroidism, adrenocorticoid insufficiency, old and debilitated patients.

Drug Interactions—CNS depressants produce additive CNS depression when used with oxymorphone.

Pharmaceutical Formulations—Available as oxymorphone hydrochloride in 1 mg/ml; 1.5 mg/ml solutions for injection and in 5 mg suppository.

OXYTETRACYCLINE

Oxytetracycline

Proprietary Names—Terramycin˙, Berkmycen˙, Uri-Tet˙, Linquamycin˙, Medamycin˙, Oxylag˙, Oxyne˙, Tetran˙, Ursocyclin®, Kepro Oxytet®; Oxycare®; Oxymeda Q®; Tetroxy®; Neoxytetramycin®; Oxyject® Oxycline®; Adamycin®; Tetrasol® (Oxytetracycline dihydrate); Altracycline®; Oxyvet®.

Chemical Class—A polycyclic naphthacenecarboxamide derivative.

Pharmacological Class—Broad spectrum bacteriostatic antibiotic.

Source—Natural; Elaborated by *Streptomyces rimosus*, a soil mold.

Solubility, Stability and Storage—Oxytetracycline is very slightly soluble in water and sparingly soluble in alcohol. Oxytetracycline IM formulations should be stored preferably between 15-30°C. Do not freeze oxytetracycline injection.

Pharmacological Actions—Oxytetracycline is bacteriostatic to a wide range of microorganisms including Gram-positive and Gram-negative bacteria, *Rickettsia*, *Chlamydia* and many spirochaetes.

Mechanism of Action—Oxytetracycline inhibits protein synthesis by binding principally to the 30s subunit of ribosome to prevent access of aminoacyl tRNA to the acceptor site of the mRNA-ribosome complex thereby preventing the addition of amino acids to the growing peptide chain. Selective action for bacterial cell is due to lack of active transport through the inner cytoplasmic membrane to the ribosome in mammalian cells as well as to differences in sensitivities of the ribosomes of bacterial and mammalian cells. It has also been shown to reduce the ability of bacteria to adhere to mammalian epithelial cells *in vitro*.

Indications—Treatment of infections involving respiratory, urinary, gastrointestinal and soft tissues caused by susceptible Gram positive and Gram negative bacteria, rickettsia and mycoplasma. These include conditions such as pneumonia, scours, metritis, mastitis, leptospirosis, erysipelas, secondary bacterial infections, infected wounds and abscesses. It is also used in prophylaxis after surgical operation.

Dosages—

Bird	200 mg/kg IM once daily (one dose). or 10-60 g/100kg of feed in poultry.
Cattle	7-11 mg/kg/day not to exceed 4 consecutive days.
Dog, cat	20 mg/kg PO, 3 times daily; 7–11 mg/kg IV, IM.
Mice	400 mg/l drinking water given continuously or 100 mg/kg SC, 2 times daily.
NHP	10 mg/kg SC, IM.
Rat	60 mg/kg SC every 72 hours of long-acting drug.
Rabbit	30-100 mg/kg in divided doses PO; 400-1000 mg/l drinking water or 15 mg/kg SC, IM three times daily for 7 days.
Reptile	6-10 mg/kg IV; IM once a day.
Sheep	7-11 mg/kg/day not to exceed 4 consecutive days.
Calf, foal	10-20 mg/kg PO
Pig	10-30 mg/kg PO; 5-10 mg/kg IV, IM.
Horse	5-10 mg/kg IV, IM.

Route(s) of Administration—Per os and intramuscular routes are appropriate. The subcutaneous and intravenous routes are also used in animals.

Absorption—Sixty to eighty percent is absorbed from the stomach and small intestine in a fasting state. Peak plasma concentration is attained within 2-4 hours. Unabsorbed drug increases with increasing dose. The presence of food or dairy products reduces the rate and extent of absorption. Absorption from IM site is poor.

Bioavailability—Oral bioavailability is 60-80%.

Distribution—Vd = 2.1 L/kg (small animals); 1.4 L/kg (horse); 0.8 L/kg (cattle). Oxytetracycline is concentrated in the liver. It undergoes enterohepatic circulation, crosses uninflamed meninges to varying levels depending on route of administration, penetrates into body fluids and tissues and crosses the placenta.

Plasma Protein Binding—20 to 40%.

Metabolism—Small amounts of oxytetracycline are metabolized in the liver.

Plasma Half-Life—8.5 to 9.6 hours (higher in renal and hepatic impairment, and during obstruction of common bile duct) in humans, 4-6 hours (dogs and cats), 10.5 hours (cattle), 6.7 hours (horses), 3.6 hours (sheep).

Residue Limit: 0.10 ppm in uncooked edible tissue of pig, cattle, catfish, lobsters); 3 ppm in uncooked kidneys of chicken or turkeys); 1 ppm in uncooked muscle, liver, fat or skin of chicken and turkey).

Withdrawal Period—This varies with species and drug formulations. The values currently set are 15-22 days (cattle), 20-26 days (pig), 5 days (chicken and turkey) and 8 days (milk). Specifically, the set values in cattle are 28 days following treatment with 200 mg/ml injection formulation and 7 days with oral formulation.

Route(s) of Excretion—Urine and feces. About 10 to 25% of a dose is eliminated in urine.

Dialysis Status—Not dialyzable.

Toxicity and Adverse Effects—Epigastric burning, abdominal discomfort, nausea, vomiting, indigestion and diarrhea in humans and animals may follow oral administration of oxytetracycline. High doses may cause renal toxicity, discoloration of teeth and depression of bone growth in the young and hepatotoxicity (characterized by cytoplasmic changes, increase in fat, jaundice, azotemia, acidosis especially during pregnancy). Oxytetracycline produces a kind of Faconi syndrome (characterized by nausea, vomiting, polyuria, polydipsia, proteinuria, acidosis, glycosuria and gross aminoaciduria following administration of outdated and degraded drug. It causes pain and thrombophlebitis following parenteral administration. The drug may also cause increased intracranial pressure in infants, superinfection and hypersensitivity reactions. High doses cause depression of ruminal microflora and ruminoreticular stasis in cattle. Cats are intolerant and may show signs of colic, fever, hair loss and depression. Rapid IV injection has caused transient collapse and cardiac arrhythmia.

Management of Overdose/Toxicity—Give symptomatic and supportive therapy.

Contraindications—Hypersensitivity to oxytetracycline or other tetracyclines; first half of pregnancy; growing animals.

Precautions—Reduce oxytetracycline dose in hepatic or renal impairment. Do not administer simultaneously with milk and antacids. Also do not administer with calcium, magnesium and iron salts.

Drug Interactions—Absorption of oxytetracycline is impaired by concurrent administration of dairy products, bismuth subsalicylate, aluminum hydroxide gel and also Ca, Mg and Fe salts. Tetracyclines interfere with the bactericidal actions of penicillins, cephalosporins and aminoglycoside antibiotics.

Pharmaceutical Formulations—The drug is available as oxytetracycline hydrochloride in 250 mg capsules; 50 mg/ml, and 125 mg/ml formulations with lidocaine for intramuscular injection in humans. Available in 250 mg boluses, aerosol spray (in combination with gentian violet), soluble powder (for administration in drinking water and feed), ointment, ophthalmic and intramammary preparations for use in animals. Oxytetracycline dihydrate complexed with magnesium is available in solution of 50 mg/ml for depot injection in animals.

OXYTOCIN

Proprietary Names—Pitocin ®; Syntocinon ®.

Chemical Class—Peptide.

Pharmacological Class—Ecbolic.

Source—Natural; extracted from the posterior lobe of the pituitary glands of cattle). Commercial forms of oxytocin are prepared synthetically.

Solubility, stability and Storage—Commercially available oxytocin is soluble in water. Oxytocin injection should be stored at temperatures less than 15-25°C and should not be frozen. Pitocin˙ should be refrigerated at 2-8°C but may be exposed to room temperatures for not more than 30 days. Oxytocin injection is physically incompatible with fibrinolysin, norepinephrine bitartrate, prochlorperazine edisylate, and warfarin sodium.

Pharmacological Actions—Oxytocin stimulates contraction of uterine smooth muscle. The contractions produced by oxytocin at term (end of pregnancy) are similar to those occurring during spontaneous labor. At term oxytocin increases the amplitude and frequency of uterine contractions. This tend to decrease cervical activity and cause dilation and effacement of the cervix and also to transiently impede uterine blood flow. High estrogen concentration lowers the threshold for uterine response to oxytocin. Uterine response to oxytocin increases with the duration of pregnancy and is greater in patients who are in labor than those not in labor. Only very large doses elicit contractions in early pregnancy. Oxytocin also causes the contraction of the myoepithelial cells which surrounds the alveolar channels in the mammary glands forcing milk from the alveoli into the larger ducts to cause milk let-down. Other peripheral actions of oxytocin include slight reduction in urine excretion, natriuresis (increased sodium excretion from the kidneys), and facilitation of sperm transport following ejaculation. Oxytocin also has actions as a central neurotransmitter. Several central actions have been attributed to oxytocin. For instance, oxytocin is secreted into the blood at orgasm in both males and females. It is known to increase maternal behavior, sexual bonding, trust and reducing fear. Oxytocin reduces blood pressure and cortisol levels, increasing tolerance to pain, and reducing anxiety. Oxytocin may play a role in encouraging "tend and befriend", as opposed to "fight or flight", behavior, in response to stress.

Mechanism of Action—Oxytocin interacts with specific high affinity G-protein-coupled receptors. It stimulates contraction of uterine smooth muscle by increasing the sodium permeability of uterine myofibrils.

Indications—To induce or augment parturition in small animals when fetal position and presentation are normal and the cervix dilated; control postpartum uterine atony and hemorrhage; stimulate uterine contraction after caesarian section or other uterine surgery; aid the expulsion of the last fetus(s) in multi-fetal species and of mummified fetuses in small animals; assist expulsion of retained placenta in mares, sows, bitches, and queens; express infected milk from udder in cases of mastitis before introducing chemotherapeutic agents; stimulate milk let-down in recently farrowed sows, cows and bitches exhibiting agalactia; aid replacement of prolapsed uterus in cows and mares.

Dosages—

Intramuscular. 10-40 IU (horse and cow); 2.5-10 IU (sheep, goat and pig); 1-10 IU (dog); 0.5-5 IU (cat).

Intravenous. 2.5-10 IU (horse and cow); 0.5-2.5 (sheep, goat and pig); 0.5 IU (dog). NOTE. It is better to give repeated small doses.

Route(s) of Administration—Intramuscular and intravenous routes are used in animals.

Distribution—Oxytocin administered intravenously does not enter the brain in significant quantities. It is excluded from the brain by the blood-brain-barrier.

Plasma Protein Binding—30%

Plasma Half-Life—5 to 12 minutes.

Withdrawal Period—Zero days.

Toxicity And Adverse Effects—Large amounts of oxytocin may cause severe decreases in maternal systolic and diastolic blood pressure. Increases in heart rate, systemic venous return and cardiac output, and arrhythmia may occur. Excessive dosage may cause hyperstimulation of the uterus, with strong (hypertonic) and/or prolonged (tetanic) contractions. Excessive dose may also cause resting uterine tone of 15-20 mm H_2O between contractions possibly resulting in uterine rupture, cervical and vaginal lacerations, postpartum hemorrhage, impaired uterine blood flow, amniotic fluid embolism, and fetal trauma including intracranial hemorrhage. Anaphylactic and other allergic reactions have occurred in human patients receiving oxytocin and may rarely be fatal.

Management of Overdose/Toxicity—The tocolytic agent atosiban (Tractocile®) acts as an antagonist of oxytocin receptors.

Contraindications—Undilated cervix; malpresentation.

Precautions—Give oxytocin by deep IM injection. Dilute the preparation 1:10 for IV injection.

Pharmaceutical Formulations—The drug is available as synthetic oxytocin injection containing 10 USP units/5 ml, oxytocin nasal spray containing 40 USP units/ml and oxytocin citrate tablets containing 200 IU.

PANCURONIUM

Pancuronium

Proprietary Names—Pavulon®.

Chemical Class—Ammonio Steroid.

Pharmacological Class—Competitive neuromuscular blocker; Non depolarizing neuromuscular blocker; Long-acting competitive neuromuscular blocker.

Source—Synthetic.

Solubility, Stability and Storage—Pancuronium is freely soluble in water and very soluble in alcohol. Refrigerate pancuronium solution for injection but product may be stable for 6 months at room temperature. The drug is incompatible with diazepam. Watch for precipitates if pancuronium is mixed with barbiturates. Pancuronium adsorbs onto plastics.

Pharmacological Actions—Pancuronium causes skeletal muscle paralysis. Unlike tubocurarine, pancuronium has no ganglion blocking effects and it rarely releases histamine.

Mechanism of Action—Pancuronium competes with acetylcholine for the nicotinic receptors at the motor endplate. It does not activate the receptors but prevent access of acetylcholine molecules to the receptors. Thus, acetylcholine-induced end plate potential are reduced to sub threshold levels or abolished. Consequently, impulse transmission is blocked and the muscle becomes paralysed without preceding stimulation.

Indications—Pancuronium is used as adjunct to general anesthesia to induce muscle relaxation. It is also used to facilitate endotracheal intubation and relax skeletal muscle during mechanical ventilation.

Dosages—0.044-0.11 mg/kg.

Route(s) of Administration—Intravenous.

Absorption—Poorly absorbed from the GIT.

Onset of Action—1 to 5.2 minutes (dose dependent).

Peak Action—2 to 3 minutes.

Duration of Action—40 to 80 minutes (dose dependent).

Distribution—Vd = 0.26-0.28 L/kg (humans).

Plasma Protein Binding—87% (humans).

Metabolism—Substantially metabolized in the liver.

Plasma Half-life—114-140 min (humans); higher in renal failure.

Clearance—1.8 to 1.9 (ml/min/kg).

Route(s) of Excretion—Urine with 55%-70% as unchanged drug.

Dialysis Status—Pancuronium is nondialyzable.

Toxicity and Adverse Effects—Mild tachycardia, hypertension, and hypersalivation are common. Overdose causes respiratory depression and circulatory collapse.

Management of Overdose/Toxicity—Pancuronium effects can be reversed by anticholinesterase agents e.g. neostigmine (0.022mg/kg). Atropine (0.04mg/kg) should be administered prior to or in conjunction with neostigmine to circumvent the muscarinic effect of neostigmine.

Contraindications—Hypersensitivity to pancuronium.

Precautions—Use pancuronium cautiously in patients with myasthenia gravis and in those patients with hepatic and renal impairment.

Drug Interactions—The concurrent use of pancuronium and another competitive neuromuscular blocker results in additive effect. Some general anaesthetic agents (e.g. halothane, enflurane and isoflurane) synergize with the neuromuscular blocking action of pancuronium. Verapamil, quinidine, furosemide, magnesium sulphate, local anaesthetics, and immunodepressants enhance its blocking action. Aminoglycoside antibiotics are potential neuromuscular blockers. Hence, their actions are synergistic with those of pancuronium.

Pharmaceutical Formulations—The drug is available as pancuronium bromide in 1 mg/ml and 2 mg/ml solution for injection.

PARACETAMOL

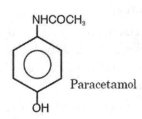

Synonyms—Acetaminophen, APAP, N-Acetyl—P-amino phenol.

Proprietary Names—Panadol˚ Tylenol˚, Anacin˚, Valedol˚, Paracin˚, Pyrigesic˚, Aceta˚, Acephen˚, Ultragin˚, Apacet˚, Banesin˚, Tempra˚, Halenol˚, Neomol˚, Metacin˚.

Chemical Class—Para-amino phenol derivative.

Pharmacological Class—Nonsteroidal anti-inflammatory drug; coal tar analgesic; analgesic-antipyretic; non-opioid analgesic; simple analgesic; aspirin-like analgesic.

Source—Synthetic.

Pharmacological Actions—Paracetamol has analgesic and antipyretic properties comparable to those of aspirin. It has weak anti-inflammatory action peripherally. The drug is most effective in relieving low intensity pain of nonvisceral origin. It does not have antirheumatic actions or depress prothrombin levels. It produces a lower incidence of gastric irritation, erosion, or bleeding than do salicylates.

Mechanism of Action—Paracetamol interferes with the conversion of endoperoxide intermediates of arachidonic acid in an environment low in peroxides. Its poor anti-inflammatory action may be due to the high concentration of peroxides at the sites of inflammation. Peripherally, it blocks pain impulse generation. The drug produces antipyresis by inhibition of the heat regulating center at the hypothalamus.

Indications—Control of mild to moderate pain; control of severe pain usually in combination with codeine; treatment of degenerative myelopathy. Used in rodents to control low grade nociception.

Dosage—1 to 2mg/ml of drinking water for rabbits and rodents.

Route(s) of Administration—Per os.

Absorption—Paracetamol is rapidly and almost completely absorbed. Peak plasma concentration is attained within 10-60 minutes.

Bioavailability—70-90 % (humans).

Duration of Action—2 to 3 hours (humans).

Distribution—Vd = 0.9 ± 0.12 L/kg (humans). It is uniformly distributed.

Plasma Protein Binding—Variable (20% to 50%).

Metabolism—Paracetamol is usually conjugated in the liver with glucuronic acid and sulfate. A small proportion is metabolized by mixed functional oxidase to a highly reactive metabolite, N-acetyl-p—benzoquinoneimine (NABQI) which is detoxified by conjugation with glutathione. Following a large dose of paracetamol, glucuronidation is saturated and more NABQI is formed leading to exhaustion of glutathione stores. Excess NABQI then binds and oxidizes thiol (-SH) groups of key enzymes in hepatic and renal tubular cells causing necrosis. Cats are unable to conjugate paracetamol with glucuronic acid.

Plasma Half-Life—2.0 ± 0.4 hours in humans.

Plasma Clearance—5.0 ± 1.4 ml/min/kg.

Toxicity and Adverse Effects—Paracetamol is safe and well tolerated at normal dose and isolated use. However, nausea and occasional skin rash may be observed. Overdose (> 150 mg/kg) or chronic use can result in severe hepatic and renal damage. Depression, methemoglobinemia, and vomiting have been reported in dogs at 0.1 g /kg dose.

Management of Overdose/Toxicity—Give general antidotal and supportive therapy. Administer acetylcysteine.

Contraindications—Hypersensitivity to paracetamol; cats.

Precautions—Use paracetamol cautiously in impaired hepatic and renal function. Avoid chronic use. Avoid use of paracetamol in dogs.

Drug Interactions—Refampicin may reduce paracetamol analgesic potency. Barbiturates, carbamazepine, hydatoins, and sulfinpyrazone may increase its hepatotoxic potential. Large doses may potentiate the effects of coumarin anticoagulants. Doxorubicin may enhance paracetamol hepatic effect by depleting hepatic glutathione.

Pharmaceutical Formulations—Commonly available in 500 mg tablets and 125 mg/5 ml syrup.

PENICILLIN G

Penicillin G

Synonyms—Benzyl penicillin; Crystalline penicillin; Sodium penicillin G; Potassium penicillin G.

Proprietary Names—Pfizerpen˙, Benzapen˙, Crystapen˙.

Chemical Class—6-aminopenicillanic acid derivative.

Pharmacological Class—Beta-lactam antibiotic; Narrow spectrum antibiotic.

Source—Natural (produced by fermentation of *Penicillium chrysogenum* in a medium containing phenylacetic acid).

Solubility, Stability and Storage—Penicillin G potassium is very soluble in water, normal saline and dextrose solutions. It is sparingly soluble in alcohol. Penicillin G sodium has an approximate solubility of 25 mg/mL in water at 25°C. Both salts of penicillin are moderately hygroscopic and dry powders of the drugs should be protected from moisture to prevent hydrolysis. Commercially available penicillin G potassium or penicillin G sodium powders for injection may be stored at room temperature. Following reconstitution of the powders for injection, penicillin G potassium or penicillin G sodium solutions are stable for 7 days at 2-8°C. Penicillin may become hydrolyzed when mixed in the same syringe with other drugs.

Pharmacological Actions—Penicillin G is bactericidal to most Gram-positive organisms. Some Gram-negative organisms like *Neisseria gonorrhea*; some anaerobes and spirochaetes are susceptible. Its action is unaffected by blood and tissue breakdown products such as pus, although, these may hinder diffusion.

Mechanism of Action—Penicillin G binds to one or more of the penicillin binding proteins to inhibit transpeptidase enzyme action thus blocking the synthesis of peptidoglycan, a component of bacteria cell wall. This may be followed by activation of autolytic enzymes in the cell wall which causes lysis of the bacteria.

Indications—Treatment of infections caused by Gram-positive and non penicillinase producing organisms. These conditions include streptococcal bovine mastitis, anthrax, erysipelas, strangles and joint ill of horses, some clostridial diseases such as tetanus and blackleg. It is used in dog bite as prophylaxis against gas gangrene and blackleg.

Dosages—.

Bird	Benzathine penicillin G: 100 mg/kg IM once a day.
	Note. May cause death if given IV.
	Procaine penicillin G: 100 mg/kg IM every 24-48 hours
	Note. Never use procaine in parrots or passerines.
Bovine	Procaine penicillin G: 20,000-40,000 U/kg IM every 12 hours.
	Procaine penicillin G and Benzathine penicillin G: 20,000-40,000 U/kg SC every 48 hours.
Cat	Procaine penicillin G: 40,000 U/kg IM every 24 hours.
Dog	Potassium penicillin G: 20,000 U/kg IM, IV (drip) every 4-6 hours.
	Procaine penicillin G: 40,000 U/kg IM once a day.
Guinea pig	May cause enterotoxic cecitis.
Mouse	Potassium penicillin: 100,000 IU/kg IM twice daily (do not use procaine penicillin) or
	Potassium penicillin: 60,000 U/mouse IM
NHP	Procaine penicillin G: 20,000 U/kg IM twice daily Benzathine penicillin G: 40,000 U/kg IM every 3 days.
Rat	Potassium penicillin: 100,000 IU/kg IM twice daily Penicillin, oral. 15,000 IU/20 ml drinking water
Rabbit	Procaine penicillin G and Benzathine penicillin G: 42,000 or 84,000 IU/kg SC once each week for 3 weeks.
	Procaine penicillin G: 60,000 U/kg IM daily for 10 days
Reptile	Procaine penicillin G and Benzathine penicillin G: 10,000 U total penicillin activity/kg IM at 24—to 72-h intervals
	Potassium penicillin: 10,000-20,000 U/kg IM, SC 3-4 times daily.
Sheep	Procaine penicillin G and Benzathine penicillin G. 10,000 or 20,000 U/kg IM every 3 or 6 days, respectively
Pig	Procaine penicillin G and Benzathine penicillin G: 10,000-40,000 U/kg IM every 3 days.

Route(s) of Administration—Intramuscular and intravenous infusion depending on formulation.

Absorption—Benzyl penicillin is rapidly absorbed. Peak plasma concentration is attained within 30 minutes of IM injection. Penicillin G potassium is labile to stomach acid and only about 15–30% of an orally administered dose of the drug is absorbed. Procaine penicillin G is slowly absorbed from IM site.

Distribution—Vd = 0.35L/kg. The drug is widely distributed but to varying concentrations in tissues and fluids. It attains about 1% of plasma concentration in CSF with normal meninges and about 5% with inflamed meninges. Significant amounts are found in liver, kidney, bile, semen, joint fluid, lymph, milk and intestine. Penicillin crosses the placenta.

Plasma Protein Binding—65%.

Metabolism—Small amounts are metabolized into penicilloic acid.

Plasma Half-Life—30 minutes (higher in renal and hepatic dysfunction).

Route(s) Of Excretion—Urine, bile and saliva. About 50-80% of a dose appear in urine as active drug.

Dialysis Status—Penicillin G is dialyzable.

Toxicity and Adverse Effects—Hypersensitivity reaction ranging from mild transitory skin reaction to anaphylactic shock are common. Direct toxic effects are low; LD_{50} in mice is 3.5 million units/kg. Penicillin G can cause CNS stimulation, twitching and convulsions. Bone marrow depression, granulocytopenia and hepatitis have been reported. It causes pain and sterile inflammatory reactions at intramuscular sites of injection.

Management of Overdose—Set up hemodialysis. Give supportive and symptomatic treatment.

Contraindications—Hypersensitivity to penicillin, penicillin breakdown products, procaine, or cephalosporins.

Precautions—Do not administer penicillin intravascularly or near a nerve to avoid damage due to its irritant property. Reduce dosage in patients with renal impairment. Do not use in pre-existing seizure disorders or in cases with history of hypersensitivity to cephalosporins.

Drug Interactions—Probenecid increases the plasma half-life of penicillins. In uremia, other organic acids compete for transport with penicillin secretion from the CSF. Tetracycline and other bacteriostatic antibiotics decrease its effectiveness. Aminoglycoside antibiotics (e.g. streptomycin) produce synergistic effects with penicillin G.

Pharmaceutical Formulations—The drug is available as the sodium or potassium salts in powder for reconstitution to aqueous solution for injection. Penicillin G is also available in combination with procaine.

PENTAZOCINE

Proprietary Names—Pentazocine˚; Talwin˚; Lexir˚; Talwin-NX˚ (pentazocine hydrochloride and naloxone hydrochloride).

Chemical Class—Benzomorphan derivative.

Pharmacological Class—Narcotic analgesic; Opioid analgesic; Partial opioid agonist.

Source—Synthetic.

Solubility, Stability and Storage. Pentazocine hydrochloride is sparingly soluble in water and freely soluble in alcohol. Store its formulations at room temperature protected from light. Do not mix pentazocine hydrochloride with barbiturates, aminophylline, flunixin meglumine and glycopyrrolate.

Pharmacological Actions—The actions of pentazocine are similar to those of morphine-like opioids i.e. analgesia, sedation, reduced GI motility, and respiratory depression. Its analgesic potency is one-half that of morphine and five times that of pethidine. It possesses antitussive effects. Pentazocine causes transient hypotension in dogs. It precipitates withdrawal syndromes in morphine-dependent human subjects.

Mechanism of Action—Pentazocine is either a weak antagonist or a partial agonist at the mu (μ) opioid receptors in addition to a powerful agonist property at the kappa (κ) opioid receptors.

Indications—Used in preanesthetic medication; control of colicky pain in horses and painful conditions in all species.

Dosages—

    Dog: 1.7-3.3 mg/kg IM

    Cat: 2.2-3.3 mg/kg parenterally

    Horse: 0.33 mg/kg IV followed in 15 minutes by 0.33 mg/kg IM for colic or 0.9 mg/kg IV for preanesthetic medication.

Route(s) of Administration—Per os; intramuscular; subcutaneous; and intravenous.

Absorption—Pentazocine is well absorbed from oral, subcutaneous and intramuscular sites. Peak plasma concentrations are reached in 15 minutes in dogs, goats, and pigs; 30 minutes in horses and 1 hour in cats after IM administration. Peak plasma concentration is attained within 1-3 hours after oral administration.

Bioavailability—Oral bioavailability is 47 ± 15% in humans. Bioavailability rises in patients with severe liver impairment.

Onset of Action—15 to 30 minutes (Per os; IM, SC); 2-3 minutes (IV).

Peak Action—30 to 60 minutes in humans.

Duration of Action—2 to 3 hours (parenteral route) and 4-5 hours (oral route) in humans. Duration of action is 48 minutes in horses and 3 hours in dogs.

Distribution—Vd = 7.1 ± 1.4 L/kg (humans); 5.09 L/kg (horse); 5.77 L/kg (goat); 4.76 L/kg (pig); 3.66 L/kg (dog); 2.78 L/kg (cat). Pentazocine distributes slowly but widely. It crosses the placenta.

Plasma Protein Binding—65% (humans); 80% (horse).

Metabolism—Undergoes oxidation and glucuronide conjugation.

Plasma Half-Life—4.6 ± 1.0 hours (humans); 97.1 minutes (horse); 51 minutes (goat); 48.6 minutes (pig); 22.1 minutes (dog) 83.6 minutes (cat).

Clearance—17 ± 5 ml/min/kg in humans.

Route(s) of Excretion—Urine with 15 ± 7% as unchanged drug in humans; 30% of dose appear in horse urine as glucuronide conjugates.

Toxicity and Adverse Effects—Pentazocine causes salivation in dogs. Higher doses produce marked respiratory depression, hypertension and tachycardia. High doses also produce convulsions, tremors, increased muscular tone and increased sensitivity to noise. Pentazocine may cause dysphoria in cats.

Management of Overdose/Toxicity—Naloxone is a specific antidote. Initiate general antidotal therapy if the drug was administered orally.

Contraindications—Hypersensitivity to pentazocine; narcotic dependence; respiratory depression; traumatic injuries of the head; raised intracranial pressure.

Precautions—Avoid repeated IM or SC injections. Administer pentazocine cautiously in pregnancy, impaired renal, hepatic or respiratory function. Avoid concurrent administration of pentazocine with barbiturates and monoamine oxidase inhibitors. Use pentazocine cautiously in cats.

Drug Interactions—CNS depressants may produce additive CNS depression when used with pentazocine. Naloxone antagonizes the respiratory depression and other effects caused by pentazocine.

Pharmaceutical Formulations—The drug is available as pentazocine lactate in solution for injection. Tablets containing both pentazocine hydrochloride (equivalent to 50 mg of the base) and naloxone hydrochloride (equivalent to 0.5 mg of the base) are available for oral use.

PHENOBARBITAL

Synonyms—Phenobarbitone; Sodium phenylethylbarbiturate; Soluble phenobarbitone.

Proprietary Names—Solfoton®; Luminal Sodium®.

Chemical Class—Barbiturate; Oxybarbiturate.

Pharmacological Class—Sedative-Hypnotic; Anticonvulsant.

Source—Synthetic.

Solubility, Stability and Storage—Phenobarbital is very slightly soluble in water and soluble in alcohol. The sodium salt is very soluble in water, freely soluble in propylene glycol, and soluble in alcohol. Phenobarbital is unstable in solution. Parenteral solutions are stabilized with propylene glycol. Do not use colored or unclear solutions and do not mix with acidic solutions to avoid precipitation of phenobarbital. Phenobarbital solutions are highly alkaline. Do not mix with ranitidine or benzquinamide in a syringe.

Phenobarbitone

Pharmacological Actions—Phenobarbital depresses the activity of muscle tissues, the heart, and the brain. Within the brain, phenobarbital act mainly at the RAS (reticular activating system), limbic system and cerebral cortex but it is able to produce all levels of depression. It has the greatest impact on awareness and respiration because of its action on the RAS and medulla oblongata respectively. As an anticonvulsant, phenobarbital increases seizure threshold and decreases the spread of seizure discharge. Phenobarbital acts as either a sedative or as a hypnotic depending on dose.

Mechanism of Action—The depressant and anticonvulsant effects of phenobarbital may be related to its ability to increase and/or mimic the inhibitory activity of GABA on nerve synapses. It appears to bind to GABA receptors and decrease excitability of membrane. Phenobarbital may also act by inhibiting the release of acetylcholine, noradrenaline and glutamate.

Indications—Control of all types of epilepsy in dogs and cats; treatment of status epilepticus and prevention of seizures in dogs, cats and horses; emergency control of acute seizure disorders such as meningitis, tetanus, eclampsia, and toxicity of local anesthetics. Also used as a sedative or hypnotic (short-term) or as anesthetic premedication in dogs and cats. Phenobarbital may be used in organochlorine toxicity to speed up the metabolism of the toxicant.

Dosages—

Dog	Sedation: 2-4 mg/kg body weight IV or 2-4 mg/kg body weight orally every six hours.
	Anesthesia: 10–30 mg/kg IV administered to effect.
	Epilepsy: 12 mg/kg loading dose.
Cat	Sedation: 2-4 mg/kg body weight IV or 2-4 mg/kg body weight orally every six hours.
	Anesthesia: 25–35 mg/kg IV.
	Epilepsy: 4 mg/kg orally every 12 hours. A total daily IV dose of 15–60 mg per day.
Horse	4-10 mg/kg PO, twice daily.

Route(s) of Administration—Per os; intravenous; intramuscular.

Absorption. Almost completely (88-95%) absorbed from the GIT. Peak plasma concentration is attained within 4-6 hours. Absorption takes about 6.4 hours.

Bioavailability—Oral bioavailability is 100 ± 11% in humans.

Effective Concentration—15-40 mcg/ml (for anticonvulsant activity).

Onset of Action—30 to more than 60 minutes in humans.

Peak Action—Up to 15 min in humans (after IV).

Duration of Action—10-16 hours in humans.

Distribution—Vd = 0.7 ± 0.15L/kg (dog); 0.96 ± 0.060L/kg (horse). Phenobarbital is distributed more slowly than other barbiturates due to lower lipid solubility. The drug is distributed throughout the body and affects all body tissues. Serum steady-state concentration is attained within 8-15 days of multiple dosing.

Plasma Protein Binding—50-60% in humans and 45% in dogs.

Metabolism—Metabolized by oxidative hydroxylation to weakly active hydroxyphenobarbital which is rapidly conjugated with glucuronic acid.

Plasma Half-life—Varies within species and individual animal. It also depends on single or multiple dosing. Values are 53-140 hours (humans); 53 ± 15 hours (dog with multiple dosing); 92.6 ± 23.7 hours (dog with a single dose); 24.2 ± 4.7 hours (single dosing in horses); 11.2 ± 2.3 hours (multiple dosing in horses; 12.8 ± 2.1 hours (foal).

Clearance (ml/min/kg)—5.6-6.6 (single dosing in dogs); 28.2 ± 5.1 (single dosing in horses); 57 ± 9.6 (multiple dosing in horses).

Route(s) of Excretion—Twenty-five percent eliminated unchanged in the urine (humans and dogs).

Dialysis Status—Dialyzable.

Toxicity and Adverse Effects—Polyuria, polyphagia and polydipsia are common following phenobarbital therapy. Phenobarbital may cause hepatotoxicity in animals whose metabolic processes have been induced. This is due to increased metabolic products. Phenobarbital causes reduced brain size in neonates. Treatment with phenobarbital during pregnancy may result in reproductive and endocrine malfunction in the offspring. Overdose causes cortical and respiratory depression, anoxia, peripheral vascular collapse, feeble, rapid pulse, pulmonary edema, decreased body temperature, clammy cyanotic skin, depressed reflexes, stupor, and coma. After initial constriction, the pupils become dilated. Death results from respiratory failure or arrest followed by cardiac arrest.

Management of Overdose/Toxicity—Initiate general antidotal therapy by using standard measures to limit absorption or enhance elimination of already absorbed drug. However, do not induce emesis if animal is unconscious to avoid aspiration of vomitus. Also, if the dose of barbiturate is high enough, the vomiting center may be depressed. Give adequate supportive and symptomatic therapy.

Contraindications—Hypersensitivity to barbiturates; severe trauma; pulmonary disease when dyspnea or obstruction is present; edema; uncontrolled diabetes; history of porphyria; impaired liver function; patients in whom barbiturates produce excitatory response.

Precautions—Use the minimum therapeutic dose of phenobarbital during pregnancy. Use cautiously in patients with CNS depression, hypotension, porphyria, fever, anemia, hemorrhagic shock, cardiac, hepatic or renal damage. Reduce the dose in debilitated animals, as well as those with impaired hepatic or renal functions.

Drug Interactions—Phenobarbital stimulates the activity of enzymes responsible for the metabolism of a large number of other drugs by a process known as enzyme induction. Hence phenobarbital may reduce the therapeutic effectiveness or even abolished the effects of such drugs. Many drugs, especially CNS depressants may potentiate the CNS depressant effect of the barbiturates with the result that concomitant administration may result in coma or fatal CNS depression. Barbiturate dosage should either be reduced or eliminated when other CNS depressants are given. Alkalinization of urine increases excretion of phenobarbital.

Pharmaceutical Formulations—Available as phenobarbital sodium in 64.8 mg/ml solution for injection. Various human formulations are available.

PHENOXYBENZAMINE

Phenoxybenzamine

Proprietary Names—Dibenzyline®.

Chemical Class—Haloalkylamine.

Pharmacological Class—Alpha-adrenergic blocking agent.

Source—Synthetic.

Solubility, Stability and Storage—Phenoxybenzamine hydrochloride has solubilities of approximately 40 mg/mL in water and 167 mg/mL in alcohol at 25°C. The capsules should be stored in well-closed containers at room temperature.

Pharmacological Actions—Phenoxybenzamine causes no appreciable change in blood pressure if administered into a normal patient. In a patient with compromised cardiovascular function such as in hypovolemia, in which sympathetic discharge is enhanced, phenoxybenzamine will cause marked hypotension. Similarly, it reduces the pressor responses resulting from administration of catecholamines. It prevents reflex hypertension caused by anoxia and occlusion of carotid arteries. It also decreases arrhythmia caused by catecholamines especially after sensitization of the myocardium by halogenated hydrocarbon anesthetic agents. Phenoxybenzamine causes relaxation of the nictitating membrane, urethra and increases opening of the bladder. It increases cutaneous blood flow and may enhance epinephrine release due to blockade of alpha$_2$ receptors.

Mechanism of Action—Phenoxybenzamine blocks the actions of α-adrenergic agonists irreversibly. It may inhibit neuronal and extraneuronal uptake mechanisms of norepinephrine. At higher concentrations, it inhibits responses to 5-HT, histamine and acetylcholine.

Indications—To reduce increased urethral sphincter tone in dogs and cats; treat secretory diarrhea and prevent or treat early stage laminitis in horses; treat tumors of the adrenal medulla and sympathetic neurons (pheochromocytoma) that secrete large quantities of catecholamines; prevent ischaemia of microvasculature during shock following adequate fluid replacement; and treat hypertensive crisis caused by sympathomimetic amines.

Dosages—

Dog	Increased urethral sphincter tone: 5-15 mg orally once a day.
	Hypertension associated with tumors of the adrenal medulla: 0.2-1.5 mg/kg orally twice daily. Use in conjunction with beta-adrenergic blockers to prevent severe hypertension.
Cat	Increased urethral sphincter tone: 0.5 mg/kg up to a maximum of 10 mg orally once daily.
Horse	1.2 mg/kg orally followed by half the dose after 12 and 24 hours. Profuse watery diarrhea: 200-600 mg every 12 hours.

Route(s) of Administration—Per os; intravenous.

Absorption—20 to 30% of administered dose is absorbed from the GIT.

Bioavailability—Oral bioavailability is 20-30% in humans.

Onset of Action—Prolonged (~2 hours) apparently because of conversion to active intermediates.

Peak Effect—4 to 6 hours.

Duration of Action—Duration of action is prolonged (3-4 days) due to irreversible nature of its action.

Distribution—Phenoxybenzamine is lipid soluble and may be localized in the adipose tissue.

Plasma Half—Life—About 24 hours in humans.

Route(s) of Excretion—Urine and feces.

Toxicity and Adverse Effects—The major adverse effect of phenoxybenzamine is hypotension followed by reflex tachycardia. The drug is also known to inhibit ejaculation, cause weakness, nausea and vomiting. It causes local irritation if administered intramuscularly. It may cause constipation in horses.

Management of Overdose/Toxicity—Give adequate fluids in hypovolemic patients. Only α-adrenergic agents such as norepinephrine may be used to reverse the hypotension.

Contraindications—Hypersensitivity to phenoxybenzamine or any component in the formulation; shock; horses with colic.

Precautions—Use phenoxybenzamine cautiously in patients with chronic heart failure or other heart diseases to avoid drug-induced tachycardia. Also use with caution in patients with renal impairment.

Drug Interactions—α-adrenergic agonist decreases the effects of phenoxybenzamine. β-adrenergic blockers increase its toxic potential by accentuating the hypotension and tachycardia produced by phenoxybenzamine overdose.

Pharmaceutical Formulations—The drug is available as phenoxybenzamine hydrochloride in 10 mg capsules.

PHENYLBUTAZONE

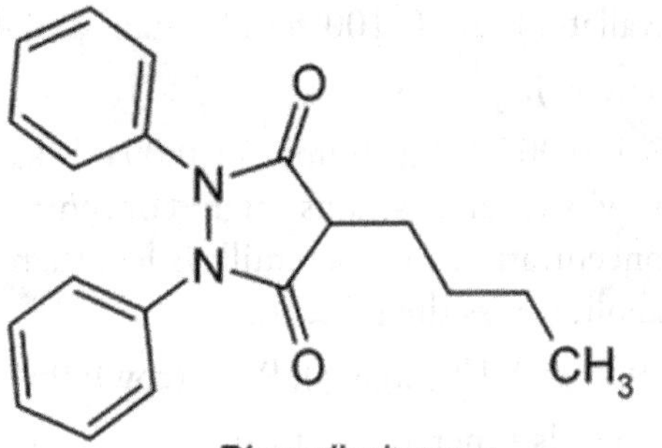

Phenylbutazone

Proprietary Names—Butazolidin®, butacote®, phenbuzone®.

Chemical Class—Pyrazolone derivative.

Pharmacological Class—Nonsteroidal anti-inflammatory drug; coal tar analgesic; analgesic antipyretic; non-opioid analgesic; simple analgesic; aspirin-like analgesic.

Source—Synthetic.

Solubility, Stability and Storage—Phenylbutazone is practically insoluble in water but soluble 1 in 28 of ethanol. It is soluble in alkaline solutions. Store phenylbutazone preparations at room temperature.

Pharmacological Actions—Phenylbutazone has prominent anti-inflammatory properties. It also has analgesic and antipyretic properties that are inferior to those possessed by salicylates. Phenylbutazone enhances uric acid excretion at high doses. At low doses the drug inhibits tubular excretion of uric acid and causes retention of urates. It causes sodium and chloride ion retention that may increase plasma volume as well as reduce urine volume and cause edema. Phenylbutazone reduces the uptake of iodine by the thyroid gland causing goiter and myxedema.

Mechanism of Action—Phenylbutazone nonselectively inhibits cyclooxygenase-1 and—2 (Cox-1 and Cox-2) and prevents the synthesis of prostaglandins and thromboxanes.

Indications—Short-term management of inflammatory and painful conditions associated with the musculoskeletal system such as lameness, osteoarthritis or non-articular rheumatism. It is frequently, although illegally, used to enhance performance of race horses.

Dosages—

Dog	14 mg/kg/ orally three times daily up to a maximum of 800 mg/day.
Cat	25 mg/kg for up to 5 days; reduce dose to 25 mg daily or on alternate days.
Horse	2 g two times a day for four days followed by 2 g/day for 4 days orally; or 2-4 mg/kg daily for 5 days maximum.
Cattle	4 mg/kg orally or IV every 24 hours.
Pig	4 mg/kg orally or IV every 24 hours.

Route(s) of Administration—Per os; intravenous (horse and dog).

Absorption—Phenylbutazone is rapidly and completely absorbed from the GIT in humans. Peak plasma concentration is attained within 2 hours. Oral absorption is slow in ruminants. Rate and extent of absorption is affected by food and dosage form in horses.

Bioavailability—Oral bioavailability is 80-100% in humans and 41.9-95.5% in ruminants.

Bioavailability (IM)—89% (cow).

Distribution—Vd = 0.097 ± 0.005 L/kg (humans); 0.091 L/kg (ruminants); 0.25 l/kg (horses). Phenylbutazone distributes widely and attains high concentrations in liver, heart, lungs and kidneys. Phenylbutazone concentration in cows' milk is less than 1% of its plasma concentration. Parent drug and active metabolite cross the placenta.

Plasma Protein Binding—96.1 ± 1.1 (humans); 93% (cow); 96-99% (horse).

Metabolism—Phenylbutazone is metabolized to oxyphenbutazone which is active and γ-hydroxyphenylbutazone.

Plasma Half-Life—56 ± 8 hours (humans); 3.5-6 hours (horses); 3 hours (rabbits); 2.5-6 hours (dogs and rats); 55 ± 6 hours (ruminants); 2-6 hours (pigs). Elimination is dose-dependent in horses and dogs.

Clearance—0.023 ± 0.003 ml/min/kg (humans); 1.24 ± 0.14 ml/kg/hour (ruminants).

Withdrawal Period—30 days, 35 days and 40 days before slaughter following 1, 2 and 3 doses respectively.

Route(s) of Excretion—Urine with 1% unchanged. Excreted more in alkaline urine.

Toxicity And Adverse Effects—Toxicity begins with inappetence, depression and weight loss. Gastrointestinal effects characterized by erosion and ulceration of buccal mucosa and GI tract are common in horses. Bone marrow effects characterized by agranulocytosis and aplastic anemia are of serious concern in humans than in animals. Intramuscular and subcutaneous injection cause irritation, leading to swelling necrosis and sloughing. Sodium retention with edema has been reported in dogs. Necrosis of hepatic vein, hepatitis, and nephritis have also been reported. In horses, toxicity can occur weeks after drug discontinuation.

Management of Overdose/Toxicity—Initiate general antidotal therapy. Stop further administration if adverse signs appear. Administer antiulcer drugs such as sucralfate, cimetidine, misoprostol etc. to control gastrointestinal erosions.

Contraindications—Congestive heart failure; at least 8 days before a race by a race horse; animals meant for food; cardiac, renal or hepatic dysfunction.

Precautions—Prolonged administration induces microsomal enzymes. Administer phenylbutazone with meals and for short durations. Avoid perivascular, intramuscular or subcutaneous administration.

Drug Interactions—Phenylbutazone can displace drugs (e.g. warfarin, sulfonamides, oral hypoglycemic drugs, other anti-inflammatory drugs etc.) from protein binding sites. Its metabolism is enhanced by inducers of microsomal enzymes e.g. barbiturates. It increases the effect of insulin.

Pharmaceutical Formulations—Phenylbutazone is available in 100 mg, 400 mg, and 1 gram tablets; 2 gram and 4 gram boluses; and 200 mg/ml solution for injection.

PHENYLEPHRINE

Phenylephrine

Synonyms—β-phenyliosopropylamine.

Proprietary Names—Neo-Synephrine®.

Chemical Class—Amine.

Pharmacological Class—α_1-Adrenergic receptor agonist; Direct-acting sympathomimetic drug.

Source—Synthetic.

Solubility, Stability and Storage—Phenylephrine hydrochloride is freely soluble in water and in alcohol. The drug is readily oxidized. Solutions containing the drug should be stored in tight, light-resistant containers. Phenylephrine hydrochloride solutions must not be used if they are brown or contain a precipitate. However, oxidation of the drug resulting in loss of activity may occur without color change being evident. Phenylephrine HCl oral tablets and injections may be stored at room temperature up to 30°C in light resistant container.

Pharmacological Actions—Phenylephrine causes peripheral vasoconstriction with resultant increases in peripheral resistance, diastolic and systolic blood pressures. It also causes arteriolar vasoconstriction in the nasal mucosa and conjunctiva. It contracts the dilator muscle of the pupil resulting in mydriasis. Phenylephrine can cause contraction of pregnant uterus and constriction of uterine vasculature. It does not stimulate the heart except at high doses. It may actually cause small decreases in cardiac output and reflex bradycardia due to pressor activation of baroreceptor-vagal reflex (this can be blocked by atropine).

Mechanism of Action—Phenylephrine activates postsynaptic α_1-adrenergic receptors at therapeutic doses. Beta-adrenergic receptors are activated by phenylephrine at higher doses.

Indications—Phenylephrine is used in the control of hypotension and shock especially in cases that do not require cardiac stimulation such as during anesthesia and in the presence of myocardial sensitizing drugs. It is useful in drug-induced hypotension as in overdose of phenothiazines, adrenergic blocking agents, and ganglion blockers. It is widely used in humans to decongest the nasal and ophthalmic mucous membranes and to produce mydriasis.

Dosages—

Dog, cat	1-3 mcg/kg/minutes as a constant rate infusion; 0.088 mg/kg administered by bolus IV injection. Double the dose if IM or SC routes are used.
Horse	5 mg intravenous bolus administration.

Route(s) of Administration—Constant intravenous infusion, intravenous bolus administration, intramuscular, subcutaneous, and topical.

Absorption—Phenylephrine is readily absorbed from parenteral sites.

Bioavailability—Phenylephrine does not attain therapeutic blood level following oral administration due to extensive first pass metabolism.

Onset of Action—Immediate (IV); 10-15 minutes (I.M. and S.C).

Duration of Action—20 minutes (IV); 30 minutes to 2 hours (IM in humans); 1 hour (SC).

Metabolism—Phenylephrine is metabolized by monoamine oxidase in the liver and intestine. Its action is partially terminated by tissue uptake.

Plasma Half-Life—2.5 hours.

Route(s) of Excretion—Urine.

Toxicity and Adverse Effects—Phenylephrine causes reflect bradycardia, restlessness and excitement at therapeutic doses. Ocular application may cause photosensitivity and conjunctival hyperemia. Overdose may cause hypertension, palpitations, paresthesia, and ventricular extra systoles. Extravasation into the tissue during infusion or injection may cause severe ischaemic necrosis and sloughing.

Management of Overdose/Toxicity—Give symptomatic and supportive therapy. Phentolamine may be administered intravenously in extreme cases. Infiltrate the site of extravasation with saline containing 5-10 mg of phentolamine.

Contraindications—Hypertension; ventricular tachycardia; known hypersensitivity to phenylephrine or any component such as sodium bisulfite.

Precautions—Avoid injecting phenylephrine into the tissue. Use with caution in aged animals and in patients with hyperthyroidism or myocardial diseases.

Drug Interactions—Monoamine oxidase inhibitors may potentiate the effect of phenylephrine. Similarly oxytocic agents may potentiate its pressor effect. Alpha-adrenergic receptor blockers (e.g. phentolamine) will reduce the pressor effect of phenylephrine. Concurrent use of phenylephrine with halothane and digitalis may induce cardiac arrhythmia.

Pharmaceutical Formulations—The drug is available as phenylephrine hydrochloride in 1% solution for injection; 0.12%, 2.5% and 10% solution for ophthalmic use; 0.125%, 0.16%, 0.2% and 0.25% solution for nasal application; 0.25%, 0.5% and 1% solution for nasal spray; 0.5% jelly for nasal application. No specific formulation is available for veterinary use. The solution for injection contains sodium metabisulfite, an antioxidant.

PHENYLPROPANOLAMINE

Phenylpropanolamine

Synonyms—dl-Norephedrine.

Proprietary Names—Propalin®; Urilin®; Propagest®; Acutrim®; Dexatrim®; Prolamine® Propadrine®.

Chemical Class—Amine.

Pharmacological Class—α_1-adrenergic receptor agonist; Indirect-acting sympathomimetic drug; Anorexiant; Nasal decongestant.

Source—Synthetic.

Solubility, stability and Storage—Do not store preparations of phenylpropanolamine above 25°C. Do not refrigerate.

Pharmacological Actions—The actions of phenylpropanolamine are similar to those of ephedrine but causes less CNS stimulation. Specifically, phenylpropanolamine increases peripheral resistance and blood pressure. it also stimulates heart rate and cardiac output. It causes mild CNS stimulation, decreased nasal congestion and reduced appetite. The drug increases urethral sphincter tone and causes closure of the bladder neck. Frequent dosing or prolonged administration results in tachyphylaxis. However, tachyphylaxis has not been documented in dogs and cats.

Mechanism of Action—Phenylpropanolamine causes the release of norepinephrine from storage vesicles. Norepinephrine then activates α—and β-adrenergic receptors.

Indications—Treatment of urinary incontinence associated with urethral sphincter hypotonus in dogs and cats. Efficacy has only been demonstrated in ovariohysterectomised bitches.

Dosages—1mg/kg bodyweight 3 times daily. One 75 mg sustained-release capsule orally once daily is also adequate in cats.

Route(s) of Administration—Per os.

Absorption—Readily absorbed from the GIT.

Bioavailability—Oral bioavailability is about 100%.

Onset of Action—15 to 30 minutes in humans.

Duration of Action—About 3 hours in humans.

Distribution—Widely distributed to tissues and fluids, including the CNS.

Metabolism—Partly metabolized in the liver to norephedrine.

Plasma Half-Life—4.6 to 6.6 hours.

Route(s) of Excretion—Urine (80-90% as unchanged drug.

Toxicity and Adverse Effects—Loose stools, liquid diarrhoea, decrease in appetite, arrhythmia and collapse have been reported in some dogs. It may cause symptoms of excessive stimulation of the sympathetic nervous system such as hypertension, palpitations, insomnia, restlessness, dry mouth and nausea at therapeutic doses. Overdose may cause aggravation of these signs in addition to paresthesia, seizures and vomiting. Anorexia may be pronounced.

Management of Overdose/Toxicity—Give general antidotal and supportive therapy. Treatment should be symptomatic. α-Adrenergic blockers may be appropriate in cases of severe overdose.

Contraindications—Hypersensitivity to phenylpropanolamine or any component; pregnancy; lactating bitches or queens.

Precautions—Do not administer phenylpropanolamine concurrently with other sympathomimetic agents or within two weeks of the administration of MAO inhibitor. Use phenylpropanolamine with caution in animals with cardiovascular diseases, severe renal or hepatic insufficiency, diabetes mellitus, hyperadrenocorticism, glaucoma, hyperthyroidism or prostatic hypertrophy.

Drug Interactions—Phenylpropanolamine effects are antagonistic to those of antihypertensive drugs. Mono amine oxidase inhibitors and β-adrenergic blockers enhance the pressor effects of phenylpropanolamine. Concurrent administration with NSAIDs, reserpine, tricyclic antidepressants, or ganglion blocking agents may increase the likelihood of hypertension. Administration of phenylpropanolamine in animals under anesthesia induced with halogenated hydrocarbon anesthetic agents may cause cardiac arrhythmias.

Pharmaceutical Formulations—The drug is available as phenylpropanolamine hydrochloride in solution for oral use containing 50 mg/ml.

PILOCARPINE

Pilocarpine

Proprietary Names—Adsorbocarpine˙; Akarpine˙; Isopto˙ Carpine; Ocusert Pilo˙; Pilocar˙; Piloptic˙; Pilostat˙.

Chemical Class—Alkaloid.

Pharmacological Class—Parasympathomimetic agent; Natural cholinomimetic alkaloid.

Source—Natural; obtained from the leaves of *Pilocarpus jaborandi* and *Pilocarpus microphyllus*.

Solubility, Stability and Storage—The nitrate salt of pilocarpine is water soluble. The gel formulation should be refrigerated while the solution may be stored at 8-30⁰ C.

Pharmacological Actions—Pilocarpine stimulates the secretion of exocrine glands such as salivary, mucous, gastric, and pancreatic glands and contracts the GI smooth muscle. It causes miosis by contraction of the iris sphincter and also causes loss of accommodation by constriction of ciliary muscle. Pilocarpine reduces intraocular pressure.

Mechanism of Action—Pilocarpine predominantly activates muscarinic receptors. Its action on nicotinic receptors is minimal.

Indications—Treatment of glaucoma and keratoconjunctivitis sicca (dry eye syndrome in dogs). Pilocarpine is used alternatively with mydriatics like atropine to prevent synechiation (adhesions between the iris and the lens in cases of iridocyclitis).

Dosages. Instill 1-2 drops topically into the conjunctiva.

Route(s) of Administration—Topical.

Onset of Action—10 to 15 minutes (miosis).

Duration of Action—6 to 8 hours (miosis); 6 hours (reduced ocular pressure); 1-2 hours (accommodation).

Toxicity and Adverse Effects—Pilocarpine causes local irritation characterized by conjunctiva hyperemia and blepharospasm within a few minutes following instillation into the conjunctiva.

Its systemic side effects include salivation, severe colic, diarrhea, and bronchospasm. Death results from hypotension, bradycardia, increased bronchial secretion, and bronchoconstriction with obstruction of airways.

Management of Overdose/Toxicity—Atropine is the specific antidote.

Contraindications—Iridocyclitis; heart failure; respiratory impairment; pregnancy; colic; hypersensitivity to pilocarpine.

Drug Interactions—The action of pilocarpine is synergistic with carbonic anhydrase inhibitors (e.g. acetazolamide), adrenergic agents, and systemic hyperosmotic agents.

Pharmaceutical Formulations—The drug is available as pilocarpine nitrate and hydrochloride in various topical ophthalmic solutions of 0.25-10%. Slow release and 4% gel formulations are also available.

PIPERAZINE

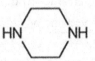

Piperazine

Proprietary Names—Antepar*; Ascalix*; Eraverm*; Piperasol*; Piperzool;* Coopane*; Assiazine*; Ascapil*; Anivermin*; Vermizine*.

Chemical Class—A heterocyclic nitrogen compound.

Pharmacological Class—Anthelmintic.

Source—Synthetic.

Solubility, Stability and Storage—Piperazine is soluble in water and ethanol. The drug is unstable. It is available for use in form of simple salts which are stable. The salts are adipate (37%), citrate (35%), phosphate (42%), sulfate (46%), chloride (48%), dihydrochloride (50-53%), and hexahydrate (44%). The numbers in parenthesis indicate the amount of active piperazine base present in the particular salt form.

Pharmacological Actions—Piperazine causes flaccid paralysis and subsequent expulsion of round worms especially ascarids and modular worms of all species of domestic animals and man.

Mechanism of Action—The drug causes hyper polarization at the myoneural junction of the worm apparently by altering the permeability of cell membrane to ions which are responsible for the maintenance of resting potential. Thus, the drug renders the muscle unexcitable by acetylcholine and causing flaccid paralysis. The worms are then expelled by peristaltic action.

Indications—Treatment of ascarids and nodular worm infections in all species.

Dosages—

Piperazine (adipate and citrate):

Bird	100-500 mg/kg PO once; repeat in 10-14 days.
Cattle	110 mg/kg. PO.

Dog, Cat	200 mg/kg. Repeat treatment at 3 monthly intervals for adults. Treat puppies and kittens at 2 weeks of age and every 2 weeks until 12 weeks of age.
Goat	110 mg/kg PO.
Guinea pig	Piperazine adipate: 4-7 mg/ml drinking water.
Mouse	Piperazine adipate: 4-7 mg/ml drinking water for 3-10 days.
	Piperazine citrate: 200 mg/kg daily in drinking water for 7 days, off 7 days, repeat for 7 days.
Non Human Primate	65 mg/kg. PO once daily for 10 days.
Rat	200 mg/100 ml drinking water.
	Piperazine adipate: 250 mg/50-60 g in drinking water for 3 days.
Rabbit	Piperazine adipate: 0.5 mg/kg PO for 2 days.
	Piperazine citrate: 100 mg/ml drinking water for 1 day
	Piperazine powder: 200 mg/kg PO.
Reptile	Piperazine citrate: 40-60 mg/kg. PO; not more often than once every 2 weeks.
Sheep	110 mg/kg PO.
Pig	110 mg/kg PO.

Piperazine base:

110m g/kg body weight in large animals; 45-65 mg/kg body weight in small animals; 32 mg/kg body weight in feed or water for 2 days in poultry.

Route(s) of Administration—Per os.

Absorption—Rapidly absorbed from the GIT.

Route(s) of Excretion—Urine with 20-40% as unchanged drug.

Toxicity and Adverse Effects—Piperazine is almost nontoxic under normal circumstances. LD_{50} in mice is 11.4g/kg body weight. However, occasional gastrointestinal upset, transient neurological effects and urticaria reactions has been observed in humans. Large oral doses occasionally produce emesis, diarrhea and incoordination in dogs and cats. Transient neurological effects and urticarial reactions have occasionally been noted.

Contraindications—Chronic renal and hepatic diseases; known hypersensitivity to piperazine.

Precautions—Do not administer a purgative and pyrantel concurrently with piperazine. No fasting is needed with piperazine therapy. Reinfection is easy because the eggs within voided worms are viable.

Drug Interactions—Piperazine action is antagonistic to that of pyrantel.

Pharmaceutical Formulations—The drug is available in 250-500 tablets and 100-150 mg/ml syrup for humans and small animals. It is also available as suspension and powder for administration in feed or drinking water for livestock and poultry.

PIROXICAM

Proprietary Names—Feldene®, proponol®.

Chemical Class—Oxicam derivative.

Pharmacological Class—Nonsteroidal Anti-inflammatory Drug.

Source—Synthetic.

Solubility, Stability and Storage—Piroxicam is sparingly soluble in water and slightly soluble in alcohol and in alkaline aqueous solution. Store piroxicam preparations below 30⁰C. Protect products from light and moisture.

Piroxicam

Pharmacological Actions—Piroxicam possesses analgesic, antipyretic and anti-inflammatory actions with long duration of action. It reduces edema, erythema, fever, pain and tissue proliferation irrespective of etiology. Piroxicam has immunomodulatory properties.

Mechanism of Action—Piroxicam blocks prostaglandin synthesis by reversibly inhibiting cyclooxygenase. It also inhibits other processes like the activation of neutrophils, release of lysosomal enzyme from activated leucocytes, and superoxide generation by neutrophils.

Indications—Treatment of osteoarthritis in dogs; control of postoperative pain and pain arising from trauma. Piroxicam has been shown to reduce the size of some tumors (e.g. transitional cell tumors) in dogs.

Dosages—0.3 mg/kg orally daily (for adjunctive treatment of tumor) or every other day (for analgesic and anti-inflammatory action).

Route(s) of Administration—Per os.

Absorption—Piroxicam is rapidly and completely absorbed from the GIT. Peak plasma concentration is attained within 2-4 hours. Foods have effect on rate but not the extent of absorption. Antacids have no effect on rate and extent of absorption.

Bioavailability—Oral bioavailability is 100% in dog.

Onset of Action—Onset of analgesia is timely.

Peak Action—Piroxicam produces maximum therapeutic response in 2 weeks.

Distribution—Vd = 0.15 ± 0.03 L/kg in humans and 0.34 L/kg in dogs. Piroxicam may attain 40% of its plasma level in the synovial fluid but it attains low levels in milk.

Plasma Protein Binding—99.3 ± 0.2%.

Metabolism—Piroxicam is extensively degraded to inactive hydroxylated and conjugated metabolites.

Plasma Half-Life—48 ± 8 hours in humans and 40-45 hours in dogs. Piroxicam undergoes enterohepatic circulation.

Clearance—0.036 ± 0.008 (ml/min/kg) in humans. Clearance decreases in cirrhosis.

Route(s) of Excretion—Urine and feces. About 5% appear in urine as unchanged drug.

Toxicity and Adverse Effects—Piroxicam causes gastrointestinal irritation, prolonged bleeding time, and renal papillary necrosis. Papillary necrosis is prominent in the dog but rare in monkeys. Dogs are particularly sensitive to piroxicam. The inhibition of prostaglandin synthesis by NSAIDs has been associated with increased incidence of dystocia and delayed parturition in pregnant animals when treatment is given during late pregnancy.

Management of Overdose/Toxicity—Initiate general antidotal therapy. Activated charcoal reduces absorption. Give supportive and symptomatic treatment.

Contraindications—History of allergy to the drug or other NSAIDs; late pregnancy; lactating animals.

Precautions—Concurrent use of piroxicam and other NSAIDs is not recommended because there are no data to support that the additive beneficial effects outweigh the adverse effects. Use piroxicam with caution in animals with heart disease because the drug may cause sodium, potassium and fluid retention.

Drug Interactions—Piroxicam is highly protein bound and may displace or be displaced by other protein bound drugs (such as anticoagulants, sulfonamides, phenylbutazone, hydatoins etc.) from binding sites. This may increase the free portion of displaced drugs in plasma. Piroxicam increases blood concentration, half-life and likelihood of toxicity of methotrexate. Gastrointestinal bleeding or ulceration may be severe if used with drugs that alter hemostasis (e.g. heparin, warfarin) or cause ulceration (e.g. aspirin, phenylbutazone, corticosteroids etc.). Concomitant use of piroxicam and aspirin may cause 80% reduction in the plasma levels of piroxicam.

Pharmaceutical Formulations—Piroxicam is available in 10 and 20 mg capsules; 20 mg tablets and 20 mg/ml solution for injection.

POLYMYXIN B

Proprietary Names—Aerosporin˙.

Chemical Class—Peptide.

Pharmacological Class—Narrow spectrum antibiotic.

Source—Natural; obtained from *Bacillus polymyxa*.

Solubility, Stability and Storage—The drug is freely soluble in water and in 0.9% sodium chloride solution. It is slightly soluble in alcohol. Polymyxin B sulfate is inactivated by strong acidic or alkaline solutions. The drug is chemically incompatible with many drugs including amphotericin B, chloramphenicol sodium succinate, chlorothiazide sodium, heparin sodium, penicillins, prednisolone sodium phosphate, and tetracyclines. Polymyxin B sulfate in solution is also incompatible with the salts of calcium and magnesium. Polymyxin B sulfate sterile powder should be stored at room temperature and protected from light.

Pharmacological actions—Polymyxin is bactericidal to Gram-positive bacilli, particularly *Pseudomonas* and coliform organisms. It inactivates bacterial endotoxin. Its spectrum of activity is similar to that of colistin derivatives. There is complete cross-resistance between colistin derivatives and polymyxin B.

Mechanism of Action—Polymyxin B binds to phosphate groups in the lipids of bacterial cytoplasmic membrane and acts as a cationic detergent. It penetrates into and disrupts the structure, osmotic properties and transport mechanisms of cell membranes thereby altering the osmotic barrier of the membrane and causing leakage of macromolecules and death of the cell.

Indications—Treatment of bovine mastitis due to *Pseudomonas aeruginosa*; infection caused by *Pseudomonas* spp in other animals and canine otitis external. The drug is used as semen additive to inhibit the growth of *Pseudomonas*.

Dosages—

Cattle	40,000 units/kg orally or 10,000 units/kg parenterally in divided doses.
Bird	50,000 IU/l water.
Rabbit	3 mg/300—to 400-g animal PO bid for 5 days.

Route(s) of Administration—The oral, intramuscular, intravenous routes are appropriate. The drug may also be applied topically.

Absorption—Polymyxin B is absorbed from IM site. Peak plasma concentration is attained within 2 hours. It is minimally absorbed from the GIT, mucous membranes and intact skin.

Distribution—Polymyxin B is widely distributed into body tissues but poorly distributed into body fluids. It does not appear in synovial fluid, aqueous humor of the eye and the CSF (even when the meninges are inflamed. Polymyxin B does not cross the placenta. Approximately 50% of a dose is reversibly bound to phospholipids of cell membranes in the liver, kidneys, heart, muscle, brain, and probably other tissues. The drug is also strongly bound by cell debris and purulent exudates.

Plasma Protein Binding—Polymyxin B does not appear to be highly bound to serum protein.

Plasma Half-Life—4.3 to 6 hours in adult humans with normal renal function.

Route(s) of Excretion—Urine (60% as unchanged drug).

Maximum Residue Limit—4.0 mcg/ml of milk.

Toxicity and Adverse Effects—Large oral dose may cause nausea, vomiting and diarrhea. Neurotoxicity (characterized by paresthesia, dizziness, flushing and incoordination) and nephrotoxicity (characterized by proteinuria and hematuria) are associated with parenteral administration in humans and animals. Overdose may cause renal failure, neuromuscular paralysis and even death. Polymyxin causes local irritation at injection site. It causes neuromuscular blockade especially when given soon after anesthesia or muscle relaxants.

Management of Overdose/Toxicity—Discontinue therapy if adverse effects are serious. Give symptomatic and supportive treatment.

Contraindications—Concurrent use with neuromuscular blockers; known hypersensitivity to polymyxin B.

Precautions—Reduce the dose in cases of renal impairment. Administer intramuscularly if the drug is required for systemic infection. Avoid concurrent or sequential use of other neurotoxic and nephrotoxic drugs such as bacitracin, colistin and the aminoglycosides antibiotics.

Drug Interactions—The actions of polymyxin B are blocked by bivalent metallic ions. It increases or prolongs the effects of neuromuscular blocking drugs.

Pharmaceutical Formulations—Polymyxin is available as polymyxin sulfate in solutions for ophthalmic, otic and topical uses in combination with other antibiotics or drugs. Solutions containing 500,000 units are available for parenteral use. The drug is also available in ointments, and intramammary formulations with other antibiotics such as oxytetracycline for intramammary infusion. Polymyxin B sulfate contains not less than 6,000 units of polymyxin B activity per mg, calculated on the dried basis, and each mg of pure polymyxin B is equivalent to 10,000 units of polymyxin B activity.

POLYSULFATED GLYCOSAMINOGLYCAN

Synonyms. PSGAG.

Proprietary Names. Adequan®.

Chemical Class. A sulfated polysaccharide.

Pharmacological Class. Antiarthritic agent.

Source. Natural; obtained from bovine trachea.

Solubility, Stability and Storage. Store PSGAG products at 8-15⁰C. Do not mix with other drugs. Discard unused portion.

Pharmacological Actions. PSGAG promotes synthesis of matrix components, retards catabolic processes, relieves pain and inflammation, and restores the functioning and consistency of synovial fluid. PSGAG also has anti-inflammatory properties.

Mechanism of Action. Its mechanism of action is uncertain. It is thought to cause chondrocyte proliferation and matrix biosynthesis as well as inhibit the actions of proteolytic enzymes and complement activity. Its anti-inflammatory action is associated with inhibition of prostaglandin E_2 that is released following joint injury.

Indications—PSGAG is indicated in degenerative and traumatic joint diseases in humans and animals.

Dosages—

Horse	Ten doses of 500 mg IM per dose every 4 days or 5 doses of 250 mg intra-articularly per dose every week.
Dog, Cat	Six doses of 3-5 mg/kg every 4 days.

Route(s) of Administration—Intra-articular (in joint disease only); intramuscular (in joint disease and tendonitis).

Absorption—PSGAG is absorbed readily from IM site and attains peak levels at the joint within 48 hours.

Distribution—The drug attains high levels at the joints where it is deposited in all layers of articular cartilage.

Metabolism—PSGAG is minimally degraded.

Route(s) of Excretion—Urine.

Dialysis Status—Nondialyzable

Toxicity and Adverse Effects—PSGAG is well tolerated. Increased bleeding time may be possible since PSGAG is chemically related to heparin.

Management of Overdose/Toxicity—Treat post injection inflammation of the joint with anti-inflammatory drugs.

Contraindications—Hypersensitivity to PSGAG.

Precautions—Use with caution in breeding animals and during pregnancy since the effects of PSGAG on reproductive performance is unknown. Do not use PSGAG in animals with septic joint disease. Adopt strict aseptic measures during intra-articular injection to avoid post injection inflammation of the joint. Since PSGAG is chemically related to heparin, its concurrent use with other drugs capable of increasing bleeding time or altering hemostasis should be avoided.

Drug Interactions—No specific interactions have been documented.

Pharmaceutical Formulations—Available in 250 mg/ml in 1 ml ampoules for intra-articular injection, and 100 mg/ml in 5 ml ampoules for IM injection

PRALIDOXIME

Pralidoxime

Synonyms—2-PAM; 2-Pyridine Aldoxime Methochloride.

Proprietary Names—Protopam®.

Chemical Class—Quaternary ammonium oxime.

Pharmacological Class—Cholinesterase reactivator.

Source—Synthetic.

Solubility, Stability and Storage—Pralidoxime is freely soluble in water. Store powder at room temperature. Reconstitute with preservatives free sterile water. Use reconstituted solution within a few hours. The drug can be diluted with normal saline.

Pharmacological Actions—Pralidoxime reactivates phosphorylated cholinesterase enzymes consequently increasing the LD_{50} of organophosphates and the survival rate of patients poisoned by organophosphates.

Mechanism of Action—Organophosphates phosphorylates acetylcholinesterase enzyme by interacting irreversibly at the esteratic site of the enzyme. Pralidoxime binds electrostatically at the anionic site of the phosphorylated acetylcholinesterase enzyme and to the phosphorus atom of the organophosphate. The resulting oxime-phosphonate complex is then split off thereby releasing the cholinesterase enzyme. Aged phosphorylated enzymes are resistant to reactivation. Pralidoxime may be ineffective in reactivating carbomylated enzymes.

Indications—Treatment of organophosphate poisoning (in combination with atropine and supportive measures) and control of drug overdose in the treatment of myasthenia gravis. Pralidoxime appears to be most effective when given within 24 hours of poisoning. It is usually not effective after 36–48 hours have elapsed.

Dosages—

Dog	20 mg/kg 3 times a day. Give initial dose by slow IV infusion; subsequent doses may be given IM or SC.
Cattle	10-40 mg/kg.
Horse	20 mg/kg.

Route(s) of Administration—Intravenous; intramuscular; subcutaneous.

Absorption—Poorly absorbed from the GIT. Peak plasma concentrations are attained within 2-3 hours after oral, 5-15 minutes after IV, and 10-20 minutes after IM administration.

Effective Concentration—Minimum therapeutic plasma concentration of pralidoxime is estimated to be 4 mcg/mL.

Distribution—It distributes mainly in the ECF.

Plasma Protein Binding—Not bound.

Metabolism—Metabolized in the liver.

Plasma Half-life—0.8-2.7 hours in humans.

Route(s) of Excretion—80-90% excreted in urine as unchanged drug and metabolites.

Dialysis Status—Nondialyzable.

Toxicity and Adverse Effects—Pralidoxime is free of significant adverse effects at therapeutic doses. It causes pain at the local site of intramuscular injection. Rapid intravenous injection may produce cardiovascular signs characterised by tachycardia, hypertension, respiratory (hyperventilation, laryngeospasm) signs and transient neuromuscular blockade. An overdose may produce blurred vision, dizziness, nausea and tachycardia in humans; muscle weakness, ataxia, seizures and respiratory arrest in dogs.

Management of Overdose/Toxicity—Give supportive therapy and mechanical ventilation.

Contraindications—Known hypersensitivity to pralidoxime or any component. Pralidoxime is contraindicated in the treatment of toxic exposure to carbaryl since it appears to increase the toxicity of carbaryl.

Precautions—Reduce the dose of pralidoxime in patients with renal impairment. Use the drug cautiously in patients receiving treatment for myasthenia gravis and in patients receiving theophylline, succinylcholine, phenothiazines and respiratory depressants.

Drug Interactions—Cimetidine delays the metabolism of organophosphates. Morphine, theophylline, succinylcholine, phenothiazine and reserpine increase organophosphate toxicity.

Pharmaceutical Formulations—The drug is available as pralidoxime chloride in vials containing 1g for reconstitution with 20 ml diluent, and in 2 ml vials of 300 mg/ml. It is also available in 500 mg tablets. There are no specific veterinary formulations.

PRAZIQUANTEL

Proprietary Names—Droncit*; Biltricide*.

Chemical Class—A pyrazinoisoquinoline derivative.

Pharmacological Class—Anthelmintic.

Source—Synthetic.

Solubility, Stability and Storage—Praziquantel is very slightly soluble in water but freely soluble in alcohol. Praziquantel tablets should be stored in tight containers at room temperature.

Pharmacological Actions—Praziquantel has broad spectrum of anthelmintic activity. The drug has activity against many trematodes, as well as adult, juvenile, and larval stages of certain cestodes including *Dipylidium caninum*, *Taenia* species, and *Echinococcus granulosus*.

Praziquantel

Mechanism of Action—The mechanism is uncertain. The drug may be causing increased muscular activity, followed by contraction and spastic paralysis at low effective concentration. At higher concentration, praziquantel causes vacuolation and vesiculation of the tergument of susceptible parasites leading to activation of host defense mechanism.

Indications—Treatment of cestode and trematode infections in dogs and cats.

Dosages—3.5 to 7.5 mg/kg as single dose in dogs and cats.

Route(s) of Administration—Per os, subcutaneous and intramuscular.

Absorption—More than 80% of a dose is rapidly absorbed after oral administration. Peak plasma concentration is achieved within 1-2 hours in humans and 30-60 minutes in dogs and cats.

Bioavailability—Limited due to pronounced first-pass effect.

Distribution—Praziquantel is distributed into the CSF. It is also distributed into milk.

Metabolism—The drug is extensively metabolized in the liver to hydroxylated and conjugated products.

Plasma Half-Life—1.5 hours.

Route(s) of Excretion—Urine, mainly as metabolites.

Toxicity and Adverse Effects—Praziquantel is nontoxic at therapeutic doses. In humans, transient abdominal discomfort, headache and dizziness may be observed shortly after administration. Fever, skin rashes and eosinophilia may also be observed.

Contraindications—Known hypersensitivity to praziquantel.

Precautions—Treat female cats at least 8 days before delivery and kittens before and 14 days after sale.

Drug Interactions—Carbamazepine and phenytoin have been reported to reduce the bioavailability of praziquantel. Dexamethasone reduces plasma concentrations of praziquantel. Cimetidine has been reported to increase praziquantel bioavailability.

Pharmaceutical Formulations—Praziquantel is available in solution for injection containing 56.8 mg/ml praziquantel as active substance, 5 mg/ml chlorbutol as a preservative and 75 mg/ml benzyl alcohol as a solvent. Praziquantel is also available in tablets and fixed dose combinations with other anthelmintics including pyrantel, milbemycin oxime, levamisole and ivermectin.

PRAZOSIN

Synonyms—Furazosin.

Proprietary Names—Minipress®.

Chemical Class—Piperazinyl quinazoline derivative.

Pharmacological Class—α_1-Adrenergic receptor blocker.

Source—Synthetic.

Solubility, Stability And Storage—Prazosin is slightly soluble in water and alcohol. Store prazosin hydrochloride formulations at room temperature in well covered containers.

Pharmacological Actions—Prazosin reduces peripheral vascular resistance and blood pressure by causing dilatation of arterioles and veins. It decreases cardiac preload and causes less cardiac excitation and orthostatic hypotension, as does non-selective α-adrenergic receptor blockers. It may act centrally to depress sympathetic outflow. It increases cardiac output in patients with congestive heart failure. Prazosin inhibits cyclic nucleotide phosphodiesterase.

Mechanism of Action—Prazosin blocks postsynaptic α_1 adrenergic receptors.

Indications—Treatment of systemic hypertension or pulmonary hypertension in dogs. Prazosin may be valuable for reducing cardiac workload without reflex tachycardia in chronic congestive heart failure.

Dosages—1 mg/15 kg body weight orally three times daily.

Route(s) of Administration—Per os.

Absorption—Variable; peak plasma concentration is attained within 1-3 hours.

Bioavailability—50-70%.

Onset of Action—Within 2 hours.

Peak Effect—4 to 5 hours.

Duration of Action—10 hours.

Distribution—Vd = 0.5 L/kg. Prazosin distributes rapidly to most tissues. It has predilection for blood vessels.

Plasma Protein Binding—95 ± 1.0%.

Metabolism—Prazosin is extensively metabolized in the liver.

Plasma Half-Life. 2.9 ± 0.8 in humans (higher in chronic heart failure, aged and pregnancy).

Clearance—3.0 ± 0.3 ml/min/kg in humans (lower in chronic heart failure and pregnancy).

Route(s) of Excretion—Excreted in urine and bile with 6-10% as unchanged drug in urine.

Toxicity and Adverse Effects—In humans, prazosin produces a first-dose phenomenon characterized by postural hypotension and syncope. These adverse effects may appear 30-90 minutes after the first dose. Prazosin may also cause CNS effects such as lethargy and dizziness. Gastrointestinal effects (nausea, vomiting, diarrhea and constipation have been reported.

Management of Toxicity/Overdose—Give symptomatic and supportive treatment.

Contraindications—Pre-existing hypotensive condition; known hypersensitivity to prazosin or related drugs.

Precautions—Use cautiously in cases with chronic renal impairment. First dose phenomenon occurs most commonly in patients receiving beta-blockers, diuretics, or large doses of prazosin.

Drug Interactions—Highly protein-bound drugs may displace prazosin, or be displaced by prazosin from binding site. NSAIDs may decrease the effect of prazosin. Calcium channel blockers (e.g. verapamil and nifedipine) may give synergistic effect when used concomitantly with prazosin. Beta-adrenergic blockers such as propranolol may enhance the postural hypotensive effects of prazosin while antihypertensive agents may give additive response when used concomitantly.

Pharmaceutical Formulations. Available as prazosin hydrochloride in 1 mg, 2 mg, and 5 mg capsules. No specific veterinary formulation is available.

PREDNISONE/PREDNISOLONE

Synonyms—1,2-Dehydrohydrocortisone; Deltahydrocortisone; Δ^1-Hydrocortisone; Hydroretrocortine; Metacortandralone.

Proprietary Names—Codelcortone*; Cortalone*; Decaprednil*; Decortin H*; Delta-Cortef*; Deltacortril*; Deltasolone*; Flamasone*; Hydeltra*; Hydrodeltalone*; Klismacort*; Meticortolone*; Paracortol*; Precortilon*; Precortisyl*; Prednelan*; Solone*; Sterolone*.

Chemical Class—Glucocorticoid; Corticosteroid.

Pharmacological Class—Anti-inflammatory drug.

Source—Synthetic.

Solubility, Stability and Storage—Prednisolone is slightly soluble in water and sparingly soluble in alcohol but prednisolone acetate is practically insoluble in water and slightly soluble in alcohol. Prednisolone sodium succinate is highly water soluble. Prednisolone formulations should be stored at temperature less than 40°C, preferably between 15–30°C. Freezing of the oral solutions should be avoided.

Prednisone

Prednisolone

Pharmacological Actions—Prednisolone and prednisone have similar actions. Prednisone is metabolized by the liver to prednisolone. Like other corticosteroids, both drugs regulate protein, carbohydrate, lipid and nucleic acid metabolism. They also regulate inflammation and immune response, distribution and excretion of water and solutes, and secretion of adrenocorticotrophic hormone (ACTH) from the pituitary gland. Prednisolone is particularly effective as an immunosuppressant and affects virtually all of the immune system.

Mechanism of Action—Prednisolone and prednisone activate specific glucocorticoid receptors at the cytosol and the hormone-receptor complex is then transported into the cell nucleus where it binds with glucocorticoid response elements (GRE) on various genes and alters their expression. An opposite mechanism is called transrepression in which the activated hormone receptor interacts with specific transcription factors and prevents the transcription of targeted genes. Glucocorticoids are able to prevent the transcription of any of immune genes, including the IL-2 gene. For anti-inflammatory and immunomodulating actions, glucocorticoids induce the lipocortin-1 (annexin-1) synthesis, which then binds to cell membranes preventing phospholipase A2 from coming into contact with its substrate arachidonic acid. This prevents the synthesis of prostaglandins and leukotrienes. Glucocorticoids also stimulate the lipocortin-1 binding to the leukocyte membrane receptors and inhibit various inflammatory events such as epithelial adhesion, emigration, chemotaxis, phagocytosis, respiratory burst and the release of various inflammatory mediators such as lysosomal enzymes, cytokines, tissue plasminogen activator, chemokines etc. from neutrophils, macrophages and mastocytes.

Indications—The drugs are used principally as an anti-inflammatory or immunosuppressant agents in cases such as anaphylaxis, arthritis, itchy skin, spinal cord trauma, endotoxemic or septic shock and other severe allergic reactions.

Dosages—

Prednisolone

Cat	For prolonged use, 2-4 mg/kg PO four times a day.
	For immune suppression, 3 mg/kg IM, PO q12h
	For allergy; 1 mg/kg IM, PO q12h.
Dog	For prolonged use, 0.5-2 mg/kg PO four times a day
	For immune suppression, 2 mg/kg IM, PO q12h
	For allergy, 0.5 mg/kg IM, PO q12h.

Prednisolone sodium succinate

Bird	10-20 mg/kg IV, IM every 15 mm to effect
Dog	5.5-11 mg/kg IV, then repeat at 1, 3, 6, or 10 h
NHP	1-15 mg/kg PO total dose.
	10 mg/kg IV.
Reptile	5-10 mg/kg IM, IV as needed.

Route(s) of Administration—Per os, intravenous and intramuscular.

Distribution—The drugs distribute into breast milk.

Metabolism—Prednisone is converted by the liver to prednisolone. Animals with hepatic failure should receive prednisolone instead of prednisone. Systemic prednisolone is preferred for use in cats over prednisone because there is some question if cats are able to convert prednisone to prednisolone. Prednisolone should be used in horses rather than prednisone because horses do not absorb prednisone.

Toxicity and Adverse Effects—Adverse effects due to corticosteroid treatment usually occur with long-term administration of the drug, especially when high doses are used. Chronic or inappropriate use of corticosteroids including prednisolone can cause life threatening hormonal and metabolic changes, specifically iatrogenic Cushing's disease, or Addison's disease. Corticosteroids can cause or worsen gastric ulcers. Short-term side effects, as with all glucocorticoids, include mineralocorticoid effects such as fluid retention, high blood glucose levels, especially in patients who already have diabetes mellitus or are on other medications which increase blood glucose (such as tacrolimus). Long term side effects include Cushing's syndrome, weight gain, osteoporosis, glaucoma, and type II diabetes mellitus.

Contraindications—Herpes simplex virus infection of the eye; infection of the joint or surrounding tissue (joint injection only); systemic infection unless treated with specific anti-infectives; hypersensitivity to prednisolone or other glucocorticoid; pregnancy.

Precautions—Animals receiving systemic corticosteroids may be more susceptible to bacterial or viral infections. Systemic corticosteroids can mask signs of infection such as elevated temperature. Corticosteroids such as prednisolone should not be used in animals with systemic fungal infection. Prednisolone should not be stopped abruptly but tapered down, especially when taken for longer than 3 weeks. Use prednisolone with caution in chronic liver disease, decreased kidney function, decreased liver function, diabetes, epilepsy, glaucoma, heart failure, high blood pressure, hypothyroidism, osteoporosis and peptic ulcer. Administer prednisolone with food or after food.

Drug Interactions—Glucocorticoids may increase blood glucose concentrations. Patients with diabetes mellitus receiving concurrent insulin and/or oral hypoglycemic agents may require adjustments in the dosage of such therapy. Concomitant administration of ulcerogenic drugs such as indomethacin, aspirin etc. during corticosteroid therapy may increase the risk of GI ulceration. Because of its immunodepressant action, prednisolone may cause diminished response to toxoids, live or inactivated vaccines.

Pharmaceutical Formulations—Prednisolone and prednisone are available in tablets and solution for injection.

PRIMIDONE

Primidone

Synonyms—Desoxyphenobarbital; Primaclone.

Proprietary Names—Cyral*; Liskantin*; Midone*; Mylepsin*; Mylepsinum*; Mysoline*; Prysoline*; Resimatil*; Sertan*.

343

Chemical Class—Barbiturate.

Pharmacological Class—Anticonvulsant.

Source—Synthetic; closely related structurally to phenobarbital.

Solubility, Stability and Storage—Primidone is very slightly soluble in water and slightly soluble in alcohol. Primidone tablets should be stored in well-closed containers at room temperature.

Pharmacological Actions—Primidone shares the actions of the barbiturate-derivative anticonvulsants and has sedative properties similar to phenobarbital.

Mechanism of Action—Primidone appears to bind to GABA receptors and decrease the excitability of membranes.

Indications—Treatment of nervous disorders including epilepsy, epileptiform convulsions and hysteria in dogs; prevention of nervous complications in canine distemper.

Dosages—Dosage depends on severity of the disease; starting dose is 15-30 mg/kg daily in divided doses given 12 hours apart; increase gradually every two or three days until the required effect is obtained. The usual daily dose is 50 mg/kg. However, doses of up to 100 mg/kg/day may be required to give adequate control of convulsions in individual cases.

Route(s) of Administration—Per os.

Absorption—Approximately 60–80% of an oral dose of primidone is absorbed from the GIT. Peak serum concentration is attained within 4 hours.

Effective Concentration—5 to 12 mcg/mL. Concentrations of the active metabolites (phenobarbital and PEMA) accumulate during chronic treatment.

Distribution—Primidone is widely distributed in all organs and tissues. It crosses the blood-brain-barrier and placenta. It is distributed into milk.

Plasma Protein Binding—Less than 20%.

Metabolism—Primidone is slowly metabolized by the liver to phenylethylmalonamide (PEMA), phenobarbital and p-hydroxyphenobarbital. Both PEMA and phenobarbital are active metabolites. Although PEMA has weak anticonvulsant action, it potentiates the anticonvulsant activity of phenobarbital and is more toxic than primidone.

Plasma Half-life—10 to 12 hours for primidone; 24 to 48 hours for PEMA; 50 to 150 hours for phenobarbital.

Route(s) of Excretion—Urine with 15 to 25% as unchanged drug.

Dialysis Status—Dialyzable.

Toxicity and Adverse Effects—Occasionally, animal may show slight ataxia or polydipsia at the beginning of treatment, even at low dosage. Higher doses may cause incoordination. These symptoms are usually transitory and generally disappear within a few days even though treatment is continued. Hepatotoxicity has been observed in small proportion of dogs following prolonged medication.

Management of Overdose/Toxicity—Give symptomatic and supportive treatment.

Contraindications—Pregnancy; known hypersensitivity to primidone and its metabolites.

Drug Interactions—Other CNS depressants may potentiate the CNS depressant effect of primidone.

Pharmaceutical Formulations—Primidone is available in 50 mg and 250 mg tablets.

PROCARBAZINE

Procarbazine

Synonyms—Benzmethyzin; N-Methylhydrazine.

Proprietary Names—Matulane®; Natulan®.

Chemical Class—A hydrazine derivative.

Pharmacological Class—Antineoplastic drug; Anticancer drug; Cytotoxic drug.

Source—Synthetic.

Stability and Storage—Protect procarbazine products from light.

Pharmacological Actions—Procarbazine has antineoplastic activity. It also has leukemogenic, teratogenic, mutagenic, carcinogenic, high emetogenic, and myelosuppressive properties. It is cell-cycle nonspecific. Procarbazine does not appear to exhibit cross resistance with other antineoplastic drugs. It causes infertility in male recipients.

Mechanism of Action. Procarbazine is activated to cytotoxic reactants. Following activation, it reacts to release a methylating agent that methylates DNA, producing chromosomal damage. This is responsible for its mutagenic and carcinogenic properties. It also inhibits DNA, RNA and protein synthesis.

Uses—Adjunctive treatment of lymphoreticular tumors.

Route(s) of Administration—Per os.

Absorption—Procarbazine is rapidly and almost completely absorbed from the GIT.

Bioavailability—Oral bioavailability is high.

Distribution—The drug crosses the blood-brain-barrier readily and enters the CSF.

Metabolism—Procarbazine is metabolized in the liver in an elaborate process first to active products. Some metabolism occurs in the kidney. The main final metabolite is N-isopropylterephthalamic acid.

Plasma Half-life—1 hour in humans.

Route(s) of Excretion—The drug is excreted mainly in urine with <5% as unchanged drug and secondarily through the lungs.

Toxicity and Adverse Effects—Bone marrow depression characterized by anemia, leukopenia and thrombocytopenia is most prominent. Other adverse effects are gastrointestinal effects characterized by nausea, vomiting, diarrhea and stomatitis. Central nervous system depression, myalgia, and arthralgia have been reported.

Management of Overdose/Toxicity—Give general antidotal therapy.

Contraindications—Preexisting bone marrow depression; hypersensitivity to procarbazine.

Precautions—Use cautiously in cases with renal impairment. Avoid sympathomimetic drugs during procarbazine therapy. Exclude cheese, liver and other tyramine-rich foods from diet during therapy.

Drug Interactions—Concomitant use of sympathomimetic agents with procarbazine may cause hypertensive reactions. Barbiturates, phenothiazines and other CNS depressants enhance the CNS depressant effects of procarbazine. In humans, procarbazine produces a disulfiram-like reaction following consumption of alcohol. Phenobarbital and other enzyme inducers may enhance the rate of production of active metabolites of procarbazine.

Pharmaceutical Formulations. Procarbazine is available as the hydrochloride salt in 50 mg capsules.

PROGESTERONE

progesterone

Proprietary Names—Progestaject*; Progestasert* (intrauterine device); Protormone*; Piaponin*; Progestin*.

Chemical Class—Steroid.

Pharmacological Class—Progestational hormone.

Source—Semi synthetic.

Pharmacological Actions—Progesterone induces the development of secretory endometrium, suppresses menstruation (in human females) and uterine contractility to create a favourable environment for the implantation of the fertilized ovum and maintenance of pregnancy. It acts with estrogen to cause the development and filling of the acini of the mammary gland. Progesterone causes slight rise in body temperature, tends to delay the onset of parturition in animal species like the rabbit and blocks the release of pituitary gonadotropin.

Mechanism of Action—Progesterone binds to specific receptors distributed in the female reproductive tract and influence the transcription of a limited number of genes in the synthesis of functional proteins which express the drug action in the cells.

Indications—Suppression and synchronization of estrus to enable insemination at a predetermined fixed time without the need for oestrus detection; control of habitual and threatened abortion; induction of estrus with ovulation in ewes.

Dosages—

Cow: 50-100 mg daily or 8 x 100 mg subcutaneous implants. Sheep: 10-50 mg IM or SC daily.

Dog: 25-50 mg daily or 4 x 25 mg implants.

Cat: 2.5-5 mg daily.

Route(s) of Administration—Intramuscular and subcutaneous (in animals).

Absorption—Progesterone is poorly absorbed by oral ingestion unless micronised and in oil, or with fatty foods. It undergoes extensive first-pass metabolism in the liver. It is also rapidly absorbed and quickly metabolized when administered intramuscularly.

Metabolism—Progesterone undergoes conjugation reaction to produce glucuronide and sulfate conjugates of pregnane derivatives.

Route(s) of Excretion—Urine, bile (in ruminants).

Toxicity And Adverse Effects—Progesterone causes pain on injection. It prevents follicular development in large doses. It causes pyometra and endometritis in bitches and queens when administered for a prolonged period to suppress estrus. It may cause fatness in bitches, temporary temperamental changes and CNS depression with overdose.

Contraindications—Nymphomania due to cystic ovaries.

Pharmaceutical Formulations—Progesterone is available in 25-100 mg/ml of vegetable oil for intramuscular injection. It is also available as subcutaneous implants for animal use.

PROMETHAZINE

$$CH_2CH(CH_3)N(CH_3)_2$$

· HCl

Promethazine hydrochloride

Proprietary Names—Phenergan®.

Chemical Class—Phenothiazine derivative.

Pharmacological Class—Antihistamine; Histamine H_1 antagonist; Antiallergic drug.

Source—Synthetic.

Solubility, Stability and Storage—Promethazine is soluble in water and alcohol. It is photosensitive; store products in tight and light-resistant containers at room temperature.

Pharmacological Actions—Promethazine blocks the actions of histamine at the H_1 receptor sites. Hence, the histamine released during allergic conditions is unable to constrict smooth muscle, make exocrine glands secrete, or increase capillary permeability. Promethazine has marked sedative and anti-motion sickness actions.

Mechanism of Action—Promethazine competitively excludes histamine from H_1 receptor sites. It also blocks dopamine and α-adrenergic receptors in the brain; depresses the release of hypothalamic and hypophyseal hormones; reduces stimuli to brainstem reticular system.

Indications—Symptomatic control of allergic conditions involving histamine release; control of emesis and motion sickness. It is also used to induce sedation.

Dosages—

Cattle	1.1 mg/kg IV as tranquilizer; 0.44-1.0 mg/kg IV or IM.
Horse	1.1 mg/kg IV as tranquilizer; 0.44-1.0 mg/kg IV; 0.99-1.98 mg/kg PO.
Dog, Cat	2.2-6.6 mg/kg IV for Preanesthetic medication; 2.2-4.4 mg/kg IM or IV for sedation.
Pig	0.44-1.0 mg/kg IV or IM.

Route(s) of Administration—Per os, intramuscular and intravenous (with caution as it may cause CNS stimulation).

Absorption—Promethazine is readily absorbed in monogastric animals.

Onset of Action—20 to 45 minutes (oral); 3 to 5 minutes (IV).

Duration of Action—2 to 6 hours.

Metabolism—Promethazine undergoes hepatic degradation to mostly inactive products.

Route(s) of Excretion—Urine.

Dialysis Status—Not dialyzable.

Toxicity and Adverse Effects—CNS depression (characterized by somnolence and lethargy) and anticholinergic effects (characterized by dry mouth, urinary retention) are most common. Overdose is characterized by more prominent anticholinergic effects, CNS depression, respiratory depression, and death. Intravenous administration may cause nervous excitement.

Management of Overdose/Toxicity—Undertake general antidotal therapy procedures. Control CNS excitement with phenytoin. Anticholinergic effects may be controlled with physostigmine.

Contraindications—Angle closure glaucoma; hypersensitivity to promethazine or other antihistamines belonging to the phenothiazine group; bladder neck obstruction; pyloroduodenal obstruction; asthma.

Precautions—Do not mix promethazine with barbiturates, diphenhydramine, tetracycline, heparin, hydrocortisone, amphotericin B, cephalothin, phenytoin and promazine in the same syringe.

Drug Interactions—Concurrent use of promethazine with other CNS depressants may produce additive effect.

Pharmaceutical Formulations. Available as promethazine hydrochloride in 12.5 mg, 25 mg and 50 mg tablets; 25 mg/ml and 50 mg/ml solution for injection; 6.25 mg/5 ml and 25 mg/5 ml syrup; 12.5 mg and 50 mg rectal suppository. No specific veterinary formulation is available.

PROPRANOLOL

Proprietary Names—Inderal®; Betachron E-R®; Propranolol intesol®.

Pharmacological Class—Beta-adrenergic receptor antagonist.

Source—Synthetic.

Solubility, Stability and Storage—Propranolol is soluble 1 in 20 of water and ethanol. Store propranolol formulations at room temperature in light resistant containers. Injectable solutions decompose readily at alkaline pH. It is compatible with saline.

Propranolol

Pharmacological Actions—Propranolol is a nonselective antagonist of β-adrenergic receptors. It has no intrinsic sympathomimetic action, as it does not activate adrenergic receptors. Its blocking activity produces bradycardia, pronounced decrease in myocardial contraction and cardiac output when the heart is under sympathetic influence as during exercise and stress. It blocks the tachycardia and increased force of contraction produced by catecholamines on the heart. In addition, propranolol stabilizes membranes. This action affects the cardiac action potential and depresses the myocardium. It decreases sinus heart rate, and depresses AV conduction. Propranolol causes bronchoconstriction particularly during allergic reaction and bronchiolar asthma. It decreases hepatic and renal blood flow.

Mechanism of Action—Propranolol competes for, and blocks beta-adrenergic receptors. It also has a membrane-stabilizing effect.

Indications—Control of cardiac dysrhythmias in animals.

Dosages—

Dog	0.02-0.06 mg/kg by slow IV or 0.2-1.0 mg/kg orally every 8 hours for most cases.
Cat	0.04 mg/kg by slow IV or 2.5-5.0 mg/kg orally every 8-12 hours.
Horse	0.1-0.3 mg/kg by slow IV twice daily.

Route(s) of Administration—Per os and intravenous.

Absorption—Propranolol is well absorbed from oral sites but it undergoes extensive first-pass.

Bioavailability—Oral bioavailability is ~30% in humans and 2-27% in dogs. Availability increases in patients with liver cirrhosis.

Effective Concentration—≥15 ng/ml; resistant ventricular arrhythmia may require up to 1000 ng/ml.

Onset of Action—1 to 2 hours following oral administration in humans.

Duration of Action—6 hours (humans).

Distribution—Vd = 3.3-11 L/kg in dog and 4.3 ± 0.6 in humans. Propranolol is widely distributed. It is highly lipid soluble, crosses the BBB readily and is distributed into milk.

Plasma Protein Binding—87 ± 6% in humans. Binding rate decreases in patients with cirrhosis but increases during pregnancy, obesity and inflammatory conditions in humans.

Metabolism—Metabolized in the liver to active 4-hydroxypropranolol and inactive products.

Plasma Half-Life (hours)—3.9 ± 0.4 in humans, 0.77-2 in dogs and < 2 in horses.

Clearance—16 ± 5 (ml/min/kg) in humans.

Route(s) of Excretion—Urine with 1% as unchanged drug.

Dialysis Status—Nondialyzable.

Toxicity and Adverse Effects—Old animals are more prone to the adverse effects of propranolol. The most common adverse effects at therapeutic doses include bradycardia, lethargy, depression, chronic heart failure, hypotension, hypoglycemia and bronchospasm. Gastrointestinal effects characterized by nausea, vomiting, stomach discomfort and diarrhea have been reported. Overdose may cause pronounced hypotension, bradycardia, and CNS effects ranging from depression to seizure. Hypoglycemia and hyperkalemia may be observed.

Management of Toxicity/Overdose—Give symptomatic treatment. Empty the gut by gastric lavage and administer activated charcoal if the drug was administered orally.

Contraindications—Heart failure; sinus bradycardia; hypersensitivity to propranolol.

Precautions—Use cautiously in cases with renal and/or hepatic impairments, pre-existing heart disease, diabetes mellitus, bronchospastic disease, and in patients receiving digitalis. Propranolol and other nonselective adrenergic beta-blockers may be harmful in certain patient populations. For instance, a sudden blockade of sympathetic input to the cardiac β_1-adrenoceptors in a compensated heart, may precipitate heart failure; inhibition of β_2 receptors in lung airways may lead to bronchoconstriction; inhibition of β_2 receptors in hepatocytes may cause disruption of glucose metabolism while inhibition of those receptors in vascular smooth muscle may cause changes in blood pressure and distribution of cardiac output.

Drug Interactions—Aluminium salts, barbiturates, calcium salts, cholestyramine, colestipol, NSAIDs, penicillins, rifampicin, phenytoin and sulfinpyrazone decrease the bioavailability of propranolol and thus reduce its effects. Cimetidine and possibly ranitidine may decrease the metabolism of propranolol. Propranolol may decrease the effects of sulfonylureas while it enhances the actions of muscle relaxants such as tubocurarine and succinylcholine. Actions of β-adrenergic agonists are blocked by propranolol. Calcium channel blockers such as diltiazem, nifedipine, and felodipine increase the effects of propranolol. The hypoglycemic effects of insulin may be prolonged by propranolol.

Pharmaceutical Formulations—Available as propranolol hydrochloride in 10-, 20-, 40-, 60—and 80—mg tablets; 60-, 80-, 120—and 160 mg extended sustained-release capsules; 1 mg/ml solution for injection; 4 mg/ml, 8 mg/ml and 80 mg/ml oral solutions. No specific veterinary formulation is available.

PROTAMINE

Chemical Class—Cationic protein; it is composed of arginine, proline, serine, and valine).

Pharmacological Class—Anticoagulant; heparin antagonist.

Source—Occur naturally in the sperm of salmon and certain other species of fish. Commercially available protamine sulfate is prepared from the sperm or mature testes of salmon or related species.

Solubility, Stability and Storage—Protamine sulfate is sparingly soluble in water and very slightly soluble in alcohol. It may be physically and/or chemically incompatible with some anti-infective agents, including some cephalosporins and penicillins. Protamine sulfate injection should be stored at 15-30°C; avoid freezing.

Pharmacological Actions—Protamine has weak anticoagulant action when administered alone.

Mechanism of Action—Protamine sulfate is strongly basic. It acts by forming a complex with the strongly acidic heparin which results in a stable salt devoid of anticoagulant activity. The weak anticoagulant effect may be due to inhibition of thromboplastin production and thromboplastin activity, which prevents the conversion of prothrombin to thrombin.

Indications—Treatment of heparin overdose in all species; treatment of Bracken Fern poisoning in ruminants—

Dosages—Dosage is regulated by the dose of heparin administered, its route of administration, the time elapsed since heparin was given, and by blood coagulation studies. Generally, 1 mg of protamine sulfate will neutralize no less than 100 units of heparin sodium. As a guide, the following doses may be applied. Dogs & cats, 1mg/100 IU of heparin given. Reduce the dose as the time between heparin administration and protamine treatment increases.

Route(s) of Administration—Intravenous (slow or constant infusion).

Toxicity and Adverse Effects—Acute hypotension, bradycardia, pulmonary hypertension and dyspnoea can occur if the drug is administered rapidly by intravenous injection. A "heparin rebound" effect associated with anticoagulation and bleeding has also been reported. Hypersensitivity reactions including urticaria, angioedema, acute pulmonary hypertension, anaphylaxis, and anaphylactoid reactions have occurred in humans.

Management of Overdose/Toxicity—Give symptomatic and supportive treatment.

Contraindications—Known hypersensitivity to protamine.

Precautions—Administer by slow IV. The risk of a hypersensitivity reaction to protamine sulfate should be considered in patients that have received protamine-containing insulin.

Pharmaceutical Formulations—Protamine is presented as protamine sulphate injection containing 10 mg/ml in 5 and 25 ml ampules as well as 5 and 25 ml vials.

PYRANTEL

Pyrantel

Proprietary Names—Combantrin˚ (pyrantel pamoate); Quantrel˚ (50mg oxantel pamoate plus 50mg plus pyrantel pamoate); Banminth˚ (pyrantel tartrate).

Chemical Class—Tetrahydropyrimidine derivative.

Pharmacological Class—Anthelmintic.

Source—Synthetic.

Solubility, Stability and Storage—Pyrantel is practically insoluble in water and ethanol. Pyrantel formulations are better stored in tight, light-resistant containers at room temperature of < 30°C.

Pharmacological Actions—Pyrantel causes paralysis followed subsequently by expulsion of mature and immature forms of many gastrointestinal nematodes such as *Parascaris, Strongylus* and *Probstmayria* species in horses; *Ascaris* and *Oesophagostomum* in pigs; *Haemonchus, Ostertagia, Trichostrongylus, Nematodirus* and *Cooperia* species in cattle, sheep and goats; *Ancylostoma* and *Ascaris* species in dogs.

Mechanism of Action—Pyrantel inhibits acetyl cholinesterase thereby causing accumulation of acetylcholine. It also induces marked nicotinic activation at the neuromuscular junction as a depolarizing neuromuscular blocking agent. These two actions produce spastic paralysis of the worm. The paralyzed worms are expelled from the GI tract by normal peristalsis.

Indications—Treatment of roundworm infections in cattle, sheep, goat, pig, horses and dogs.

Dosages—

Horse	12.5mg/kg.
Pig	22mg/kg.
Cattle, sheep and goat	25 mg/kg.
Bird	4.5 mg/kg once; repeat in 10-14 days.

Route(s) of Administration—Per os.

Absorption—Pyrantel is well absorbed in monogastric animals but poorly absorbed in ruminants. Peak plasma concentration is achieved in monogastric animals within 2-3 hours.

Residue Limit—1.0 ppm (calculated as pyrantel tartrate) in pig muscle.

Withdrawal Period—Zero days (horses).

Route(s) of Excretion—Feces is the major route in animals except dog. Urine is the major route of pyrantel excretion in dogs.

Toxicity and Adverse Effects—Pyrantel is a very safe anthelmintic with therapeutic ratio greater than 1.20 in horses. LD50 in rat is 170mg/kg. Excessive overdose may cause increased respiration, profuse sweating and incoordination.

Contraindications—Severe debilitated animals; known hypersensitivity to pyrantel.

Drug Interactions—Piperazine and pyrantel pamoate have antagonistic modes of action, hence both drugs should not be administered concomitantly.

Pharmaceutical Formulations—Pyrantel is presented as pyrantel tartrate in tablets and powder (for drenching). The drug is also available as pyrantel pamoate which is commonly used in humans.

PYRIDOSTIGMINE

Pyridostigmine

Proprietary Names—Mestinon˚; Regunol˚.

Chemical Class—Quaternary ammonium compound.

Pharmacological Class—Reversible cholinesterase inhibitor; Indirect-acting cholinomimetic drug.

Source—Synthetic.

Solubility, Stability and Storage—Pyridostigmine is freely soluble in water and in alcohol. Pyridostigmine formulations are better stored at room temperature protected from light and moisture. Injection solution is unstable in alkaline media.

Pharmacological Actions—Pyridostigmine initiates and increases GI motility. It also stimulates other smooth muscles such as those of respiration and bladder. At low doses, pyridostigmine and other anticholinesterase agents augment the nervous stimulation of secretory glands including bronchial, lacrimal, sweat, salivary, gastric and intestinal glands. Higher doses produce increased secretion of these glands. Pyridostigmine may cause twitching of skeletal muscle at high doses as a result of direct nicotinic receptor activation. It causes persistent depolarization of the motor end plate if acetylcholinesterase is sufficiently inhibited resulting in neuromuscular blockade. The CNS is stimulated at low doses but depressed at high doses of pyridostigmine and other anticholinesterases. Anticholinesterase agents cause miosis, blockade of accommodation reflex and conjunctiva hyperemia if applied directly to the conjunctiva. They also reduce intraocular pressure.

Mechanism of Action. Pyridostigmine inhibits acetylcholinesterase which normally hydrolyzes acetylcholine within 200 microseconds of release. Pyridostigmine inhibition increases the residence time of acetylcholine at the synapses allowing for prolongation and exaggeration of its effect. Pyridostigmine may also directly stimulate nicotinic receptors of the motor end plate.

Indications—Treatment of myasthenia gravis; reversal of muscle relaxation caused by curare and other non-depolarizing neuromuscular blockers; treatment of curare overdose.

Dosages. 0.2-2 mg/kg orally two to three times daily.

Route(s) of Administration. Per os, intramuscular and intravenous.

Absorption—10 to 20% of dose is absorbed from the GIT.

Bioavailability—14 ± 3%.

Onset of Action—Within 15-30 min (oral); 2-5 min (IV).

Duration of Action—1 to 2 hours (IV); 2 to 4 hours (IM).

Distribution—Vd = 1.1 ± 0.3 (humans). Pyridostigmine crosses membranes poorly because of its quaternary ammonium constituent. It is excluded from the brain but it crosses the placenta.

Plasma Protein Binding—15 to 25%.

Metabolism—Pyridostigmine is partially metabolized in the liver. It is also hydrolyzed by cholinesterase.

Plasma Half-life—1.9 ± 0.2 hours in humans; t½ is prolonged in patients with renal impairment.

Clearance—8.5 ± 1.7 ml/min/kg in humans.

Route(s) of Excretion—Mainly urine with 80-90% as unchanged drug.

Dialysis Status—Nondialyzable

Toxicity and Adverse Effects—Severe muscle weakness, nausea, vomiting, diarrhea, miosis, and dyspnea are most common adverse effects caused by pyridostigmine and its congeners. They produce hypotension and bradycardia at high doses. Overdose produces signs characteristic of excessive cholinergic stimulation (cholinergic crisis). The signs include excessive salivation, sweating, miosis, lacrimation, bronchial secretion, bronchospasm, hypotension and muscle weakness. Death may result from paralysis of respiratory muscles compounded with excessive bronchial secretion.

Management of Overdose/Toxicity—Atropine is an antidote for pyridostigmine.

Contraindications—Known hypersensitivity to pyridostigmine; intestinal or urinary tract obstruction; late pregnancy; concurrent treatment with other anticholinesterase.

Precautions—Use pyridostigmine with caution in asthma, hyperthyroidism, seizure disorders, and cardiac arrhythmias.

Drug Interactions—Pyridostigmine reverses the actions of competitive neuromuscular blockers and augments those of depolarizing neuromuscular blockers. Atropine obliterates the muscarinic effects of pyridostigmine because pyridostigmine effects are attributed to the unhydrolyzed acetylcholine. The effect of pyridostigmine may be reduced by drugs that have neuromuscular blocking actions (e.g. aminoglycoside antibiotics and anesthetics).

Pharmaceutical Formulations. Pyridostigmine is presented as pyridostigmine bromide in 60 mg oral tablets; 180 mg sustained release tablet; 12 mg/ml oral syrup; and 5 mg/ml solution for injection.

PYRIMETHAMINE

Pyrimethamine

Proprietary Names—Daraprim®.

Chemical Class—Aminopyrimidine compound.

Pharmacological Class—A folic acid antagonist; Antiprotozoal drug.

Source—Synthetic.

Solubility, Stability and Storage—Pyrimethamine is practically insoluble in water and slightly soluble in alcohol. Pyrimethamine products are photosensitive; tablets should be stored in tight, light-resistant containers. Pyrimethamine is unstable in solutions containing sugars such as syrup.

Pharmacological Actions—Pyrimethamine possesses antimicrobial activity against protozoan organisms. It is similar to trimethoprim.

Mechanism of Action—It acts by inhibiting the enzyme, dihydrofolate reductase that catalyzes the conversion of dihydrofolic acid to tetrahydrofolic acid.

Indications—Treatment of toxoplasmosis in small animals (often in combination with sulfonamides); treatment of equine protozoan myeloencephalitis (equine toxoplasmosis).

Dosages—1 mg/kg once daily.

Route(s) of Administration—Per os.

Absorption—Pyrimethamine is well absorbed from the GIT.

Bioavailability—Oral bioavailability is 100%.

Distribution. Vd = 2.3 ± 0.6 L/kg in humans. Pyrimethamine is distributed primarily to the kidneys, liver, spleen, and lungs. It is excluded from the CNS but attains higher concentrations in milk than in serum. It is also slowly eliminated from milk.

Plasma Protein Binding—87 ± 1% in humans.

Metabolism—Metabolism is slow and extensive but the site(s) and mechanism(s) are uncertain.

Plasma Half-life—3 to 5 days in humans.

Clearance—0.41 ± 0.06 (ml/min/kg).

Route(s) of Excretion—Urine.

Toxicity and Adverse Effects—Anorexia, malaise, vomiting, depression and bone marrow depression characterized by anemia, thrombocytopenia and leucopenia have been reported in small animals (especially cats) and horses. Pyrimethamine is teratogenic in laboratory animals at high doses. Hematologic effects can develop rapidly hence, frequent monitoring is recommended, particularly if therapy persists longer than 2 weeks. Pyrimethamine is unpalatable to cats.

Management of Overdose/Toxicity—Oral administration of folinic acid (1 mg/kg), 5 mg/day of folic acid or Brewer's yeast at 100 mg/kg/day may alleviate adverse effects of pyrimethamine.

Contraindications—Known hypersensitivity to pyrimethamine; pre-existing hematologic disorders.

Precautions—Use pyrimethamine cautiously in pregnant animals. It may be beneficial to administer folinic acid as Ca folinate (Ca Leucovorin) concurrently with pyrimethamine if the latter is used during pregnancy.

Drug Interactions—The effect of pyrimethamine is decreased by acid. Pyrimethamine is synergistic with sulfonamides, methotrexate. p-aminobenzoic acid (PABA) is antagonistic to its actions.

Pharmaceutical Formulations—Available in 25 mg tablets. Pyrimethamine tablets may be crushed to make oral suspensions of the drug.

RAFOXANIDE

Rafoxanide

Proprietary Names—Ranide*, Ranizole* (a fixed dose combination of 14.67% thiabendazole and 2.5% rafoxanide); Flukanide*; Flukex*; Ridafluke*.

Chemical Class—Salicylamide compound.

Pharmacological Class—Anthelmintic; Trematocide.

Source—Synthetic.

Solubility, Stability and Storage—Rafoxanide is practically insoluble in water; soluble 1 in 25 of acetone, 1 in 40 of chloroform, 1 in 35 of ethyl acetate, and 1 in 200 of methanol.

Pharmacological Actions—Rafoxanide is active against almost all mature and most immature (6 weeks old) *Fasciola hepatica* and *Fasciola gigantica*. Adult *Haemonchus* species in cattle and sheep, and the parasitic larval stages of sheep nasal bot are susceptible.

Mechanism of Action—Unknown.

Indications—Treatment of fascioliasis and haemonchosis in cattle, sheep, and goats.

Dosages—7.5 mg/kg.

Route(s) of Administration—Per os.

Absorption—Rafoxanide is well absorbed after oral administration. Peak plasma concentration is attained within 24-48 hours.

Plasma Half-Life—5 to 10 days in sheep.

Withdrawal Period to 28 days before slaughter.

Toxicity And Adverse Effects—Relatively nontoxic; rafoxanide has therapeutic index of ~ 5. Doses above 45 mg/kg may cause cataract and optic nerve degeneration in sheep. A dose of 125 mg/kg may cause blindness in cattle.

Contraindications—Lactating animals.

Drug Interactions—Rafoxanide can be combined with thiabendazole (in economies where this drug is still available) for the simultaneous treatment of liver flukes and GI nematodes.

Pharmaceutical Formulations—Available as 2.5% suspension and as bolus.

ROBENIDINE

Robenidine

Proprietary Names—Cycostat®; Robenz®.

Chemical Class—Guanidine derivative.

Pharmacological Class—Anticoccidial agent.

Source—Synthetic.

Solubility, Stability and Storage—Robenidine is stable for up to 12 weeks in processed feed if stored in cool, dry condition (below 25°C).

Pharmacological Actions—Robenidine has broad-spectrum activity against *Eimeria* species of birds. It is active only against intestinal *Eimeria* spp of rabbits. Robenidine is most effective against late developing stages of first and second-generation schizonts. It exhibits some activity against gamonts (sexual stages). Its action is first coccidiostatic and then coccidiocidal.

Mechanism of Action—Robenidine interferes with energy metabolism by inhibition of respiratory chain phosphorylation and ATPase activity in mitochondria.

1. **Indications**—Prevention of coccidiosis in broiler chickens, turkeys and rabbits reared for meat. Robenidine is effective against ionophore-resistant coccidia.

Dosages—30-36 ppm in birds; 50-66 ppm in rabbits.

Route(s) of Administration—Per os (via feed).

Residue Limit—Maximum residue limit for robenidine hydrochloride in chickens are established at 0.2 ppm in skin and fat and 0.1 ppm in edible tissue other than skin and fat.

Withdrawal Period—5 days.

Contraindications—Layer birds; hypersensitivity to robenidine.

Precautions—Robenidine produces unpleasant flavor in edible tissues or eggs of treated animals if the mandatory 5 days withdrawal period is not observed or if the drug is used at higher doses.

Pharmaceutical Formulations—Robenidine is presented as robenidine hydrochloride in 6.6% premix for addition to feed.

SCOPOLAMINE

Scopolamine

Synonyms—l-Hyoscine.

Proprietary Names—Buscopan˚; Isopto˚ Hyoscine.

Chemical Class—Belladonna alkaloid.

Pharmacological Class—Parasympatholytic, Antimuscarinic, Anticholinergic, Mydriatic, Spasmolytic or Antispasmodic drug.

Source—Natural; it is usually obtained by extraction from various members of the *Solanaceae* genus of plants including *Datura metel* (datura herb), *D. stramonium* (Jimson weed), *Duboisia myoporoides*, Hyoscyamus niger (henbane), and *Scopolia carniolica*.

Solubility, Stability and Storage—Scopolamine is slightly soluble in water and very soluble in alcohol. It is unstable in acid medium. Hydrolysis occurs at pH < 3. Scopolamine hydrobromide formulations should be stored in tight, light-resistant containers at room temperature.

Pharmacological Actions—The peripheral actions of scopolamine are similar to those of atropine. Although scopolamine causes CNS depression characterized by drowsiness, amnesia, and fatigue at therapeutic doses, unlike atropine. The CNS depressant effects may be reversed occasional in the presence of severe pain. Scopolamine also causes euphoria. It has prominent action on the gastrointestinal and other smooth muscles.

Mechanism of Action. Scopolamine competitively inhibits the actions of acetylcholine and other cholinomimetic agents at muscarinic receptor sites. Thus, normal organ responses to parasympathetic stimulation or exogenous acetylcholine and muscarinic agonists are attenuated.

Indications—Treatment of intestinal spasm and hypermotility; adjunct in general anesthesia to reduce salivary and bronchial secretions; control of motion sickness. It is also used to treat gastroduodenal ulcer, toxicosis resulting from anticholinesterase and cholinomimetic agents as well as facilitate ophthalmic examination. Scopolamine is used in conjunction with a cholinesterase reactivator (e.g. pralidoxime) in the treatment of organophosphate poisoning.

Dosages—0.01 mg/kg.

Route(s) of Administration—Subcutaneous and intramuscular.

Absorption—Scopolamine is readily absorbed from subcutaneous and intramuscular routes of administration.

Bioavailability—Oral bioavailability is 27 ± 12 in humans.

Effective Concentration—40 pg/ml.

Onset of Action—30 to 60 minutes (IM, Per os); 10 minutes (IV).

Peak Action—20 to 60 minutes.

Duration of Action—4 to 6 hours (IM, Per os); 1 to 2 hours (IV). Full recovery may take from 3-7 days.

Distribution—Vd = 1.4 ± 0.7 L/kg (humans). Scopolamine crosses the blood-brain-barrier more readily than atropine.

Plasma Protein Binding—The drug is reversibly bound to plasma protein.

Metabolism—Degraded in the liver.

Plasma Half-life—2.9 ± 1.2 (humans).

Clearance—16 ± 13 (ml/min/kg) in humans.

Route(s) of Excretion—Urine with 6 ± 4% of dose eliminated as unchanged drug.

Dialysis Status—Dialyzable.

Toxicity and Adverse Effects—Scopolamine causes dilated and fixed pupil, dry mouth, dry skin, and transient bradycardia followed by tachycardia with palpitations and arrhythmias. It also causes reduction in tone and motility of the gastrointestinal smooth muscle resulting in constipation. Scopolamine causes CNS depression at therapeutic doses. Irritation at site of injection has been reported. Scopolamine poisoning is characterized by dry mouth, mydriasis, tachycardia, hyperpnoea, restlessness, hyperpyrexia, and respiratory failure.

Management of Overdose/Toxicity—Give general antidotal therapy. Anticholinesterase agents (e.g. physostigmine) are antidotes.

Contraindications—Acute angle glaucoma; tachycardia; obstruction of the GIT and/or urinary tract; cardiac ischemia; acute hemorrhage; paralytic ileus; myasthenia gravis; known hypersensitivity to atropine.

Drug Interactions—Procainamide, amantadine, quinidine, butyrophenones, phenothiazines, pethidine, benzodiazepines, and antihistamines may enhance the effect of scopolamine since they possess some anticholinergic actions. Primidone, disopyramide, prolonged use of corticosteroids may enhance the toxic potential of scopolamine. Scopolamine may enhance the actions of nitrofurantoin, thiazide diuretics and sympathomimetic agents. Large doses of muscarinic receptor agonists or agents that prevent the hydrolysis of acetylcholine (e.g. anticholinesterases) can reverse the actions of scopolamine and other antimuscarinic drugs.

Pharmaceutical Formulations—Scopolamine is available as scopolamine hydrobromide in 0.3 mg/ml, 0.4 mg/ml, 0.86 mg/ml and 1 mg/ml solutions for injection; 0.25 % ophthalmic solution; and transdermal patches of 1.5 mg/disc. It is also available as scopolamine-N-butylbromide (Buscopan°) in 10 mg sugar coated tablets, 5 mg/5 ml oral liquid, and 20 mg/ml solution for injection. No specific veterinary formulations are available.

SERUM GONADOTROPIN

Synonyms—Pregnant Mare Serum.

Proprietary Names—Antostab®; FSH®; Gonadyl®; Fostim®; Serogan®; Apocrine®; Folligon®; PG 600°.

Chemical Class—Glycoprotein.

Pharmacological Class—Gonadotropin.

Source—Natural; obtained from the serum of pregnant female horse.

Solubility, stability and Storage—Store in a refrigerator; protect from light.

Pharmacological Actions—PMS possesses follicle stimulating hormone-like action with some luteinizing hormone activity. Thus, it stimulates follicular development in the female and spermatozoa production in the male.

Mechanism of Action—It binds to specific receptors in gonadal tissues. The receptors are coupled to adenylyl cyclase by means of a guanine nucleotide-binding regulatory protein (GS). Activity results in elevation of cAMP levels, which ultimately mediates the action of the hormone.

Indications—Promotion of a fertile oestrus cycle in gilts and in sows post-weaning; treatment of suboestrus or anoestrus due to hormonal imbalance in females; treatment of impaired spermatogenesis in males. PMS is also indicated for the inducement of twining and triplets in small ruminants and also to induce estrus in these species.

Dosages—1000-2000 IU (cattle); 500-1000 IU (sheep and goats); 50-200 IU (dogs) and 100 IU (cats).

Route(s) of Administration—Parenteral.

Plasma Half-Life—26 hours.

Toxicity and Adverse Effects—PMS is antigenic; thus, it can stimulate immunologic response with repeated use. It can cause superfetation because of release of multiple ova.

Management of Overdose/Toxicity—Administer adrenaline 1:1000 solution if anaphylactic reaction occurs.

Contraindications—Known hypersensitivity to PMS.

Precautions—Do not breed monotocous animals at the induced estrus. Wait till the subsequent estrus to avoid superfetation. Do not inject PMS into subcutaneous fat.

Pharmaceutical Formulations—Available in sealed ampoules as powder to be dissolved in water. Each milligram should contain not less than 400 units of follicle stimulating activity. PG 600° is available as a freeze dried white crystalline plug for reconstitution with the solvent provided.

Each 5 ml single dose glass vial contains 400 IU Serum Gonadotrophin and 200 IU chorionic gonadotrophin.

SEVOFLURANE

Servoflurane

Proprietary Names—SevoFlo˚.

Chemical Class—Halogenated compound.

Pharmacological Class—Inhalational anesthetics agent.

Source—Synthetic.

Solubility, Stability and Storage—Do not store above 25°C; do not refrigerate; keep the container tightly closed.

Pharmacological Actions—Sevoflurane produces unconsciousness and modest increases in cerebral blood flow and metabolic rate. It may increase intracranial pressure at concentrations of 2.0 MAC and above under normal partial pressures of carbon dioxide (normocapnia). At low MAC, sevoflurane tend to increase heart rate which returns to normal with increasing MAC. It causes systemic vasodilation and produces dose-dependent decreases in mean arterial pressure, total peripheral resistance, and cardiac output. Sevoflurane depresses respiration and increases total liver blood flow. Renal blood flow falls in a linear fashion with increasing hypotension in sevoflurane anaesthetized dogs. Sevoflurane induces muscle relaxation and reduces pains sensitivity by altering tissue excitability.

Mechanism of Action—Sevoflurane induces a reduction in junctional conductance by decreasing gap junction channel opening times and increasing gap junction channel closing times. It also bind to several receptors including GABA, glutamate and glycine receptors as well as the large conductance Ca^{2+} activated potassium channel.

Indications—Induction and maintenance of general anaesthesia in dogs.

Dosages—The administration of sevoflurane must be individualized based on the dog's response. An inspired concentration of 5 to 7% sevoflurane with oxygen is recommended for mask induction.

Route(s) of Administration—Administered via a vaporizer specifically calibrated for use with sevoflurane.

Absorption—The drug is rapidly absorbed into circulation via the lungs, however, solubility in the blood is low.

Onset of Action—Anaesthetic induction is rapid.

Metabolism—1 to 5% is metabolized to hexafluoroisopropanol (HFIP) with release of inorganic fluoride and CO_2. HFIP is rapidly conjugated with glucuronic acid.

Plasma Half-life—Biphasic, with an initial rapid phase and a second, slower phase. The half-life for the slow elimination phase is approximately 50 minutes.

Route(s) of Excretion—Sevoflurane is eliminated via the lungs; its metabolites are excreted in urine.

Toxicity and Adverse Effects—Hypotension followed by tachypnoea, muscle tenseness, excitation, apnoea, muscle fasciculations and emesis are common. Sevoflurane causes dose-dependent respiratory depression. Infrequent adverse reactions include paddling, retching, salivation, cyanosis, premature ventricular contractions and excessive cardiopulmonary depression. Sevoflurane may trigger episodes of malignant hyperthermia in susceptible dogs. Like other halogenated anaesthetic agents, sevoflurane may induce liver damage. This response has been observed rarely after repeated exposure.

Management of Overdose/Toxicity—Discontinue the drug if severe cardiopulmonary depression or malignant hyperthermia develops. Appropriate supportive and symptomatic treatment should be immediately instituted. Patent airway should be ensured, and ventilation assisted or controlled with pure oxygen. Cardiovascular depression should be treated with plasma expanders, pressor agents, antiarrhythmic agents or other appropriate techniques. Bradycardia can be reversed by the administration of anticholinergic drug.

Contraindications—Known sensitivity to sevoflurane or other halogenated anaesthetic agents; pregnancy; lactating bitches; known or suspected genetic susceptibility to malignant hyperthermia; animals less than 12 weeks of age.

Precautions—Arterial blood pressure should be monitored at frequent intervals during sevoflurane anaesthesia. Facilities for artificial ventilation, oxygen enrichment and circulatory resuscitation should be on standby. Avoid prolonged episodes of hypotension in order to maintain renal blood flow. Reduce the maintenance dose by 2.8% to 3.1% in premedicated geriatric dogs and 3.2 to 3.3% in unpremeditated geriatric dogs).

Drug Interactions—Sevoflurane administration is compatible with the intravenous barbiturates, propofol, benzodiazepines and opioids However, the concurrent administration of thiopental may slightly increase sensitivity to adrenaline-induced cardiac arrhythmias. Similarly, the MAC of sevoflurane is reduced by the concurrent administration of benzodiazepines and opioids. Sevoflurane is also compatible with anticholinergic premedicants such as atropine and glycopyrrolate. Hypotensive episodes during sevoflurane anaesthesia may enhance the nephrotoxic potential of certain NSAIDs when used in the perioperative period. Sevoflurane increases both the intensity and duration of neuromuscular blockade induced by non depolarising muscle relaxants. This effect which has been observed in humans has not been fully documented in dogs. Concurrent use of sevoflurane and α_2-adrenergic receptor agonists may cause bradycardia. Also, alpha$_2$—adrenergic agonists have an anaesthetic sparing effect; hence the dose of sevoflurane should be reduced accordingly.

Pharmaceutical Formulations—Sevoflurane is available as volatile liquid.

SILVER SULFADIAZINE

Proprietary Names—Sivadene*; Thermazine*; Flamazine*.

Chemical Class—Sulfonamide.

Pharmacological Class—Antibacterial agent.

Source—Synthetic.

Solubility, Stability and Storage—Store at 8 to 25°C. Discard cream which has darkened. Keep this medication in the container it came in, tightly closed and out of the reach of children or pets. Store at room temperature away from excess heat and moisture.

Pharmacological Actions—The combination has activity against pathogenic bacteria and fungi. It releases silver slowly in concentrations toxic to microorganisms. The sulfadiazine component is also bacteriostatic for most Gram-positive and Gram-negative bacteria and some other microorganism. Silver sulfadiazine minimizes the rapid depletion of chloride and associated electrolyte from burns.

Mechanism of Action—Sulfadiazine interferes with the biosynthesis of folic acid in susceptible organisms by competing with para-aminobenzoic acid (PABA) for incorporation into dihydrofolic acid. By replacing the PABA molecule in dihydrofolic acid, sulfadiazine prevents formation of folic acid required for nucleic acid synthesis and multiplication of the cell.

Indications—Prevention and treatment of infections of second and third degree burns. Silver sulfadiazine is especially indicated in the treatment and prophylaxis of infection in serious burn victims. It is also used for the treatment of leg ulcers, burns, skin grafts, incisions, and other clean lesions, abrasions, minor cuts, and wounds.

Dosages—Silver sulfadiazine is usually applied once or twice a day.

Route(s) of Administration—Topical.

Absorption—In burned pigs, the absorption of silver was less than 1% of the applied dose while 5 to 8% of the sulfadiazine was absorbed. When treatment with silver sulfadiazine involves prolonged administration and/or large burned surfaces, considerable amounts of silver sulfadiazine are absorbed. In such cases, the mean silver serum levels are moderately higher than the normal range.

Bioavailability—Serum concentration of silver sulfadiazine may approach 8 to 12 mg % if treatment is prolonged and/or extensive.

Effective Concentration—Sulfadiazine concentration in burn wound exudate is about 20 times the MIC for sensitive bacteria (50 mg/L).

Distribution—There is very little penetration of the silver below the outer layers of the wound surface, and the largest amount of the absorbed silver is found in the liver. High concentrations of silver have been measured in the bile.

Route(s) of Excretion—The high concentrations of silver measured in the bile suggest a hepatobiliary excretion of the silver moiety. However urinary excretion of silver is markedly elevated. The sulfadiazine moiety is excreted via the kidneys.

Toxicity and Adverse Effects—Although side effects from this product are not common, they can occur. Potential symptoms include pain, burning and itching. A self-limiting leukopenia has been reported following the use of silver sulfadiazine, especially in human patients with large area burns. This often occurs 2 to 3 days after treatment has commenced. Therapy with silver sulfadiazine does not normally need to be discontinued since the WBC count usually returns to the normal range in a few days.

Contraindications—Known hypersensitivity to silver sulfadiazine or other sulfa drugs.

Precautions—Silver sulfadiazine should be used with caution in patients with significant hepatic or renal impairment. Use with caution in pregnant or lactating females.

Drug Interactions—Silver sulfadiazine may inactivate enzymatic debriding agents, thus the concomitant use of these compounds may be inappropriate. In patients with large area burns where serum sulfadiazine levels may approach therapeutic levels, the action of oral hypoglycemic agents and phenytoin may be potentiated. Coadministration of cimetidine may increase the incidence of leucopenia in cases with extensive burn. Silver sulfadiazine action is not inhibited by PABA.

Pharmaceutical Formulations—Silver sulfadiazine is available as cream in sterile jars of 500 g and sterile tubes of 50 g and 20 g. Each gram of cream contains silver sulfadiazine 1% w/w. The nonmedicinal ingredients contained in the cream include alcohol, distilled water, glycerol monostearate, liquid paraffin, polysorbate 60, polysorbate 80 and propylene glycol.

SODIUM AUROTHIOMALATE

Synonyms—Gold sodium thiomalate.

Proprietary Names—Myocrisin®; Myochrysine®.

Chemical Class—Metallic gold preparation.

Pharmacological Class—Disease-modifying antiarthritic drug.

Source—Synthetic.

Solubility, Stability and Storage—The drug is very soluble in water and insoluble in alcohol. Gold sodium thiomalate injection should be protected from light and stored at 15-30°C; freezing should be avoided. Gold sodium thiomalate injection should not be used if the color is darker than pale yellow.

Pharmacological Actions—Gold sodium thiomalate exhibit anti-inflammatory, antiarthritic, and immunomodulating effects. It suppresses or prevents the degenerative lesions associated with arthritis. It has minimal anti-inflammatory action in other circumstances.

Mechanism of Action—It is not certain. Its action may be due to its ability to inhibit the maturation and function of mononuclear phagocytes, inhibition of lysosomal enzyme release, decreased level of rheumatoid factors and immunoglobulins, and suppression of cellular immunity.

Indications—Treatment of rheumatoid arthritis.

Dosages—1 mg/kg weekly (dogs and cats).

Route(s) of Administration—Intramuscular.

Absorption—Gold sodium thiomalate is rapidly absorbed. Peak plasma concentration is attained within 2-6 hours from aqueous suspensions.

Onset of Action—The beneficial effects of gold preparations may occur only after several weeks or months of therapy and may persist long after chrysotherapy has been discontinued.

Distribution—Vd = 0.26 ± 0.05. Gold sodium thiomalate binds avidly to tissues and is concentrated in the reticuloendothelial cells of the lymph nodes, bone marrow, kidneys, liver, and spleen. It is also widely distributed throughout body tissues.

Plasma Protein Binding—95%.

Metabolism—Its metabolic fate is unclear; the drug may not be reduced to elemental form of gold.

Plasma Half-Life—25±5 days (increases with continued administration).

Plasma Clearance—7.0 ± 0.6 (ml/min/kg).

Route(s) of Excretion—Urine and feces; 70% appear in urine as unchanged drug.

Dialysis Status—Partly dialyzable.

Toxicity and Adverse Effects—The most frequent adverse effects of parenteral gold therapy involve skin and mucous membranes. Cutaneous reactions varying from simple erythema to exfoliative dermatitis and inflammation of the mucous membranes such as stomatitis, pharyngitis, vaginitis, tracheitis, gastritis, colitis and glossitis have been reported. Also, gray-to-blue pigmentation (chrysiasia) on skin and mucous membrane, renal damage, and blood dyscrasia have been observed.

Management of Overdose/Toxicity—Withdraw the drug and give symptomatic and supportive treatment.

Contraindications—Known hypersensitivity to gold sodium thiomalate.

Precautions—The drug should be used by experienced veterinarians.

Drug Interactions—Heavy metal antagonists containing sulfhydryl groups such as dimercaprol and penicillamine chelate gold and increase the excretion of gold from parenteral gold compounds.

Pharmaceutical Formulations—Gold sodium thiomalate is available in 1-, 5-, 10-, 20-, and 50—mg sterile aqueous solution for injection.

SODIUM BICARBONATE

Synonyms—Baking soda; Sodium hydrogen carbonate; Sodium acid carbonate.

Pharmacological Class—Alkalinizing agent.

Source—Synthetic.

Solubility, Stability and Storage—Sodium bicarbonate is soluble in water and insoluble in alcohol. Its formulations should be stored at room temperature. The tablets should be in tight containers; avoid freezing the solution for injection.

Pharmacological Actions—Sodium bicarbonate dissociates to provide bicarbonate ion. Bicarbonate is the conjugate base component of the principal extracellular buffer (the bicarbonate:carbonic acid buffer) in the body. Sodium bicarbonate is a potent antacid; each gram of the compound has an in vitro neutralizing capacity of about 12 mEq of acid.

Indications—Treatment of metabolic acidosis of various etiology; alkalinization of urine as in the treatment of certain intoxications (e.g., phenobarbital, salicylates) to decrease renal reabsorption of the drugs; adjunct in the treatment of hypercalcemic or hyperkalemia crises.

Dosages—Dosage is determined by severity of the acidosis, appropriate laboratory determinations and clinical condition. Estimate bicarbonate requirement using the formula:

Bicarbonate deficit (HCO3 mEq) = base deficit (mEq/L) x 0.5 x body weight (kg).

Route(s) of Administration—Per os and intravenous.

Toxicity and Adverse Effects—Sodium bicarbonate may cause metabolic alkalosis, hypokalemia, hypocalcaemia, hypernatremia, volume overload, congestive heart failure, decreased tissue oxygenation, and paradoxical CNS acidosis leading to respiratory arrest especially following high dose parenteral use. High oral and parenteral doses may contribute significant amounts of sodium and thus causing hypernatremia and volume overload. Overdose and/or rapid parenteral administration may cause severe alkalosis with irritability or tetany. Inadvertent extravasation of hypertonic solution of sodium bicarbonate causes chemical cellulitis resulting in tissue necrosis, ulceration, and/or sloughing at the site of injection.

Management of Overdose/Toxicity—Discontinue treatment if alkalosis is mild. Severe alkalosis may require intravenous calcium therapy. Sodium chloride or potassium chloride may be administered if hypokalemia is present.

Contraindications—Metabolic or respiratory alkalosis; excessive chloride.

Precautions—Use sodium bicarbonate with caution in patients with congestive heart failure or acute renal failure. Check dosages thoroughly and monitor electrolyte and acid/base status. Do not administer other drugs orally within 1-2 hours of sodium bicarbonate administration. Avoid extravasation of hypertonic sodium bicarbonate injections.

Drug Interactions—Orally administered sodium bicarbonate alters stomach pH and either increases or reduces the rate and/or extent of absorption of many orally administered drugs. When urine is alkalinized by sodium bicarbonate, excretion of certain drugs (e.g., quinidine, amphetamines, ephedrine) is decreased, and excretion of weakly acidic drugs (e.g., salicylates) is increased. The solubility of ciprofloxacin and enrofloxacin is decreased in alkaline urine produced by sodium bicarbonate. Concurrent use of sodium bicarbonate and potassium-wasting diuretics (e.g., thiazides, furosemide) may produce hypochloremic alkalosis. High dosages of sodium bicarbonate and ACTH or glucocorticoids may result in hypernatremia.

Pharmaceutical Formulations—Sodium bicarbonate is available in powder, tablets and solution for injection.

SODIUM THIOSULFATE

Synonyms—Sodium hyposulfite.

Proprietary Names—Versiclear˚; Cya-dote Injection˚.

Chemical Class—Inorganic salt.

Pharmacological Class—Antifungal agent; cyanide and arsenic antidote.

Source—Synthetic.

Solubility, Stability and Storage—Sodium thiosulfate is very soluble in water and insoluble in alcohol. Store sodium thiosulfate formulations at room temperature. Crystals should be stored in tight containers.

Pharmacological Actions—Sodium thiosulfate provides the body with sulfur which could be used in detoxification processes, especially that of cyanide.

Mechanism of Action—Sodium thiosulfate provides rhodanese (thiosulfate cyanide sulfurtransferase) with exogenous sulfur to hasten the conversion of cyanide to the relatively nontoxic thiocyanate ion which is then excreted in urine. Its action as antifungal agent may be due to slow release of sulfur.

Indications—Sodium thiosulfate is used in conjunction with sodium nitrite to treat cyanide toxicity. It is also used as topical antifungal agent in humans to treat tinea versicolor.

Dosages—For cyanide toxicity, first give sodium nitrite at a dose of 16 mg/kg IV followed with 30-40 mg/kg of 20% sodium thiosulfate solution IV. For repeat treatment, use sodium thiosulfate only.

Route(s) of Administration—Intravenous and topical.

Distribution—Following systemic administration, sodium thiosulfate distributes in the extracellular fluid.

Route(s) of Excretion. Sodium thiosulfate is rapidly excreted via urine.

Toxicity and Adverse Effects—Sodium thiosulfate is relatively non-toxic. Large oral doses may cause profuse diarrhea.

Contraindications—Lactating animals.

Precautions—Administer sodium thiosulfate by slow IV. Use the drug with caution in pregnant animals.

Pharmaceutical Formulations—Sodium thiosulfate is available in 250 mg/ml (humans approved formulation) and 300 mg/ml (veterinary formulation) solutions for injection.

SPECTINOMYCIN

Spectinomycin

Proprietary Names—Spectam*; Trobicin*.

Chemical Class—Aminocyclitol.

Pharmacological Class—Narrow spectrum antibiotic.

Source—Natural; obtained from *Streptomyces spectabilis*.

Solubility, Stability and Storage—Spectinomycin is readily soluble in water but insoluble in alcohol. Its products are stable at room temperature. Reconstitute spectinomycin powder with the supplied diluent. Reconstituted product should be used within 24 hours.

Pharmacological Actions—Spectinomycin has antimicrobial activity against a number of Gram-negative bacteria. *Escherichia coli*, and species of *Klebsiella, Proteus, Enterobacter, Salmonella, Streptococcus, Staphylococcus,* and *Mycoplasma* are susceptible. Its action is inferior to other drugs that are active against the same organisms. It is bacteriostatic.

Mechanism of Action—It inhibits protein synthesis by binding reversibly to the 30S ribosomal subunit of susceptible bacteria.

Indications—Treatment to *E. coli* infection in piglets; treatment of chronic respiratory disease of poultry (in combination with lincomycin). It is used occasionally in other species to treat susceptible infections.

Dosages—

Dog	20-40 mg/kg orally every 12 hours.
Cat	512 mg/kg IM every 12 hours.
Cattle	2233 mg/kg parenterally every 8 hours.
Horse	20 mg/kg parenterally every 8 hours.
Pig	10 mg/kg orally or IM every 12 hours
Bird	0.5 g/4.5 litres of drinking water for weight gain or 2 g/4.5 litres for control of CRD.

Route(s) of Administration—Per os (for enteric infections in animals) and intramuscular.

Absorption—Spectinomycin is rapidly absorbed from intramuscular site. Peak plasma concentration is attained within 1 hour. It is poorly absorbed from the GIT.

Bioavailability—Oral bioavailability is poor.

Duration of Action—Up to 8 hours.

Distribution—Vd = 0.2 L/kg. It penetrates tissue poorly apparently due to low lipid solubility.

Plasma Protein Binding—Less than 10%.

Metabolism—Spectinomycin is poorly metabolized.

Plasma Half-Life—1.7 hours.

Withdrawal Period—Pig, 21 days; Chicken, 5 days;

Route(s) Of Excretion—Urine (75-100% as active drug).

Dialysis Status—50% dialyzable.

Toxicity and Adverse Effects—Adverse effects have not been documented in animals. It is less likely to cause ototoxicity and nephrotoxicity than other drugs in its group. Adverse effects are few in humans and include urticaria, chills, fever, dizziness, nausea, and insomnia. Spectinomycin can cause neuromuscular blockade. Overdose has been reported to cause ataxia in turkeys.

Management of Overdose/Toxicity—Neuromuscular blockade can be reversed by administration of calcium.

Contraindications—Hypersensitivity to spectinomycin; egg-laying hens.

Drug Interactions—Concurrent use with chloramphenicol and tetracycline has resulted in antagonism.

Pharmaceutical Formulations—The drug is presented as spectinomycin hydrochloride in 2 g and 4 g sterile powder for reconstitution to solution for injection. Oral preparation for use in animals is available.

SPIRONOLACTONE

Spironolactone

Proprietary Names—Aldactone®; Xenalon®; Verospiron®; Aldactide® (fixed-dose combination); Aldactazide® (fixed-dose combination).

Chemical Class—Steroid lactone.

Pharmacological Class—Potassium-sparing diuretic; Aldosterone antagonist.

Source—Synthetic.

Solubility, Stability and Storage—Spironolactone is practically insoluble in water but soluble in alcohol. Spironolactone tablets should be stored in tight, light-resistant containers at room temperature.

Pharmacological Actions—Spironolactone causes diuresis consequent to the decreased reabsorption of sodium that is finally excreted with an iso-osmotic equivalent of water. It increases calcium excretion due to direct effect on tubular transport. It also inhibits the biosynthesis of aldosterone at high concentrations. Unlike thiazide diuretics, spironolactone does not cause potassium depletion or affect glucose metabolism or uric acid excretion. Spironolactone is a weak diuretic, but it can be combined with other diuretics. Thus, spironolactone is a useful adjunct to thiazide therapy when diuresis is inadequate or reduction of potassium excretion is necessary.

Mechanism of Action—Spironolactone inhibits the effect of aldosterone by competing for intracellular aldosterone receptor in the distal tubular cells where sodium reabsorption is related to potassium secretion. This increases the secretion of water and sodium, while decreasing the excretion of potassium. Physiologically, aldosterone is secreted in response to hyponatremia and/or hyperkalemia. Spironolactone aids tubular reabsorption of sodium and decreases that of potassium.

Indications—Management of edema associated with excessive aldosterone excretion such as idiopathic edema and edema accompanying cirrhosis of the liver, nephrotic syndrome and congestive heart failure. It is used commonly in conjunction with other diuretics.

Dosages—0.5-1.5 mg/kg alone or in combination with thiazide or other potassium wasting diuretics.

Route(s) of Administration—Per os.

Absorption—Spironolactone is fairly rapidly absorbed from the gastrointestinal tract. About 70% of oral dose is absorbed. Food increases the bioavailability of unmetabolized spironolactone by almost 100%.

Bioavailability—Oral bioavailability is 60-70%.

Onset of Action—Spironolactone has slow onset of action; its effects take several days to develop and similarly they diminish slowly.

Plasma Protein Binding—>90%.

Metabolism—Rapidly and extensively metabolized to carenone and 7-α-thiomethyl spironolactone, among others. These two metabolites are active. Spironolactone is subject to extensive first-pass metabolism and enterohepatic circulation.

Plasma Half-Life—4 to 17 hours. The wide range is due to presence of active metabolites and extensive enterohepatic circulation. Half-life for parent compound is about 10 minutes.

Toxicity and Adverse Effects—Hyperkalemia may be observed especially in severe renal insufficiency and with the use of spironolactone as sole diuretic agent. Acute overdose may cause drowsiness, maculopapular or erythematous rash, nausea, vomiting, or diarrhea. Spironolactone is tumorogenic in rats following prolonged use.

Management of Overdose/Toxicity—Discontinue therapy; start general antidotal therapy.

Contraindications—Chronic renal insufficiency; anuria; concurrent use with another potassium-sparing diuretic (e.g. amiloride).

Precautions—Do not give potassium supplements during spironolactone therapy.

Drug Interactions—Salicylates may interfere with the tubular secretion of carenone with resultant decrease in spironolactone effectiveness. Concurrent use with another potassium-sparing agent (e.g., amiloride, triamterene) may increase the risk of hyperkalemia. Indomethacin, angiotensin-converting enzyme (ACE) inhibitor (e.g., captopril) and potassium supplements or other substances containing potassium may also increase the risk of hyperkalemia if used concurrently with spironolactone. Spironolactone increases the half-life of digoxin, resulting in increased serum digoxin concentrations and subsequent cardiac glycoside toxicity.

Pharmaceutical Formulations—Tablets of 25-, 50-, and 100—mg of spironolactone alone are available. The drug is also available in fixed dose combination with hydrochlorothiazide.

STREPTOMYCIN/DIHYDROSTREPTOMYCIN

Proprietary Name	Constituents
Streptomycine*	Streptomycin sulfate.
Streptomycin*	Streptomycin sulfate
Streptopen*	Streptomycin sulfate and Penicillin G
Combiotic*	Dihydrostreptomycin sulfate and Procaine Penicillin G.
Dipen*	Dihydrostreptomycin sulfate and Procaine Penicillin G.
Penstrep*	Dihydrostreptomycin sulfate and Procaine Penicillin G.

Chemical Class—Aminoglycosidic aminocyclitol.

Pharmacological Class—Aminoglycoside antibiotic.

Source—Natural; obtained from *Streptomyces griseus*.

Spectinomycin

Pharmacological Actions—These drugs have rapid bactericidal action against Gram-negative aerobic bacilli. They produce synergistic bactericidal effect against strains of *Enterococci* and *Streptococci* when administered with penicillin. Streptomycin is bactericidal to the tubercule bacilli in vitro. It suppresses the tubercule bacilli in vivo.

Mechanism of Action—They bind to at least three proteins and perhaps the 16S molecule of RNA and the 30S ribosomal subunit to interfere with the initiation of protein synthesis leading to accumulation of abnormal initiation complexes. They may also induce misreading of the RNA template resulting in incorrect amino acid incorporation into the growing polypeptide chains.

Indications—Treatment of metritis, enteritis, cystitis, septicemia, leptospirosis, vibriosis and *Corynebacterium equi* and other infections caused by susceptible organisms.

Dosages—

Bird	10-20 mg/kg IM twice daily for 7 days.
Fish	30-40 mg/kg IP once daily.
Cattle, horse, pig, sheep	10 mg streptomycin base/kg.
Dog, cat	10-20 mg streptomycin base/kg.
Mouse	4-5 mg/adult mouse SC once a day.
Rabbit	10 mg/kg IM every 4 hours
Reptile	10 mg/kg IM twice daily.

Route(s) of Administration—Intramuscular, intravenous and per os (for treatment of enteritis in animals).

Absorption—Less than 1% of the dose is absorbed from the GIT. The drugs are absorbed from IM site. Peak plasma concentration of 25 to 50 µg/mL is attained within 1 hour.

Distribution—Vd (streptomycin) = 0.25 ± 0.02 L/kg in humans and 0.23 ± 0.041 L/kg in horses. Streptomycin distributes mainly in the ECF. It is largely excluded from cells, CNS and eyes. Concentrations in secretions and tissues are low. It attains high concentration in renal cortex, endolymph and perilymph of the inner ear. Inflammation increases its concentration in peritoneal, pericardial, and cerebrospinal fluids. Streptomycin crosses the placenta and serum levels in the cord blood are similar to maternal levels. Small amounts are excreted in milk, saliva, and sweat.

Plasma Protein Binding—48 ± 14%.

Metabolism—The drugs are probably not extensively metabolized.

Plasma Half-Life—

Streptomycin: 2.6 ± 0.4 hours in humans (higher in uremia and neonates) and 3.4 ± 0.4 hours in horses.

Dihydrostreptomycin: 1.5-9.3 hours in horses and 2.35-4.50 hours in cattle.

Clearance (Streptomycin)—1.2 ± 0.3 ml/min/kg in humans (lower in uremia) and 0.77 ± 0.14 ml/min/kg in horses.

Route(s) of Excretion—Urine (for parenterally administered drug with 50% as unchanged drug in humans); 60-100% of an oral dose of streptomycin is excreted unchanged in the feces of humans.

Dialysis Status—The drugs are dialyzable.

Residue Limit—0.125 ppm in milk; 2.0 ppm in kidneys; 0.5 ppm in other tissues.

Withdrawal Period—4 days before slaughter of chicken; 2 days before slaughter of cattle.

Toxicity and Adverse Effects—Streptomycin causes pain and development of hot tender masses at the site of injection. Varying degrees of ototoxicity which may manifest as hearing loss (cochlear damage) or vertigo, ataxia, loss of balance (vestibular damage) and nephrotoxicity are common at therapeutic doses. Hearing loss, when extensive is usually permanent. Neurotoxicity may appear as curare-like effect producing neuromuscular blockade and respiratory paralysis with high doses especially when the drug is given soon after anesthesia and the use of muscle relaxants. Streptomycin contains sodium metabisulfite, a sulfite that may cause allergic-type reactions including anaphylactic symptoms and life-threatening or less severe asthmatic episodes in certain susceptible people, especially asthmatics. This is significant in veterinarians and pharmacy technicians who may have local sensitization with dermatitis from handling of drug. It may cause deafness in the newborn if used during pregnancy. Dihydrostreptomycin is more toxic than streptomycin.

Management of Overdose/Toxicity—Hydration and force diuresis may enhance removal from blood.

Contraindications—Known hypersensitivity to streptomycin, aminoglycosides or their components; pregnancy; egg-laying hens; psittacines or passerines.

Precautions—Reduce streptomycin dose in patients with renal impairment. Use the drug with caution in patients with pre-existing hearing loss. Avoid concurrent or sequential use of other neurotoxic and/or nephrotoxic drugs particularly neomycin, kanamycin, gentamicin, cephaloridine, paromomycin, viomycin, polymyxin B, colistin, and tobramycin with streptomycin. Since streptomycin readily crosses the placental barrier, caution in the use of the drug in pregnant animals is important to prevent ototoxicity in the fetus. Do not administer streptomycin for more than 5 days.

Drug Interactions—Both drugs are synergistic with beta-lactam antibiotics. They may be inactivated by penicillin in vitro and in end-stage renal failure. Depolarizing and non-depolarizing neuromuscular blockers may prolong their effects. Concurrent use of loop diuretics and amphotericin may enhance their nephrotoxicity potential.

Pharmaceutical Formulations—Available as streptomycin sulfate either in powder or in a sterile, nonpyrogenic solution for intramuscular use. Each mL contains streptomycin sulfate equivalent to 400 mg of streptomycin base, sodium citrate dihydrate 12 mg, phenol 0.25% w/v as preservative, and sodium metabisulfite 2 mg in water for injection. The drug is also available as the hydrochloride and calcium chloride complex salts, and in fixed dose combination with penicillin and vitamins for animal treatment.

SUCCINYLCHOLINE

Succinylcholine chloride

Synonyms—Suxamethonium.

Proprietary Names—Anectine*; Quelicin*; Sucostrin*.

Pharmacological Class—Depolarizing neuromuscular blocker; Muscle relaxant.

Source—Synthetic.

Solubility, Stability and Storage—Succinylcholine is soluble to the levels of 1 g/mL in water and 2.9 mg/mL in alcohol at 25°C. Store solutions in the refrigerator but product may remain stable for up to 14 days at room temperature. Powder products are stable for indefinite periods but reconstituted products are stable for 4 weeks at 5°C, or 1 week at room temperature. Succinylcholine is compatible with normal saline. It is incompatible with sodium bicarbonate, pentobarbital and thiopental. Keep succinylcholine solutions on ice on the field.

Pharmacological Actions. Succinylcholine blocks impulse transmission at the motor-end plate and causes paralysis of skeletal muscle. The paralysis is usually preceded by muscle contraction.

Succinylcholine stimulates and then blocks ganglia; induces salivation which can be blocked by atropine. It is a weak histamine releaser. Bovines and canines are more sensitive while pigs and horses are more resistant. It releases potassium from muscle.

Mechanism of Action. Succinylcholine causes neuromuscular blockade by persistent depolarization of the endplate region which does not allow the subsynaptic membrane to completely repolarize thereby rendering the endplate non-responsive to the normal action of Ach. Succinylcholine also causes desensitization of receptors towards Ach (phase II block). Hence, it is said to produce dual blockade. Phase II block has the character of blockade caused by curare.

Indications—As an adjunct to general anesthesia to facilitate tracheal intubation and to provide skeletal muscle relaxation; to control convulsions during tetanus and trauma during status epilepticus.

Dosages—

Dog	0.3 mg/kg IV
Cat	1 mg/kg
Pig	2 mg/kg
Cattle, Sheep	0.01-0.02 mg/kg
Horse	0.088 mg/kg

Route(s) of Administration—Intravenous and intramuscular.

Absorption—Succinylcholine is poorly absorbed from the GIT.

Onset of Action—2 to 3 minutes (IM); full relaxation in 30-60 seconds following IV injection.

Duration of Action—4 to 6 minutes (IV); 10-30 minutes (IM); duration is prolonged in dogs. Duration appears to be determined by the rate of diffusion of the drug away from the motor end-plate rather than by enzymatic hydrolysis.

Distribution. Succinylcholine crosses the placenta in small amounts. This may become significant if doses are high or repeated.

Metabolism. The drug is hydrolyzed to succinyl monocholine and choline by plasma pseudo cholinesterase. Succinyl monocholine has some level of activity and is slowly metabolized by pseudocholinesterase to succinic acid and choline.

Plasma Half-life—10 minutes.

Route(s) of Excretion—Urine with 10% as unchanged drug.

Toxicity and Adverse Effects—Respiratory paralysis, prolonged apnoea, hypotension, bronchoconstriction due to histamine release, soreness of muscle, and cardiac arrhythmia in digitalized subjects are some of the known adverse effects of succinylcholine. Repeated therapy causes bradycardia, extrasystoles and even cardiac arrest. Muscle soreness is observed 1-3 days after succinylcholine administration. High doses may stimulate pregnant uterus. Succinylcholine may cause increased intraocular pressure. Overdose causes respiratory paralysis and cardiac arrest.

Management of Overdose/Toxicity—Stop drug administration and give artificial respiration. Injection of purified pseudo cholinesterase preparation hastens recovery from the effects of succinylcholine. Give a small dose of competitive neuro-muscular blocker before succinylcholine administration to prevent muscle fasciculation that usually precedes paralysis. Atropine may be used to suppress succinylcholine effect on the heart.

Contraindications—Severe liver disease; chronic anemia; hyperkalemia; disorders of plasma pseudocholinesterase; penetrating eye injury; malignant hyperthermia; myopathies associated with increased serum creatinine phosphokinase (CPK); glaucoma; known hypersensitivity to succinylcholine.

Precautions—Artificial respiration may be required for prolonged period. Phenothiazines possess some anticholinesterase activity. Therefore, the use of phenothiazines with succinylcholine in a patient exposed to organophosphates may be hazardous. Use succinylcholine cautiously in subjects with impaired liver, pulmonary and kidney functions. Use cautiously in pregnant animals and in patients with raised plasma potassium (as in severe burns and muscle trauma).

Drug Interactions—Anticholinesterase agents (organophosphates, carbamates, neostigmine etc.) augment the action of succinylcholine because they inhibit pseudocholinesterase which is responsible for breakdown of succinylcholine. Succinylcholine sensitizes the myocardium to the action of digitalis and also increases the arrhythmogenic action of epinephrine. Procaine and amethocaine increase the half-life of succinylcholine because they compete with succinylcholine for enzyme site. Immunosuppressants (e.g. cyclosporine, cyclophosphamide) may prolong the neuromuscular blocking action of succinylcholine by decreasing plasma pseudocholinesterase. Inhaled anaesthetics may increase the cardiac effects of succinylcholine.

Pharmaceutical Formulations—Available as succinylcholine chloride in solutions of 20 mg/ml, 50 mg/ml, and 100 mg/ml. The drug is also available in 100 mg, 500 mg and 1 g powder for reconstitution to injectable solution. There are no specific veterinary formulations.

SUCRALFATE

Synonyms—Aluminum sucrose sulfate.

Proprietary Names—Carafate*.

Chemical Class—Sucrose aluminum hydroxide compound; anionic sulfated disaccharide.

Pharmacological Class—Antiulcer agent; Pepsin inhibitor.

Source—Synthetic.

Solubility, Stability and Storage—Sucralfate is practically insoluble in alcohol or water. Store sucralfate tablets in tight containers at room temperature.

Pharmacological Actions—Sucralfate protects ulcerated mucosa surfaces and aid healing of ulcers. It does not appreciably affect gastric acid output or concentration.

Mechanism of Action—Sucralfate acts locally by reacting with hydrochloric acid in the stomach to form a highly condensed, viscous, adhesive, paste-like substance which binds to the proteinaceous exudates at ulcer surfaces, thus physically protecting the ulcerated surface from the actions of acid, pepsin or bile. Sucralfate may give further protection by direct inhibition of pepsin, binding of bile salts, epithelial growth factor and fibroblast growth factor. The last two enhance the growth and repair mechanism of the stomach lining. Sucralfate may also increase prostaglandin production resulting in protection of the lining of the stomach.

Indications—Adjunctive treatment of gastrointestinal ulcers; prophylaxis of drug-induced gastric erosion.

Dosages—

Dog	500-1000 mg/animal 2-3 times daily.
Cat	250 mg/animal 2-3 times daily.
Foal	2 mg/kg 3 times daily or 1-2 grams 4 times daily.

Route(s) of Administration—Per os.

Absorption—About 3-5% of oral dose is absorbed.

Duration of Action—Approximately 6 hours (oral).

Route(s) of Excretion—The absorbed portion is excreted in urine as unchanged drug. The unabsorbed portion forms sucrose sulfate which is excreted in feces.

Toxicity and Adverse Effects—Sucralfate is generally well tolerated. It is safe in pregnant animals. Constipation has been reported in dogs. **Contraindications**—No definite contraindications.

Precautions—Sucralfate should be given 30 minutes prior to the administration of antacid. Separate administration of sucralfate and other drugs whose bioavailability are crucial since sucralfate can alter the absorption of some drugs from the GI tract. Sucralfate may reduce intestinal transit time, hence use with caution in animals where decreased intestinal transit times may be deleterious.

Drug Interactions—Sucralfate reduces the bioavailability of cimetidine, digoxin, ketoconazole, phenytoin, ranitidine, tetracycline and theophylline following concurrent oral administration. Sucralfate decreases GI absorption of ciprofloxacin and norfloxacin and may result in substantial (e.g. 50% or greater) decreases in serum concentrations of the drugs. Therefore, sucralfate should not be administered within 2 hours of ciprofloxacin or norfloxacin therapy.

Pharmaceutical Formulations—Sucralfate is available in 500 mg/5 mL oral suspension and 1 g tablet.

SULFACLOZINE

Synonyms—Sulfachloropyrazine.

Proprietary Names—ESB$_3$.

Chemical Class—Sulfonamide; Sulfanilamide derivative.

Pharmacological Class—Anticoccidial drug.

Source—Synthetic.

Solubility, Stability and Storage—Sulfaclozine is freely soluble in water. Store sulfaclozine powder at room temperature protected from light and moisture.

Pharmacological Actions—Sulfaclozine has antimicrobial action against some protozoa (especially *Eimeria* species) and some bacteria including *Salmonella gallinarum*.

Mechanism of Action—Sulfaclozine interferes with the biosynthesis of folic acid in susceptible organisms by competing with para-aminobenzoic acid (PABA) for incorporation into dihydrofolic acid. By replacing the PABA molecule in dihydrofolic acid, sulfaclozine prevents formation of folic acid required for nucleic acid synthesis and multiplication of the cell.

Mechanism of Selective Toxicity—Sulfonamides are effective only in cells that must produce their own folic acid e.g. bacteria and protozoa. Mammalian cells do not synthesize folic acid, but acquire it from preformed sources such as diet.

Indications—Treatment of infections such as coccidiosis in poultry caused by *Eimeria* species, fowl typhoid caused by *Salmonella gallinarum* and fowl cholera due to infection with *Pasteurella multocida*.

Dosages—Dissolve 1g ESB$_3$ 30% per liter of water. This provides approximately 50 mg of active ingredient, or 170 mg ESB$_3$ per kg bodyweight. Treat for 3 consecutive days and repeat after a

2-day break if necessary. Shuttle programs like day 1, 3, 5, 7, 9 or 1, 2, 5, 6, 9 have also been found effective. For the treatment of cholera and typhoid, doses of 1 to 2 g ESB_3 per liter of water for at least 5 days are required.

Route(s) of Administration. Per os (through drinking water).

Withdrawal Period. Chicken: 14 days; Turkeys: 21 days (turkey meat and offal excluding skin: 14 days); Eggs: 11 days.

Contraindications—Known hypersensitivity to sulfaclozine.

Precautions—Prepare fresh solution daily.

Drug Interactions—PABA-containing compounds and local anesthetics derived from PABA (e.g. procaine, proparacaine, and tetracaine) may decrease the effect of sulfaclozine.

Pharmaceutical Formulations—The drug is available as sulfaclozine sodium monohydrate in powder containing 30 g active ingredient per 100 g.

SULFADIAZINE

Sulfadiazine

Proprietary Names—Microsulfon˙; Sulfadiazine˙.

Chemical Class—Sulfonamide; Sulfanilamide derivative.

Pharmacological Class—Antimicrobial drug.

Source—Synthetic.

Solubility, Stability and Storage—Sulfadiazine is practically insoluble in water, sparingly soluble in alcohol and slightly soluble in human serum at 37 °C. Sulfadiazine is stable in air but slowly darkens on exposure to light. Sulfadiazine formulations may be stored in well-closed, light-resistant containers at room temperature.

Pharmacological Actions—Sulfadiazine has bacteriostatic action against Gram-positive and Gram-negative bacteria. *Chlamydia, Actinomyces, Norcardia* species, and some protozoan organisms are susceptible. It is effective against *E. coli, Klebsiella, Enterobacter, Proteus mirabilis, Proteus vulgaris, Staph aureus, Toxoplasma, H. influenzae.*

Mechanism of Action—Same as for other sulfonamides. See sulfaclozine

Mechanism of Selective Toxicity—See sulfaclozine.

Indications—Treatment of post distemper bacterial infections in dogs, urinary tract infections in small animals, and infections due to susceptible organism.

Dosages—

Horse, cow, sheep, cat.	130 mg/kg in 2 divided doses every 12 hours.
Dog and Pig.	130 mg/kg in equally divided doses every 8 hours.
Chicken.	0.5% in feed.

Route(s) of Administration—Per os and intravenous (rare).

Absorption—Sulfadiazine is rapidly absorbed from the GIT; 70-100% of oral dose is absorbed. Peak plasma concentration is attained within 3-6 hours. Absorption can be variable among dogs and between different doses given to the same dog. The absorption of oral sulfadiazine in calves is slow but complete and unaffected by rumen status. Absorption of sulfadiazine in sheep is comparable to that in dogs.

Bioavailability—Oral bioavailability is ~100% (85 to 89% in pigs).

Effective Serum Concentration—Therapeutic serum concentrations is > 0.1 mcg/mL.

Distribution—Vd = 0.29 ± 0.04L/kg (human); 0.393 L/kg (ewe); 0.58 L/kg (horse); 0.54 L/kg (pig); 0.85 L/kg (ruminating calf). Sulfadiazine is widely distributed in body fluids and tissues. It attains therapeutic concentration in the CSF. Sulfadiazine sodium has good penetrability in the brain. The drug appears in milk (the milk/plasma concentration ratio for sulfadiazine is 0.5 in cows). In dogs, sulfadiazine is distributed into the aqueous and vitreous humors of the eye at concentrations that are 30 to 50% of serum concentrations. Sulfadiazine distributes into prostatic fluid at about 10% of the concurrent serum concentration. It crosses the placenta and enters fetal circulation.

Plasma Protein Binding—54 ± 4%.

Metabolism—15-40% of sulfadiazine is acetylated in the liver.

Plasma Half-Life—9.9 ± 4.3 hours (human); 3.1-4.31 hours (pig); 9.84 hours (dog); 4.1 hours (cattle).

Clearance (ml/min/kg)—0.55 ± 0.17 (human); 3.15 (ruminating calf); 1.92 (horse); 2.3 (pig).

Residue Limit—Edible tissues. 0.1 ppm.

Route(s) of Excretion—Urine with 57 ± 14% as unchanged drug. Urinary excretion is accelerated by administration of alkali.

Toxicity and Adverse Effects—Adverse effects of sulfadiazine involve several organs or systems including blood, bone marrow, skin, kidney, liver, nervous system and GIT. Gastrointestinal disturbances (anorexia, nausea, vomiting and diarrhea); neurological effects (lethargy, depression) are common. The incidence of blood dyscrasia is low but may be serious. The potential for crystalluria, hematuria and nephritis is high because of poor solubility of acetylated form. Hypersensitivity reactions involving skin and mucous membranes as well as photosensitization are common.

Management of Overdose/Toxicity—Give general antidotal therapy. Treat symptomatically.

Contraindications—Hypersensitivity to sulfadiazine or other sulfonamides; pregnancy.

Precautions—Do not administer sulfadiazine by intrathecal, subcutaneous or intramuscular routes. Adjust the dose in patients with renal or hepatic impairment. Maintain adequate fluid intake or administer $NaHCO_3$ to avoid crystalluria. Continue administration for 48 hours after disappearance of clinical signs. Do not use longer than 7-8 days in herbivores to avoid vitamin deficiency.

Drug Interactions—PABA-containing compounds and local anesthetics derived from PABA (e.g. procaine, proparacaine, and tetracaine) may decrease the effect of sulfadiazine. Anticoagulants, methotrexate, oral hypoglycemic drugs, and hydatoin anticonvulsants may be displaced from binding and/or their metabolism may be inhibited by sulfadiazine. Thus, the actions and potential toxicities of these drugs may be enhanced. Sulfadiazine may be displaced from binding sites by phenylbutazone, salicylates and probenecid. Concomitant use of sulfadiazine with ascorbic acid and hexamine can precipitate crystalluria. Sulfadiazine increases the risk of liver damage if administered concurrently with cyclosporine. It decreases the levels of folic acid if administered with pyrimethamine.

Pharmaceutical Formulations—Sulfadiazine is available in 500 mg tablets and as sulfadiazine sodium for intravenous injection. Fixed dose combination with trimethoprim (80 mg trimethoprim and 400 mg sulfadiazine) in tablets, boluses, dispersible powder, oral suspension and injection solution is available for animal treatment. Fixed dose combination with pyrimethamine is also available in suspension containing 250 mg/mL sulfadiazine (as the sodium salt) and 12.5 mg/mL pyrimethamine.

SULFADIMETHOXINE

Sulfadimethoxine

Proprietary Names—Albon*; Coxi Plus*; Combisan* (in combination with trimethoprim and colistin sulfate); Trisulmix* (in combination with trimethoprim); Sultriject* (in combination with trimethoprim); Asco Trimaxin* (in combination with trimethoprim and ascorbic acid).

Chemical Class—Sulfonamide; Sulfanilamide derivative.

Pharmacological Class—Antimicrobial agent; Antibacterial agent.

Source—Synthetic.

Solubility, Stability and Storage—Sulfadimethoxine is practically insoluble in water and slightly soluble in alcohol. Store sulfadimethoxine products at room temperature in light resistant containers.

Pharmacological Actions—Sulfadimethoxine has bacteriostatic action against Gram-positive and Gram-negative bacteria, Clamydia, Actinomyces, Norcardia species, and some protozoan organisms.

Mechanism of Action—See sulfaclozine.

Mechanism of Selective Toxicity—See sulfaclozine.

Indications—Treatment of coccidiosis, fowl cholera and infectious coryza in poultry; treatment of respiratory, genitourinary, enteric and soft tissue infections caused by susceptible organisms in dogs, cats, horses, sheep, and cattle; treatment of coccidiosis in dogs.

Dosages—55 mg/kg initially, followed with 27.5 mg/kg once daily. The dose in birds is 50mg/kg bodyweight dispensed in drinking water and administered for 5 days.

Route(s) of Administration—Per os, intramuscular, subcutaneous and intravenous.

Absorption—Sulfadimethoxine is slowly absorbed from oral route. Peak plasma concentration is attained within 8-10 hours.

Bioavailability—Oral bioavailability is 59.1% in cattle.

Duration of Action—The drug is long-acting due to tubular reabsorption.

Distribution—Vd = 0.31 L/kg (cattle); 0.17-0.33 L/kg (adult pig); 0.48 L/kg (piglet); 0.35 L/kg (growing pigs); 0.17 L/kg (sheep). Sulfadimethoxine is widely distributed into body tissues and fluids including endometrium, synovial and peritoneal fluids. It attains low concentration in the CSF.

Plasma Protein Binding—The drug is highly protein bound.

Metabolism—Sulfadimethoxine is acetylated in the liver to acetylsulfadimethoxine. It is poorly metabolized in dogs.

Plasma Half-life—12.5 hours (cattle); 16.16 (piglet); 9.35 hours (growing pig). 15 hours (sheep); 11.3 hours (horse).

Clearance (ml/min/kg)—4.21 to 7.37 (adult pig); 20.9 (piglet); 26.1 (growing pig).

Residue Limit—0.1 ppm (edible tissues of cattle); 0.01 ppm (milk).

Withdrawal Period—Varies with formulation; 5 days (slaughter) and 60 hours (milk) for injectable formulations; 7 days (slaughter) and 60 hours (milk) for oral formulations; 21 days (slaughter) for sustained release formulations; 7 days (slaughter of cattle) or 5 days (slaughter of poultry) for soluble powder dosage forms.

Route(s) of Excretion. Urine.

Toxicity and Adverse Effects. Skin rashes, photosensitization, hemolytic anemia and agranolocytosis have all been reported in animals and humans. Chronic toxicity assumes two forms namely, 1) depression of the intestinal flora and interference with vitamin B metabolism and 2) crystalluria. Crystalluria results when dosage is excessive either in quantity, frequency or duration. Crystalluria may also result if the intake of water and excretion of the drug has been restricted or the pH of urine has become acid. Sulfadimethoxine is goitrogenic to pig fetuses during late gestation.

Management of Overdose/Toxicity—Withdraw the drug; administer fluids and give symptomatic treatment.

Contraindications—Hypersensitivity to sulfonamides, thiazides or sulfonylurea agents (e.g. tolbutamide, chlorpropamide, gilbenclamide etc.); severe hepatic and renal impairment.

Precautions—Use sulfadimethoxine with caution in patients with hepatic and/or renal impairment; or in patients with urinary obstruction. Since sulfonamides are excreted primarily by the kidneys, an adequate urine volume must be maintained and alkalization of urine may be desirable in some species and individuals.

Drug Interactions—See sulfadiazine.

Pharmaceutical Formulations—Sulfadimethoxine is available in 40% solution for injection and in combination with other drugs as water soluble powder for addition to drinking water.

SULFAMETHAZINE

Synonyms—Sulfadimidine.

Proprietary Names—Sulfazine*; Samidine*; Sulfadine 333*; Sulphasan* (in combination with sulfadiazine, and sulfamerazine); Triprim* powder (in combination with trimethoprim); Clortadona-TS* (in combination with erythromycin, neomycin, trimethoprim and bromhexine); Triple sulfa* (in combination with sulfaquinoxaline and sulfamerazine); Ladsulfad* (in combination with sulfadiazine, sulfaguanidine, vitamins A and K).

Chemical Class—Sulfonamide; Sulfanilamide derivative.

Pharmacological Class—Antimicrobial agent; Antibacterial agent.

Source—Synthetic.

Sulphamethazine

Solubility, Stability and Storage—Store products at room temperature in light-resistant containers.

Pharmacological Actions—Sulfamethazine has antimicrobial activity against Gram-positive organisms such as hemolytic *Streptococci, Pneumococci* and some *Staphylococci* spp. It is also active against Gram-negative bacteria such as *Pasteurella* spp, *E. coli* and *Salmonella* spp as well as some rickettsiae.

Mechanism of Action—See sulfaclozine.

Mechanism of Selective Toxicity—See sulfaclozine.

Indications—Treatment of bacterial diseases such as bovine respiratory disease complex (shipping fever complex), necrotic pododermatitis (foot rot), calf diphtheria, colibacillosis (bacterial scours), acute mastitis and acute metritis. It is also used to treat pasteurellosis in sheep, bacteria pneumonia in sheep and pigs, bacterial pig enteritis and reduction in the incidence of cervical abscesses. Sulfadimidine is also used to control infectious coryza, coccidiosis, acute fowl cholera, and pullorum disease in poultry. It is used in combination with chlortetracycline and penicillin in food-producing animals to promote growth and increase feed efficiency.

Dosages—

Cattle, pig, sheep, and goats: 200 mg/kg stat followed by 100 mg/kg for 3-5 days.

Poultry (for control of coccidiosis): 100-200 mg/liter of drinking water.

Guinea pigs: 166-517 mg/liter of drinking water.

Route(s) of Administration—Oral and parenteral routes are appropriate.

Absorption—Sulfadimidine is rapidly absorbed from the gut. Sustained-release formulations achieve therapeutic blood levels in 6-12 hours.

Bioavailability—Sulfadimidine attains good therapeutic levels following oral administration.

Distribution—Vd = 0.24-3.7 (cattle); 0.51 (pig); 0.32 (goat); 0.41 (sheep); 0.47-0.56 (horse); 0.628 (dog); 0.394 (camel).

Metabolism—Sulfadimidine is extensively acetylated. The acetylated products are less soluble in urine, thus crystalluria is likely. The parent compound and metabolites like N^4-acetyl sulfadimidine, the N^4-glucose conjugate of sulfadimidine and desaminosulfadimidine constitute the major residues in the tissues of pigs treated with sulfadimidine. Dietary nitrite enhances the production of the desmanino metabolites.

Plasma Half-life (hours)—3.64 to 5.82 (cattle); 10-16.6 (pigs); 1.97-4.75 (goats); 3.64-10.8 (sheep); 5-6 (horses); 9.5-14.6 (old horses); 16 (dog); 7.36-13.2 (camel).

Clearance (ml/min/kg)—Clearance depends on age and dose. The values are 44-54 (cattle); 21-42 (pig); 20-70 (goat); 44.6 (sheep); 65-67 (horses); 22.4 (dogs); 40 (camel).

Residue Limit—0.1 ppm in edible tissues; 0.01 ppm in milk.

Withdrawal Period—Ten days before slaughter of cattle.

Route(s) of Excretion—Rapidly excreted in urine.

Toxicity and Adverse Effects—Sulfamethazine may cause hemorrhagic enteritis in cattle. Increased incidence of thyroid hyperplasia has been demonstrated in rats and pigs. Hypersensitivity reaction, crystalluria, and kidney damage may occur.

Management of Overdose/Toxicity—Give general antidotal therapy.

Contraindications—Liver or renal dysfunction; hypersensitivity to sulfamethazine or other sulfonamides; lactating animals; horses intended for food.

Precautions—Allergic reaction to sulfa drugs may occur sometimes. Treatment should continue 24 to 48 hours beyond the remission of disease symptoms, but not to exceed 5 consecutive days.

Drug Interactions. Sulfamethazine enhances the actions of phenytoin, tolbutamide and warfarin by inhibiting of their metabolism. It increases the toxicity of methotrexate.

Pharmaceutical Formulations—Sulfamethazine is available as 16% or 33% injectable solution and as water soluble powder or liquid for addition to drinking water. Sulfamethazine is available singly or in combination with other drugs.

SULFAMETHOXAZOLE

Proprietary Names—Gantanol˚; Urobak˚.

Chemical Class—Sulfonamide; Sulfanilamide derivative.

Pharmacological Class—Antimicrobial drug.

Source—Synthetic.

Solubility, Stability and Storage—Sulfamethoxazole is practically insoluble in water but sparingly soluble in alcohol. Store products at room temperature.

Sulphamethoxazole

Pharmacological Actions—Sulfamethoxazole has bacteriostatic action against Gram-positive and Gram-negative bacteria, *Clamydia, Actinomyces, Norcardia* species and some protozoan organisms including *Plasmodium falciparum* and *Toxoplasma gondii*.

Mechanism of Action—See sulfaclozine.

Mechanism of Selective Toxicity—See sulfaclozine.

Indications—Urinary tract infections in dogs and cats.

Dosages—45.8 mg/per kg of body weight. See product insert for details.

Route(s) of Administration—Per os.

Absorption—Sulfamethoxazole is completely but slowly absorbed from the GIT. Peak plasma concentration is attained within 3-4 hours.

Bioavailability—Almost 100%.

Distribution—Vd = 0.21 ± 0.02 L/kg (humans). It distributes readily to most tissues and fluids including pleural, synovial, peritoneal and cerebrospinal fluids. Sulfamethoxazole crosses the placenta.

Plasma Protein Binding—62 ± 5% in humans.

Metabolism—Partially acetylated in the liver.

Plasma Half-Life—10.1 ± 4.6 hours humans.

Clearance—0.32 ± 0.04 (ml/min/kg).

Route(s) of Excretion—Urine, with 14 ± 2% as unchanged drug.

Dialysis Status—Moderately dialyzable (20-50%).

Toxicity and Adverse Effects—Adverse effects involve several organs or systems including blood, bone marrow, kidney, liver, nervous system and gastrointestinal system. GI disturbances (anorexia, nausea, vomiting and diarrhea), neurological disorders (lethargy, depression), crystalluria, hematuria, nephritis, hypersensitivity reactions involving skin and mucous membranes as well as photosensitization are common. **Management of Overdose/Toxicity**—Withdraw the drug; administer fluids and give symptomatic treatment.

Contraindications—Known hypersensitivity to sulfamethoxazole or any sulfonamide; pregnancy.

Precautions—Adjust the dose in animals with renal impairment. Maintain adequate fluid intake or administer $NaHCO_3$ to avoid crystalluria. Continue administration for 48 hours after disappearance of clinical signs.

Drug Interactions—PABA-containing compounds and local anesthetics derived from PABA (e.g. procaine, proparacaine, tetracaine) may decrease the effect of sulfamethoxazole. Anticoagulants, methotrexate, oral hypoglycemic drugs, and hydatoin anticonvulsants may be displaced from binding and/or their metabolism inhibited by sulfamethoxazole. Sulfamethoxazole may be displaced from binding sites by phenylbutazone, salicylates and probenecid.

Pharmaceutical Formulations—Sulfamethoxazole is available in 500 mg and 1 g tablets and also in 500 mg/5 ml oral suspension. The drug is available in combination with trimethoprim as Co-trimoxazole˙.

SULFAQUINOXALINE

Sulphaquinoxaline

Proprietary Names—

Proprietary Name	Constituents Other Than Sulfaquinoxaline
Embazin*	None
Embazin Forte*	Diaveridine and vitamin K
Keprococ*	Amprolium and vitamin K
Quinoxipra-SP*	Diaveridine
Quinoxipra-P*	Pyrimethamine
Amprosulvit*	Amprolium and vitamin K
Coccifor*	Sulfadimidine, ethopabate, Oxytetracycline, vitamin A, and vitamin K
Ampro-sul*	Amprolium, ethopabate and vitamin K
Ancoxin*	Amprolium
Coccisan*	Amprolium and vitamin K
Assupermed*	Amprolium and vitamin K
Coccimed*	Amprolium and vitamin K
Biccocin*	Amprolium
Pluricoccin*	Pyrimethamine
Allecid*	Pyrimethamine

Chemical Class—Sulfonamide.

Pharmacological Class—Antimicrobial agent; Antibacterial agent.

Source—Synthetic.

Solubility, Stability and Storage—Sulfaquinoxaline is practically insoluble in water and very slightly soluble in alcohol. Store Sulfaquinoxaline formulations at room temperature.

Pharmacological Actions—Sulfaquinoxaline is active against coccidial organisms and certain bacteria such as *Salmonella gallinarum* and *Pasteurella multocida*.

Mechanism of Action—See sulfaclozine.

Mechanism of Selective Toxicity—See sulfaclozine.

Indications—Used singly or in combination with other drugs such as amprolium or pyrimethamine for control and treatment of coccidiosis in cattle, chickens and turkeys; control of fowl typhoid caused by *Salmonella gallinarum* in chickens and turkeys and acute fowl cholera caused by *Pasteurella multocida*. Sulfaquinoxaline is also indicated for the control of coccidiosis in rabbits.

Dosages—

Recommended dose is 0.25%-0.4% in drinking water.

For the control and treatment of coccidiosis in cattle and calves, give diluted solution for 3-5 days.

For the control of coccidiosis in chickens, give the drug for 2-3 days, skip 3 days, give 2 more days.

To control coccidiosis in turkeys, give the drug for 2 days, skip 3 days, give for another 2 days, skip 3 days, give for a final 2 more days.

Give sulfaquinoxaline for 2-3 days in cases of fowl typhoid and acute fowl cholera.

Route(s) of Administration—Per os.

Distribution—Sulfaquinoxaline attains high concentration in liver, kidney, and caecum.

Residue Limit—0.1 ppm in edible tissues of chickens, turkeys, cattle, calves, sheep, and rabbits; 0.01mcg/ml in milk.

Withdrawal Period—Treated birds must not be slaughtered for use as food for at least 12 days after the last treatment with sulfaquinoxaline.

Toxicity and Adverse Effects. Toxicity has been reported in chickens and dogs. Signs include hypothermia and pale mucous membranes. Sulfaquinoxaline causes hypothrombinemia. Pathological signs include enlarged pale livers, pale bone marrow, gangrenous dermatitis and widespread hemorrhages which may be predominant on the epicardium, kidney, intestine and caecum.

Management of Overdose/Toxicity—Treat with vitamin K.

Contraindications—Hypersensitivity to sulfaquinoxaline or other sulfonamides; laying birds.

Drug Interactions—PABA-containing compounds and local anesthetics derived from PABA (e.g. procaine, proparacaine, tetracaine) may decrease the effect of sulfaquinoxaline.

Pharmaceutical Formulations—Sulfaquinoxaline is available as soluble powder singly or in combination with other drugs.

SULFASALAZINE

Sulfasalazine

Synonyms—Salicylazosulfapyridine; Salazosulfapyridine.

Proprietary Names—Azulfidine˙; Azaline˙.

Chemical Class—Sulfonamide-salicylic acid combination.

Pharmacological Class—Antimicrobial drug; gut-active sulfonamide.

Source—Synthetic.

Solubility, Stability and Storage—Sulfasalazine is more soluble in alcohol than water. Store sulfasalazine products in tight containers at room temperature.

Pharmacological Actions—Sulfasalazine is a combination of sulfapyridine and 5-aminosalicylic acid. It has bacteriostatic action against Gram-positive and Gram-negative bacteria. It also has anti-inflammatory action.

Mechanism of Action—Sulfasalazine antimicrobial action is due to inhibition of folic acid synthesis by the sulfapyridine moiety. The 5-aminosalicylic acid moiety acts locally to reduce inflammatory response and systemically to reduce GI secretion by inhibiting prostaglandin synthesis.

Indications—Treatment of colitis in dogs and cats.

Dosages—

    Dog: 20-30 mg/kg every 8 hours for 3-6 weeks depending on the severity.

    Cat: 10-20 mg/kg every 8-12 hours for 10 days.

Route(s) of Administration—Per os.

Absorption—Sulfasalazine is very poorly (10-30%) absorbed from the intestine.

Bioavailability—Oral bioavailability is low.

Distribution—Sulfasalazine is poorly distributed. Small amounts appear in feces and milk.

Metabolism—The drug is cleaved into active sulfapyridine and 5-aminosalicylate by intestinal bacteria. Sulfapyridine is then absorbed and metabolized. The 5-aminosalicylic acid exerts its anti-inflammatory effects locally.

Plasma Half-Life—5.7 to 10 hours.

Route(s) of Excretion—Urine and feces. It is excreted as unchanged drug and metabolites in urine.

Toxicity and Adverse Effects—Keratoconjunctivitis has been observed in dogs but this is rather uncommon. Sulfasalazine is capable of disrupting tear production which may manifest as squirting of the eye or apparent eye discomfort. This is the most common side effect seen. Gastrointestinal disturbances (anorexia, nausea, vomiting and diarrhea) are common. Hematological effects characterized by leukopenia, and hemolytic anemia are potential adverse effects. Hypersensitivity reactions involving skin and mucous membranes and characterized by itching, rash, serum sickness-like reactions and photosensitization are common. Sulfasalazine may cause foliate deficiency. Decreased sperm count has been reported in dogs and laboratory animals at high doses.

Management of Overdose—Give general antidotal therapy. Urine alkalinization and forced diuresis may be necessary.

Contraindications—Hypersensitivity to sulfasalazine, or any sulfonamide; GI or genitourinary obstruction; hypersensitivity to salicylates; pregnancy.

Precautions—Use sulfasalazine cautiously in cats because of its salicylate content. Use cautiously also in renal impairment, hepatic insufficiency; urinary obstruction, and blood dyscrasia.

Drug Interactions—Iron, PABA, PABA-derived local anesthetics may decrease the effects of sulfasalazine. Digoxin may work less effectively in the presence of sulfasalazine. Drugs whose actions may be enhanced following displacement from binding site by sulfasalazine include methotrexate, warfarin, thiazide diuretics, aspirin and phenytoin.

Pharmaceutical Formulations—Sulfasalazine is available in 500 mg tablets, 500 mg enteric coated tablets and 250 mg/5 ml oral suspension.

SULFISOXAZOLE

Sulfisoxazole

Synonyms—Sulphafurazole.

Proprietary Names—Gantrisin*; Azo Gantrisin* (in combination with phenazopyridine).

Chemical Class—Sulfonamide; Sulfanilamide derivative.

Chemical Name—N'-(3,4-dimethyl-5-isoxazolyl) sulfanilamide.

Pharmacological Class—Antimicrobial drug.

Source—Synthetic.

Solubility, Stability and Storage—Sulfisoxazole has solubility of approximately 0.13 mg/mL in water at 25°C. Sulfisoxazole acetyl, the N 1-acetyl derivative, is practically insoluble in water. The relative solubility of sulfisoxazole in alkaline and slightly acidic urine makes the drug particularly useful for the treatment of urinary tract infections. Sulfisoxazole preparations should be protected from light and moisture.

Pharmacological Actions—Sulfisoxazole is bacteriostatic to Gram-positive and Gram-negative bacteria, clamydia, actinomyces, norcardia species and some protozoan organisms.

Mechanism of Action—See sulfaclozine.

Mechanism of Selective Toxicity—See sulfaclozine.

Indications—Treatment of urinary tract infections caused by *E. coli, Proteus vulgaris, Pseudomonas aeruginosa* and Gram-positive cocci in dogs and cats; aid in treatment of bacterial pneumonia and bacterial enteritis caused by organisms sensitive to sulfisoxazole.

Dosages—130-250 mg/kg daily in divided doses every 6 hours. Administration of one-half daily dosage at 12-hour intervals or one-third daily dosage at 8-hour intervals provide a more constant blood level.

Route(s) of Administration—Per os and topical.

Absorption—Sulfisoxazole is rapidly absorbed from the GIT. Peak plasma concentration is attained within 2-3 hours.

Bioavailability—96 ± 14%.

Distribution—Vd = 0.15 ± 0.02 L/kg in humans. Sulfisoxazole differs from other sulfonamides in that its distribution is largely confined to the extracellular space. It reaches 8-57% of blood concentrations in CSF when meninges are normal; higher CSF concentrations may be reached if the meninges are inflamed.

Plasma Protein Binding—91.4 ± 1.2 % in humans.

Metabolism—Sulfisoxazole is acetylated in the liver into inactive metabolites. It is also conjugated with glucuronic acid. Acetylation is less important in animals.

Plasma Half-Life—6.6 ± 0.7 hours in humans.

Clearance—0.33 ± 0.01 (ml/min/kg) in humans.

Route(s) of Excretion—Urine with 49 ± 8% as unchanged drug. Sulfisoxazole is rapidly excreted. Urinary alkalinization reduces tubular reabsorption and affects urinary excretion of sulfisoxazole.

Dialysis Status—More than 50% can be removed by hemodialysis.

Toxicity and Adverse Effects—The adverse effects observed following treatment with sulfisoxazole are similar to those of other sulfonamides and they involve several organs or systems including blood, bone marrow, skin, kidney, liver, nervous system and GIT. GI disturbances (anorexia, nausea, vomiting and diarrhea); neurological effects (lethargy, depression); hematological disorders characterized by agranulocytopenia, thrombocytopenia, aplastic anemia and hepatitis have been observed. Hypersensitivity reactions involving skin and mucous membranes as well as photosensitization are common.

Management of Overdose/Toxicity—Withdraw the drug; administer fluids and give symptomatic treatment.

Contraindications—Known hypersensitivity to sulfisoxazole or other sulfonamide; pregnancy; urinary obstruction.

Precautions—Repeat dosage at 24-hour intervals for 2 to 3 days after disappearance of clinical symptoms. Provide adequate supply of drinking water. Use sulfisoxazole cautiously in animals with renal or hepatic impairment.

Drug Interactions—PABA-containing compounds and local anesthetics derived from PABA (e.g. procaine, proparacaine, tetracaine) may decrease the effect of sulfisoxazole. Anticoagulants, methotrexate, oral hypoglycemic drugs, and hydatoin anticonvulsants may be displaced from binding and/or their metabolism may be inhibited by sulfisoxazole. Sulfisoxazole may be displaced from binding sites by phenylbutazone, salicylates and probenecid.

Pharmaceutical Formulations—Sulfisoxazole is presented in 500 mg tablets. It is also available as sulfisoxazole acetyl in 500 mg/ml suspension, 500 mg/5 ml syrup and 1 g/5ml time-release liquid as well as sulfisoxazole diolamine in 4% solution and ointment for topical use in the eye. Fixed-dose combination with phenazopyridine (500 mg sulfisoxazole and 50 mg phenazopyridine) is available.

TACROLIMUS

Proprietary Names—Prograf; Protopic.

Chemical Class—Macrolide.

Pharmacological Class—Calcineurin inhibitor; immunosuppressant.

Source—Produced by *Streptomyces tsukubaensis*.

Solubility, Stability and Storage—Tacrolimus is practically insoluble in water but soluble in alcohol.

Pharmacological Actions—Tacrolimus has anti-inflammatory and immunosuppressive or immunomodulatory properties. It stimulates tear production.

Mechanism of Action—The exact mechanism is uncertain. In the treatment of atopic dermatitis, the mechanism(s) of action of tacrolimus appears to involve inhibition of the proliferation of T—lymphocytes and cytotoxic cells by inhibition of calcium dependent pathways that effect the enzymatic action of calcineurin. Tacrolimus also has been shown to inhibit release of mediators from skin mast cells and basophils and to downregulate the expression of high-affinity receptors for immunoglobulin E (IgE) on Langerhans cells.

Indications—Primarily for treatment of keratoconjunctivitis sicca (KCS) in dogs and cats and also for treatment of immune-mediated dermatologic diseases including atopic dermatitis, pemphigus, miliary dermatitis and eosinophilic granuloma complex. Tacrolimus is considered more effective than cyclosporine in the treatment of KCS. It is useful in animals that are refractory to cyclosporine.

Dosages—Apply to affected parts every 12 hours. Animals with immune-mediated KCS will need to be on treatment for the rest of their lives.

Route(s) of Administration—Topical (for cutaneous problem and KCS); intravenous and orally (in humans for organ transplant).

Absorption—Absorption of tacrolimus after oral administration in humans is erratic and generally poor. Tacrolimus may be absorbed into systemic circulation following topical application but serum concentrations are generally low, the apparent systemic bioavailability being less than 0.5%. Broken skin theoretically may increase systemic exposure to the drug.

Bioavailability—Oral bioavailability is 5 to 67% (mean, 30%).

Distribution—Vd = 0.5 to 1.4 L/kg. Tacrolimus is primarily associated with red blood cells. It undergoes extensive tissue distribution. It is distributed in milk following systemic administration.

Plasma Protein Binding—77 to 99%.

Metabolism—Tacrolimus is extensively (>99%) metabolized in the liver and in the GI tract following IV or oral administration in humans undergoing organ transplant. Hepatic impairment causes increased plasma concentration, prolonged half-life and reduced clearance.

Plasma Half-life—43 hours in healthy human volunteers and 12 to 16 hours in transplant patients.

Clearance—0.6 to 5.4 (mean, 1.8) L/h/kg.

Route(s) of Excretion—Elimination is primarily via bile (>90% of an absorbed dose is excreted in bile as metabolites. Less than 1% of the dose is excreted in urine as the unchanged drug.

Toxicity and Adverse Effects—Tacrolimus is very well tolerated when used topically. GI symptoms may arise from ingestion of the topical ointment (licking). Animal studies using tacrolimus indicate a possible dose-related risk of lymphoma and other malignancies, particularly of the skin, possibly secondary to immunosuppressive effects of the drug. Systemic use of tacrolimus in kidney and liver transplant in human patients has been associated with development of lymphoma and skin cancers.

Contraindications—Hypersensitivity to tacrolimus.

Pharmaceutical Formulations—Tacrolimus is available in 0.03 or 0.1% ointment suitable for animal use.

TERBINAFINE

Proprietary Names—Lamasil˚.

Chemical Class—Allylamine.

Pharmacological Class—Antifungal agent.

Source—Synthetic.

Solubility, Stability and Storage—Terbinafine should be stored at room temperature and protected from light exposure.

Pharmacological Actions—Terbinafine is active *in vitro* against many fungi including *Trichophyton, Microsporum, Epidermophyton, Aspergillus, Blastomyces* as well as yeasts. Terbinafine is fungicidal to most dermatophytes but only fungistatic to *Candida*. It is more active than azole (including imidazole) derivatives (e.g. ketoconazole, itraconazole) against dermatophytes but is less active than these drugs against *Candida* species.

Terbinafine

Mechanism of Action—Terbinafine inhibits squalene epoxidase, thus blocking the biosynthesis of ergosterol, an essential component of fungal cell membranes.

Mechanism of Selective Toxicity—Mammalian squalene epoxidase is only inhibited at higher (4000 fold) concentrations than is needed for inhibition of the dermatophyte enzyme.

Indications—Treatment of dermatophytosis (ringworm infection).

Route(s) of Administration—Per os and topical.

Absorption—Terbinafine is readily absorbed from gastrointestinal tract.

Distribution—It concentrates in the skin and fat tissues of the body.

Plasma Protein Binding—>99%.

Plasma Half-life—36 hours.

Toxicity and Adverse Effects—The most common side effect is upset stomach. More rarely but also more seriously, there have been cases of liver failure, skin reactions, and bone marrow suppression.

Contraindications—Kidney or liver disease; pregnancy; lactating animal; known hypersensitivity to terbinafine.

Precautions—Oral terbinafine works best when given with food.

Pharmaceutical Formulations—Terbinafine is presented in 250 mg tablets as well as a 1% gel for topical use.

TERBUTALINE

Terbutaline

Proprietary Names—Brethine®; Bricanyl®.

Pharmacological Class—Sympathomimetic agent; Beta$_2$-adrenergic agonist.

Source—Synthetic.

Solubility, Stability and Storage—Terbutaline is soluble in water and slightly soluble in methanol. Terbutaline sulfate is stable in solutions of pH 1-7 and is sensitive to excessive heat and light. Store products at room temperature and protect from light. Discolored solutions of terbutaline sulfate should not be used.

Pharmacological Actions—Terbutaline selectively inhibits smooth muscle contraction thereby causing smooth muscle relaxation or dilatation. It causes bronchodilation and vasodilatation.

Mechanism of Action—Terbutaline activates beta$_2$-adrenergic receptors.

Indications—Adjunctive treatment of tracheobronchitis, collapsing trachea, pulmonary edema and allergic bronchitis in small animals.

Dosages—0.01 mg/kg subcutaneously every 4 hours or 0.03 mg/kg orally every 8 hours.

Route(s) of Administration—Per os and subcutaneous.

Absorption—Terbutaline is poorly (33-50%) absorbed from the GIT in humans. It is well absorbed from the subcutaneous site.

Bioavailability—Oral bioavailability is 14 ± 4 % in humans.

Effective Concentration—2.3 ± 1.8 ng/ml.

Onset of Action—Oral, 30-45 minutes in humans; SC, 6-15 minutes in humans.

Peak Action—SC, 30-60 minutes; Oral, 2-3 hours in humans.

Duration of Action—SC, 4 hours; Oral, 8 hours in humans.

Distribution—Vd = 1.8 ± 0.2 L/kg (humans).

Plasma Protein Binding—20-25% (humans).

Metabolism—Terbutaline is partly metabolized in the liver to inactive sulfate products.

Plasma Half-life—11-16 hours (humans).

Clearance—3.4 ± 0.6 ml/min/kg in humans.

Route(s) of Excretion—Urine with 56 ± 4% as unchanged drug in humans.

Dialysis Status. Nondialyzable.

Toxicity and Adverse Effects. CNS excitement, tachycardia, tremors and dizziness have been reported. These effects are dose related and may be transient. Terbutaline causes sweating and CNS excitement in horses. Overdose may cause cardiac arrhythmias, hypertension, vomiting, seizures, mydriasis and CNS stimulation.

Management of Overdose/Toxicity—Give supportive and symptomatic therapy. Cardio selective β-adrenergic blocker (e.g. atenolol) may be used with caution.

Contraindications—Hypersensitivity to terbutaline or any component.

Precautions—Use terbutaline with caution in patients with diabetes, hyperthyroidism, hypertension, seizure disorders or cardiac diseases.

Drug Interactions—Concurrent use of terbutaline with other sympathomimetic agents may increase the likelihood of cardiovascular adverse effects. Monoamine oxidase inhibitors and tricyclic antidepressants may enhance the pressor effects of terbutaline. Administration of terbutaline to animals under anesthesia induced with halogenated hydrocarbon anesthetic agents may enhance the potential of terbutaline to cause cardiac arrhythmias. Concurrent use with digitalis may induce cardiac arrhythmia. Bronchodilation may be enhanced by concomitant administration of methylxanthine (e.g. aminophylline) in patients that have experienced receptor down regulation due to prolonged terbutaline administration.

Pharmaceutical Formulations. Terbutaline is presented as terbutaline sulfate in 2.5 mg and 5 mg tablets as well as 1 mg/ml solution for injection. Metered-dose inhaler is available for humans. No specific veterinary formulation is available.

TESTOSTERONE

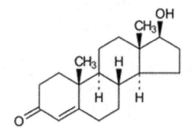

Testosterone

Proprietary Names—Testoject-50˙; Aquaviron˙; Testosterone implants˙; Delatestryl˙; Durateston˙.

Chemical Class—Steroid.

Pharmacological Class—Androgen.

Source—Testosterone is a naturally occurring hormone. It may be obtained from animal testes but is usually prepared synthetically from cholesterol.

Solubility, Stability and Storage—Testosterone and its esters are insoluble in water, freely soluble in alcohol and soluble in vegetable oils. Testosterone enanthate injection should be stored at room temperature. It may form precipitate if stored at a low temperature.

Pharmacological Actions—Testosterone promotes the development of the male phenotype in the fetus and initiates the development and maintenance of accessory sex organs, secondary sexual characteristics, sex drive and spermatogenesis at puberty in the male. It has anabolic effects which include nitrogen retention, protein sparing, increased muscle mass, electrolyte retention, bone metabolism and erythropoiesis. Testosterone regulates gonadotropin output by a feedback mechanism on the hypothalamus.

Mechanism of Action—Testosterone acts by activation of the cytoplasmic androgen receptor [directly or through its metabolite, 5α-dihydrotestosterone (DHT)] and also by conversion to estradiol and activation of certain estrogen receptors. DHT binds more avidly to androgen receptors than testosterone. The hormone-receptor complex undergoes a structural change that allows it to move into the cell nucleus and bind directly to hormone response elements (HREs) and influence transcriptional activity of certain genes, producing the androgen effects.

Indications—Reversion of feminization in male dogs which could occur in patients with Sertoli cell tumors; suppression of oestrus in bitches and queens; treatment of pseudopregnancy in bitches; treatment of certain skin conditions in dogs and cats (e.g. endocrine alopecia, alopecia due to hypogonadism in male dogs and senile alopecia in male dogs); prophylaxis of urethra calculi in castrated male cat; deficient sex drive and infertility due to hypogonadism.

Dosages—10 mg every 10-14 days in bitches and queens to delay estrus; 25-50 mg in dogs for infertility.

Route(s) of Administration—Parenteral.

Absorption—Testosterone is rapidly absorbed from IM sites. Approximately 10% of the dose applied on the skin surface is absorbed into systemic circulation.

Plasma Protein Binding—Approximately 40% of testosterone in plasma is bound to sex hormone-binding globulin and 2% remains unbound and the rest is bound to albumin and other proteins.

Metabolism—Testosterone is metabolized to 17-keto steroids through two different pathways. The major active metabolites are estradiol and dihydrotestosterone (DHT).

Plasma Half-Life—10 to 100 minutes.

Route(s) of Excretion—Urine and feces.

Toxicity and Adverse Effects—The administration of androgens to prepubertial animals may result in early epiphyseal closure. Testosterone causes exacerbation of pre-existing seborrhoeic dermatitis in bitches and queens. Medication may be associated with sodium and water retention which may aggravate cardiac insufficiency. Undesirable virilisation such as clitoral enlargement and a low grade vaginitis can occur from overdose in some human females. Testosterone may cause azoospermia in normal men; sustained erection in hypogonadal males at the beginning of therapy; masculinization in women and female animals. It may cause damage to female fetus in utero and also exacerbate prostrate hypertrophy.

Management of Overdose/Toxicity—Should unwanted virilisation occur, medication should be discontinued until symptoms regress. After which reduced dosage may then be introduced.

Contraindications—Cardiac insufficiency or prior history of liver or kidney disease; pregnancy; prostrate hypertrophy; androgen dependent neoplastic conditions.

Precautions—Use testosterone cautiously in cardiac and renal insufficiency.

Pharmaceutical Formulations—Testosterone is commercially available as the base, and as the cypionate, enanthate, and propionate esters. It is presented in aqueous suspension for injection.

TETRACYCLINE

Tetracycline

Synonyms—TCN.

Proprietary Names—Hostacycline˚; Idilin˚; Achromycin˚; Panmycin˚; Sumycin˚; Tetralan˚; Nor-Tet˚, Robitet˚; Teline˚; Tetracyn˚; Latycin˚; Mysteclin˚; Latycin˚; Nyacycline˚; Racycline˚; Steclin˚; Tetrafect˚; Tetrasuiss˚; Tetrivo˚; Unimycin˚; Upcyclin˚.

Chemical Class—Polycyclic naphthacenecarboxamide derivative.

Pharmacological Class—Broad spectrum bacteriostatic antibiotic.

Source—Semisynthetic (from chlortetracycline).

Pharmacological Actions—TCN is bacteriostatic to a wide range of microorganisms including Gram-positive and Gram-negative bacteria, rickettsia, chlamydia and many spirochaetes. Some protozoa are susceptible. TCN may be bactericidal at high doses.

Mechanism of Action—TCN inhibits protein synthesis by binding principally to the 30s subunit of ribosome to prevent access of aminoacyl tRNA to the acceptor site of the mRNA-ribosome complex thereby preventing the addition of amino acids to the growing peptide chain.

Indications—Treatment of infections involving respiratory, urinary, gastrointestinal and soft tissues caused by susceptible Gram-positive and Gram-negative bacteria, rickettsia and mycoplasma such as pneumonia, scours, metritis, mastitis, leptospirosis, erysipelas and ehrlichiosis.

Dosages—

Large animals	2-4 mg/kg IM.
	11-22 mg/kg in 3 or 4 divided doses orally/day.
Small animals	4-11 mg/kg IM at a strength of 50 mg/ml in two divided doses/day.
	33-110 mg/kg in 3 or 4 divided doses orally/day.
Birds	10g soluble powder/4.5 liters of drinking water for 5-10 days.

Route(s) of Administration—Per os, intramuscular (in animals) and topical.

Absorption—About 60-80% of tetracycline is absorbed from the GIT. Peak plasma concentration is attained within 2-4 hours. Food or dairy products reduce GI absorption of oral preparations of tetracycline by 50% or more. It is poorly absorbed from the IM site (plasma level is poorer than with oral absorption).

Bioavailability—77% (oral); <40% (IM).

Distribution—Vd (L/kg) = 1.5 ± 0.08 in humans and 1.2 to 1.3 in small animals. TCN is concentrated in the liver. It undergoes enterohepatic circulation, crosses uninflamed meninges, penetrates into body fluids and tissues and crosses the placenta. It is distributed into milk.

Plasma Protein Binding—65 ± 3% in humans.

Metabolism—Not metabolized.

Plasma Half-Life (hours)—Humans, 10.6 ± 1.5 (57-108 in end stage renal disease); dogs and cats, 5-6.

Clearance—1.67 ± 0.24 (ml/min/kg).

Residue Limit—0.25 ppm in edible tissues of cattle, pigs, sheep, chickens and turkeys.

Withdrawal Period—

Calf: 4 days (soluble powder) and 12 days (oral bolus).

Sheep: 5 days (oral bolus).

Pig: 7 days (soluble powder).

Route(s) of Excretion—Urine and feces; 58 ± 8% appear in urine as unchanged drug.

Dialysis Status—Not dialyzable.

Toxicity And Adverse Effects—Oral administration of tetracycline may cause nausea, vomiting and diarrhea in humans and animals. The drug may cause hepatotoxicity (characterized by cytoplasmic changes, increase in fat, jaundice, azotemia, acidosis especially during pregnancy). Renal toxicity, discoloration of teeth and depression of bone growth in the young are also produced by tetracycline. It causes pain and thrombophlebitis following parenteral administration.

Management of Overdose/Toxicity—Give symptomatic and supportive therapy.

Contraindications—Hypersensitivity to oxytetracycline or other tetracyclines; latter half of pregnancy; growing animals.

Precautions—Reduce the dose of tetracycline in patients with hepatic or renal impairment. Do not administer tetracycline simultaneously with milk, antacids, calcium, magnesium and iron salts. Give oral dose when the stomach is not full. Do not use expired drug so as to avoid nephropathy.

Drug Interactions—Absorption of tetracycline is impaired by concurrent administration of dairy products, aluminum hydroxide gel, bismuth subsalicylate, Ca, Mg and Fe salts. Concurrent use with methoxyflurane may cause fatal nephrotoxicity. TCN potentiates the action of warfarin.

Pharmaceutical Formulations—Tetracycline is obtainable as the base and hydrochloride salt in 100 mg/ml oral suspension, 500 mg oral boluses, and in 10g, 25g soluble powder for addition to drinking water.

THIOGUANINE

Thioguanine

Synonyms—Tioguanine; 6-Thioguanine; 2-Amino-6-Mercaptopurine; TG; 6-TG; 2-aminopurine-6-thiol.

Proprietary Names—Thioguanine®.

Chemical Class—Purine analog.

Pharmacological Class—Antineoplastic drug; Anticancer agent; Antimetabolite.

Source—Synthetic.

Solubility, Stability and Storage—Thioguanine is insoluble in water and in alcohol. It is stable when stored at room temperature in tight containers.

Pharmacological Actions—Thioguanine has anticancer and moderate myelosuppressive actions. It inhibits DNA and RNA syntheses.

Mechanism of Action—Thioguanine is converted to the corresponding monoribonucleotide, 6-thioguanosine-5'-phosphate, which inhibits the conversion of inosine monophosphate to adenine and guanine nucleotides.

Indications—Adjunctive treatment of acute leukemia in dogs and cats.

Dosages—

　　Dog:　40 mg/m^2 orally every 24 hours initially, then every 3 days.

　　Cat:　25 mg/m^2 orally every 24 hours initially, and then every 30 days as needed.

Route(s) of Administration—Per os.

Absorption—Oral absorption of thioguanine is variable and usually incomplete; about 30% is absorbed in humans. Peak plasma concentration is attained within 2-4 hours of administration.

Bioavailability—Oral bioavailability is variable.

Distribution—Thioguanine crosses the placenta. It is detectable in DNA and RNA of bone marrow.

Metabolism—Thioguanine is metabolized extensively in the liver to both active and inactive metabolites.

Plasma Half-life—11 hours in humans.

Route of Excretion—Urine.

Dialysis Status—Non dialyzable.

Toxicity and Adverse Effects—Thioguanine has low therapeutic index. Its myelosuppressive effect is moderate at therapeutic dose and is characterized by gradual onset, anemia, leucopenia and less severe thrombocytopenia. Overdose causes bone marrow depression, nausea and vomiting.

Management of Overdose/Toxicology—Give supportive therapy. There is no antidote.

Contraindications—Hypersensitivity to thioguanine; evidence of previous resistance to thioguanine or mercaptopurine; pregnancy.

Precautions—Reduce thioguanine dose in animals with hepatic or renal impairment. Thioguanine is potentially carcinogenic and teratogenic hence pregnant women must avoid handling this and other antineoplastic agents. Use cautiously in animals with history of urolithiasis.

Drug Interactions—Cross-resistance exists between mercaptopurine and thioguanine. Thioguanine may produce additive bone marrow depression with other antineoplastic agents and bone marrow depressants such as chloramphenicol, flucytosine, amphotericin B, and colchicine. Azathioprine, cyclophosphamide, corticosteroids and other immunodepressants may increase the risk of infection when used concurrently with thioguanine. Halothane, ketoconazole, primidone, valproic acid and other hepatotoxic drugs may increase the hepatotoxic potential of thioguanine.

Pharmaceutical Formulations. Thioguanine is available in 40 mg tablets. No specific veterinary formulation is available.

THIOPENTONE

Synonyms—Thiopental.

Proprietary Names—Pentothal ˚; Intraval sodium ˚.

Chemical Class—Barbiturate; Thiobarbiturate.

Pharmacological Class—Intravenous Anesthetic Agent; Central Nervous System Depressant; General Anesthetic Agent; Sedative–Hypnotic; Ultrashort-acting CNS depressant.

Source—Synthetic.

Solubility, Stability and Storage—Thiopentone is soluble in water and alcohol and highly soluble in lipids. Thiopental sodium powder for injection should be stored at controlled room temperature of 15-30°C. The powder for injection may be reconstituted with sterile water for injection, 0.9% sodium chloride or 5% dextrose injection. The 2-5% solutions of thiopental sodium are physically and chemically stable for 3 days at room temperature or 7 days when refrigerated. However, solutions should be stored in tight containers under refrigeration to maximize stability. Thiopentone is physically incompatible with acids, acidic salts and oxidizing agents; do not mix with these agents. Use only water for injections or physiological saline as solvent.

Thiopentone sodium

Pharmacological Actions—Thiopentone causes CNS depression which rapidly results in hypnosis and anesthesia without analgesia or excitement. It causes profound respiratory depression.

Mechanism of Action—Thiopentone prolongs the post-synaptic inhibitory effect of gama aminobutyric acid in the thalamus by binding at a distinct binding site associated with Cl^- ion pore at the $GABA_A$ receptor and increasing the duration of time for which the Cl^- ion pore is opened.

Indications—Induction and maintenance of general anaesthesia in horses, dogs and cats. It may be used as the sole anesthetic agent for brief (15 minute) procedures or for induction of anesthesia prior to administration of other anesthetic agents such as inhalational agents.

Dosages—25-30 mg per kg in young healthy dogs and cats. Administer thiopental to effect. The first 5 mg per kg of the computed dose should be injected over a period of 10 seconds. After waiting for 30-40 seconds, further small increments are given until the required depth of anaesthesia is reached. A pause of 30-40 seconds should be made between injections to allow the effects of each increment to be observed. In very young, elderly or debilitated animals the initial dose must be reduced by 50% and the administration time increased to about one minute. The use of premedicants has the effect of reducing the required dosage of thiopentone to 10 mg/kg bodyweight or less. The recommended dose in horses is 10 mg/kg. The dose is given intravenously by rapid injection into the jugular vein and the dose volume should not exceed 50 ml. Injection should be completed in 8-10 seconds.

Route(s) of Administration—Intravenous.

Effective Concentration—19 ± 7 mcg/ml.

Distribution—$Vd = 2.3 \pm 0.5$ L/kg. Thiopentone is rapidly distributed to the vascular tissues of the brain and other organs because of its high lipid solubility. This is followed by redistribution to lean tissues such as muscle and finally very slowly to fat.

Plasma Protein Binding—$85 \pm 4\%$. Binding is reduced in the aged, cirrhosis, renal disease and cardiopulmonary bypass surgery.

Metabolism—Thiopentone is metabolized in the liver to pentobarbitone and inactive products.

Plasma Half-Life—Biphasic; initially 9 minutes as a result of redistribution and then 9.0 ± 1.6 hours. Half-life is higher in old animals, obesity, cirrhosis and neonates.

Clearance—3.9 ± 1.2 (ml/min/kg).

Duration of Action—5 to 30 minutes.

Route(s) of Excretion—Thiopentone is excreted via urine as inactive metabolites, with small amounts as unchanged drug.

Withdrawal Periods—Horse meat: 28 days.

Toxicity and Adverse Effects—Rapid administration of a bolus dose of thiopentone may cause serious hypotension and has resulted in death from circulatory failure. Hypothermia may arise in foals younger than 12 weeks and puppies and kittens below 8 weeks of age due to delayed recovery. Accidental injection into the perivenous tissues may cause severe tissue reaction. Local extravasation can cause extensive necrosis and sloughing. Intra-arterial injection causes intense pain. Overdose causes respiratory depression and hypotension.

Management of Overdose/Toxicity—Inject procaine through the same needle in case of extravasation of thiopentone. Administer plasma volume expanders and pressor agents in cases of overdose. Respiratory stimulants may be used in cases of mild respiratory depression. Artificial respiration, with the administration of oxygen may be necessary in deeper levels of depression.

Contraindications—Shock or hypovolemia, valvular disease and pericarditis in dogs and cats; hypersensitivity to barbiturates.

Precautions—Administer thiopentone under expert supervision. Facilities for resuscitation and endotracheal intubation should be on standby. Avoid accidental injection into tissues other than veins. Provide intravenous access. Use thiopentone cautiously in hepatic or renal disease and in hypotension. Administer the drug singly. It is safer to tolerate slight limb movements or respiratory irregularities caused by surgical stimulation than to administer supplementary doses of thiopentone. Avoid intra-arterial injection.

Drug Interactions—CNS depressants may enhance thiopentone depressant action. Antihypertensive drugs and diuretics may enhance its hypotensive effect. Salicylates and sulfisoxazole may increase its toxicity. Thiopentone solution is alkaline and is incompatible with acidic drugs such as succinylcholine, atropine sulfate etc.

Pharmaceutical Formulations—Thiopentone **is** available as powder in vials of 250 mg, 400 mg, 500 mg, 1 g, 2.5 g and 5 g.

THIOPHANATE

Thiophanate

Proprietary Names—Nemafax*.

Chemical Class—Probenzimidazole.

Pharmacological Class—Anthelmintic.

Source—Synthetic.

Pharmacological Actions—Thiophanate is extremely effective in removing the adult and larval forms of the main gastrointestinal nematodes in cattle, sheep and goats. It is also effective against worms causing parasitic bronchitis in sheep and goats, adult and larval stomach worms, and nodular worms in pigs. It is active against worm eggs.

Mechanism of Action—Thiophanate binds selectively to beta-tubulin and inhibit microtubule formation. This action results in progressive energy depletion, inhibition of waste products and degenerative alteration in the integument and intestinal cells.

Indications—Treatment and prophylaxis of helminthiasis in cattle, sheep, goat and pig.

Dosages—50-100mg/kg body weight as a drench or premix.

Route(s) of Administration—Per os.

Absorption—Rapidly absorbed; peak plasma concentration is achieved within 8 hours.

Metabolism—Thiophanate is converted by cyclisation to benzimidazole carbamates.

Route(s) of Excretion—Faces (major) and urine.

Withholding period—Seven days (slaughter); 3 days (milk).

Toxicity and Adverse Effects—It is a very safe drug; 20 times the therapeutic dose did not produce toxic effects.

Contraindications—None.

Pharmaceutical Formulations—Thiophanate is available as 20% w/v suspension; 22.50% w/v premix; 70% w/w wettable powder; 22.5% w/w premix and bolus.

THIOTEPA

Synonyms—Triethylenethiophosphoramide; TESPA; TSPA; Thiophosphoramide.

Proprietary Names—Thiotepa®.

Chemical Class—Ethyleneimine; Alkylating agent.

Pharmacological Class—Antineoplastic drug.

Source—Synthetic.

Solubility, Stability and Storage—Thiotepa is soluble in water and freely soluble in alcohol. Keep thiotepa formulations refrigerated. Reconstituted powder is stable for 5 days if refrigerated. At higher temperatures thiotepa is inactivated by polymerization which occurs faster in warm and moist conditions. Do not use reconstituted product with precipitate or that has become opaque. Protect products from light.

Thiotepa

Pharmacological Actions—Thiotepa has cytotoxic actions due to disruption of nucleic acid function by interfering with DNA replication, RNA transcription and replication. It is cell cycle nonspecific and it possesses immunosuppressive properties.

Mechanism of Action—Protonation of the aziridine ring nitrogen causes the ring to open resulting in the formation of reactive molecule that reacts with DNA phosphate groups to produce cross-linking of the DNA strands leading to inhibition of DNA, RNA and protein synthesis.

Indications—Adjunctive treatment of carcinomas, neoplastic effusions and transitional cell tumors in dogs.

Dosages—0.2-0.5 mg/m².

Route(s) of Administration—Intravenous and intracavitary.

Absorption—Thiotepa is poorly absorbed from the GIT. Absorption from intramuscular and intracavitary sites are variable.

Distribution—Distribution characteristics are not known.

Metabolism—Thiotepa is rapidly converted by hepatic mixed function oxygenase to triethylenephosphoramide (TEPA).

Plasma Half-life—1.2 to 2 hours for the parent drug and 3-24 hours for the primary metabolite (TEPA) in humans.

Route(s) of Excretion—Urine with < 10% as parent drug.

Toxicity and Adverse Effects—These include bone marrow depression with prominent leukopenia and GI toxicity characterized by vomiting, diarrhea, stomatitis and intestinal ulceration. Uric acid may precipitate in kidney tubules with overdose. Thiotepa causes pain at injection site.

Management of Overdose/Toxicity—Give supportive therapy.

Contraindications—Hypersensitivity to thiotepa; severe bone marrow depression; pregnancy.

Precautions—Use thiotepa with caution in patients with infection and bone marrow depression. Reduce the dose in patients with renal and/or hepatic impairment. Use milk replacers if administered to nursing bitches. Handle thiotepa with extreme caution.

Drug Interactions—Simultaneous use of thiotepa with other alkylating agents or irradiation enhances toxicity. The risk of infection may increase if used with other immunodepressants.

Thiotepa inhibits plasma pseudocholinesterase and prolongs the actions of neuromuscular blockers such as succinylcholine.

Pharmaceutical Formulations. Available in 15 mg powder for injection.

THYROGLOBULIN

Proprietary Names—Proloid*.

Chemical Class—Iodinated thyronine derivative.

Pharmacological Class—Thyroid hormone.

Source—Natural; a purified extract of pig thyroid.

Pharmacological Actions—Thyroglobulin possesses the actions of thyroxine and triiodothyronine. Thus, it causes normal growth and development as well as increased basal metabolic rate and cholesterol metabolism.

Mechanism of Action—The exact mechanism is uncertain.

Indications—Treatment of thyroid hypofunction manifesting as hairless calf, hairless piglet, and big neck; treatment of goiter, myxedema, unthritiness, slow growth, poor hair color and lethargy.

Route(s) of Administration—Per os.

Absorption—Variable and incomplete.

Plasma Half-Life—6 to 7 days; 3-4 days in hyperthyroidism.

Route(s) of Excretion—Bile and feces.

Toxicity and Adverse Effects—Elevated and irregular heart rate, forceful heartbeat, prominent arterial pulse, increased appetite, loss of weight, flushed moist and warm skin, weak and tremulous muscles, insomnia, restlessness and increased bowel movement are early manifestations of overdose. Excessive dosage results in iatrogenic thyrotoxicosis.

Management of Overdose/Toxicosis—Withdraw the drug if adverse effects become serious and give symptomatic treatment.

Contraindications—Hypersensitivity to thyroglobulin.

Drug Interactions—Estrogens increase the level of protein binding by thyroglobulin but binding to plasma protein is inhibited by salicylate and dicoumarol.

Pharmaceutical Formulations—Thyroglobulin for clinical use is available in tablets.

THYROTROPIN

Synonyms—Thyroid-stimulating hormone; thyrotrophic hormone; TSH.

Proprietary Names—Thytropar*.

Chemical Class—Glycoprotein.

Source—Natural; obtained from bovine pituitary glands.

Solubility, Stability and Storage. Thyrotropin lyophilized powder for injection may be stored at room temperature. Reconstituted product is stable for up to 3 weeks if refrigerated.

Pharmacological Actions—Thyrotropin stimulates the formation and secretion of thyroid hormones.

Mechanism of Action—Thyrotropin binds to specific receptors and activates adenylate cyclase resulting in accumulation of cAMP and phosphorylation of various cellular proteins. These cellular activities result in increased thyrocyte iodine uptake, thyroid hormone organification and secretion.

Indications—Differential diagnosis of hypothyroidism in dogs, cats and horses.

Dosage—

Dog: 0.1 unit/kg (maximum of 5 units).

Cat: 1 unit/kg.

Horse: 5-10 units.

Route(s) of Administration—Intravenous (favored in animals), intramuscular and subcutaneous.

Absorption—Thyrotropin is well absorbed from muscular and subcutaneous sites.

Metabolism—The drug is degraded in the liver.

Half-Life—Approximately 1 hour depending upon thyroid state.

Route(s) of Excretion—Urine.

Toxicity and Adverse Effects—Adverse effects are relatively few. Tachycardia, hyperthermia, nausea, and vomiting have been observed. Repeated administration may cause anaphylaxis. Local soreness at the site of injection is common. An overdose may cause weight loss, sweating, and tachycardia. Prolonged use may cause thyroid hyperplasia.

Management of Overdose/Toxicity—Give symptomatic treatment.

Contraindications—Known hypersensitivity to thyrotropin or any component in its preparation.

Precautions—Use thyrotropin cautiously in patients with heart disease, adrenocortical insufficiency/suppression or hypopituitarism.

Pharmaceutical Formulations—Thyrotropin for clinical use exist in vials containing 10 units in the lyophilized form for reconstitution.

TIAMULIN

Proprietary Names—Tiamutin˙.

Chemical Class—Pleuromutilin.

Pharmacological Class—Antimicrobial agent.

Solubility, Stability and Storage—Store at room temperature (25ºC). Protect from light and moisture.

Pharmacological Actions—Tiamulin is a broad spectrum bacteriostatic agent. It is active against *Klebsiella pneumonia, Staphylococcus, Streptococcus, Pasteurella, Actinobacillus, Haemophilus, Fusobacterium, Bacteroides,* and *Campylobacter* species. Tiamulin has an exceptional overall activity against the mycoplasmas being the most active antibiotic against *M. gallisepticum* with almost 100% sensitivity. It is also highly active against *M. synoviae, M. meleagridis* and is also capable of preventing losses from many secondary infections. The rate of development of resistance to tiamulin is very slow, especially in comparison with tylosin. Tiamulin is suitable for use in breeding and laying birds.

Mechanism of Action—Tiamulin prevents protein synthesis in susceptible organisms.

Indications—Treatment and prevention of mycoplasma infections such as enzootic pneumonia of pigs; chronic respiratory diseases and infectious synovitis of chickens and turkeys; treatment and prevention of pig dysentery, porcine colonic spirochetosis and porcine proliferative enteropathy. The drug is also used in conjunction with tetracyclines against other primary (*A. pleuropneumoniae*, *B. bronchiseptica*) and secondary (*P. multocida*) respiratory pathogens. Tiamutin at 50 ppm and chlortetracycline at 150 ppm, in both feed and water, is very effective for prevention (100ppm/300ppm for treatment) of *M. gallisepticum* infections in broilers.

Dosages—

Chicken	Treatment of chronic respiratory disease (CRD) and infectious synovitis: 25-50mg tiamulin/kg bodyweight (inclusion level of 500ppm tiamulin in feed or 250 mg per litre water) daily for 3-5 consecutive days.
	Prevention and control of CRD in broilers: 3mg tiamulin/kg bodyweight (inclusion level of 30ppm tiamulin in the feed or 125 mg/litre) daily administered for the period of risk e.g. 1-5 weeks.
	Prevention and control of CRD in breeders and layers and improvement in egg production: 3mg tiamulin/kg bodyweight (inclusion level of 50ppm tiamulin in the feed) daily administered one week per month throughout the laying period.
Turkey	1g of 45% Water Soluble Powder/1.8 L drinking water (0.025%, 250 mg /litre) for 5 consecutive days.
Pig	Treatment of pig dysentery: 6-7.5mg/kg body weight.
	Prevention of pig dysentery: 1.5-2.0mg/kg body weight.
	Prevention and treatment of respiratory diseases: 8-10mg/kg BW

Route(s) of Administration—Per os (via drinking water or feed).

Absorption—Over 90% of tiamulin is absorbed from the GIT. Peak plasma concentrations are attained within 2 hours after administration.

Distribution—Tiamulin is well distributed throughout body tissues. It attains up to 40 times blood levels in the lungs. This is a kind of pharmacokinetic reservoir, to maintain tiamulin concentrations in the extracellular fluid where the mycoplasmas live. Tiamulin can also concentrate into polymorphs at 5-10 times the surrounding antibiotic concentration. This may play an additional role in combating the mycoplasmas that are engulfed by these immuno-defensive cells. Tiamulin penetrates into eggs in the laying hen at levels in excess of most strains of *M. gallisepticum* MIC for up to 9 days following medication for 3 days at 0.0125% or 0.025% in drinking water or at 200 and 400 ppm in feed.

Metabolism—Tiamulin is metabolised in the liver.

Withdrawal Period—Two days before slaughter of chicken; 5 days for turkey; 7 days for pigs; zero for eggs.

Route(s) of Excretion—Urine.

Toxicity and Adverse Effects—Water intake may be depressed during the administration of tiamulin to birds. This appears to be concentration dependent with 0.025% tiamulin reducing intake by approximately 15%. Severe growth depression or even death may result if administered concurrently with monensin, salinomycin, maduramycin, or narasin. The situation is transient and recovery normally occurs within 3-5 days following withdrawal of tiamulin treatment.

Management of Overdose/Toxicity—Stop tiamulin feed medication immediately and replace with fresh feed if interaction with ionophore (polyether) anticoccidial drugs like monensin, salinomycin, maduramycin, or narasin occurs.

Contraindications—Known hypersensitivity to tiamulin; concomitant administration with monensin, narasin or salinomycin.

Precautions—Do not administer products containing monensin, narasin or salinomycin, during or for at least seven days before or after treatment with therapeutic doses of tiamulin. People with known hypersensitivity to tiamulin should administer the product with caution. When mixing with feed, direct contact with mucous membranes or skin should be avoided as it may cause irritation.

Drug Interactions—Tiamutin has synergistic activity with the tetracyclines. Tiamulin interferes with the metabolism of the ionophore anticoccidial drugs (e.g. monensin, salinomycin, maduramycin and narasin). Concomitant use of tiamulin and the ionophore anticoccidial drugs may cause severe growth depression or even death.

Pharmaceutical Formulations—Tiamulin is presented as tiamulin hydrogen fumarate in 45% water soluble powder; 12.5% solution; 10% and 80% premix.

TICARCILLIN

Proprietary Names—Ticar®, Timetin® (ticarcillin and clavulanic acid), Ticilin®.

Chemical Class—6-aminopenicillanic acid derivative.

Pharmacological Class—Carboxypenicillin; Extended-spectrum penicillin; Antipseudomonas penicillin.

Source—Semisynthetic.

Pharmacological Actions—Ticarcillin is bactericidal to *Pseudomonas aeruginosa*, indole positive *Proteus* and *Enterobacter*. It is more active than carbenicillin.

Mechanism of Action—The mechanism is same as for other penicillins. See penicillin G.

Indications—Treatment of endometritis caused by beta hemolytic streptococci in horses and systemic infections caused by *Pseudomonas aeruginosa*. Also effective in combination with clavulanate potassium for the treatment of infections caused by, or suspected of being caused by, susceptible β-lactamase-producing strains of *Citrobacter, Enterobacter, Escherichia coli, Haemophilus influenzae, Klebsiella, Serratia,* and *Staphylococcus* when an extended-spectrum penicillin alone would be ineffective.

Ticarcillin

Dosages—

Dog, cat	75-100 mg/kg every 6-8 hours.
Horse	44-50 mg/kg every 6-8 hours.
	6g intrauterine/day for 3 days during estrus for treatment of endometritis.
Bird	200 mg/kg every 8 hours.

Route(s) of Administration—Intramuscular and intravenous.

Absorption—Up to 86% is absorbed from intramuscular site. Peak plasma concentration is attained within 30-75 minutes(IM).

Bioavailability (IM): 65% in horses.

Distribution—Vd (L/kg) = 0.21 ± 0.03 (human), 0.22-0.25 (horse), 0.34 (dog). The drug is distributed to milk, pleural fluid, interstitial fluid and bile. It is almost excluded from CSF except when meninges are inflamed. Concentration of ticarcillin in milk rises with mastitis.

Plasma Protein Binding—65% in humans.

Metabolism—10 to 15% of ticarcillin is hydrolyzed to inactive products in humans.

Plasma Half-Life—Human, 1.3 ± 0.1 hours (higher in uremia); dogs and cats, 45-80 minutes; horses, 54 minutes.

Clearance—(ml/min/kg)—Human, 2.0 ± .02 (lower in uremia); dogs, 4.3; horses, 2.8 to 3.2.

Withdrawal Period—2 days (milk).

Route(s) of Excretion—Urine with 92 ± 2% as unchanged drug.

Dialysis Status—Dialyzable.

Toxicity and Adverse Effects—Hypersensitivity reaction ranging from skin rash to anaphylaxis. Convulsion, electrolyte imbalance, hemolytic anemia, interstitial nephritis and myoclonus of muscles have been observed in less than 1% of humans at therapeutic doses. Overdose may cause neuromuscular hypersensitivity reaction (characterized by agitation, seizures and confusion), electrolyte imbalance and renal failure.

Management of Overdose/Toxicity—Set up hemodialysis; give supportive and symptomatic treatment.

Contraindications—Hypersensitivity to ticarcillin, the penicillins, their products or components.

Precautions—Reduce ticarcillin dose in animals with renal impairment. Use ticarcillin cautiously in animals with seizures. Do not use the milk of treated animals for human food within 2 days after treatment has stopped. Refrigerate ticarcillin or use within 30 minutes after reconstitution. Do not mix ticarcillin physically with aminoglycoside antibiotics.

Drug Interactions—Tetracyclines decrease ticarcillin efficacy. High concentration of ticarcillin inactivates aminoglycoside antibiotics physically, otherwise there is synergism between ticarcillin and aminoglycoside antibiotics. Probenecid increases ticarcillin plasma level. Ticarcillin increases the duration of action of neuromuscular blockers. Concurrent administration of ticarcillin with clavulanic acid results in a synergistic bactericidal effect which expands the spectrum of activity of ticarcillin against many strains of β-lactamase-producing bacteria that are resistant to ticarcillin alone.

Pharmaceutical Formulations—The drug is used clinically as ticarcillin disodium formulated in 1-, 3-, 6-, 20-, and 30—g powder in vials for injection with each gram containing about 5mEq of Na⁺. It is also available in combination with clavulanic acid.

TILMICOSIN

Tilmicosin

Proprietary Names—Pulmotil˚; Micotil˚.

Chemical Class—Macrolide.

Pharmacological Class—Antibiotic.

Source—Semi-synthetic.

Solubility, Stability and Storage—Tilmicosin remains stable in animal feed for 1 month. Store tilmicosin formulations at room temperature, preferably below 25°C. Protect them from direct sunlight and humidity.

Pharmacological Actions. Tilmicosin is active primarily against Gram-positive bacteria, although some Gram-negative bacteria are affected. *Mycoplasma* and *Pasteurella haemolytica* are sensitive to tilmicosin.

Mechanism of Action—Uncertain.

Indications—Treatment of bovine respiratory diseases (BRD) caused by *Pasteurella haemolytica*; treatment of pneumonia caused by *Actinobacillus pleuropneumoniae, Mycoplasma hyopneumoniae, Haemophilus parasuis, Pasteurella multocida* and other organisms sensitive to tilmicosin in growing fattening pigs.

Dosages—

Growing fattening pigs: 8-16 mg/kg bodyweight (200-400g tilmicosin activity per tonne of feed) for 15 days.

Cattle: 10 mg/kg.

Route(s) of Administration—Per os (in pig feed) and subcutaneous.

Distribution—Tilmicosin apparently concentrates in lung tissue. At 3 days post injection, the lung:serum ratio is about 60:1.

Withdrawal Period. The periods before slaughter are 14 days for pigs and 28 days for cattle.

Toxicity and Adverse Effects—Tilmicosin has low safety margin. It may cause local tissue reaction at IM injection site. Edema may be noted at the site of subcutaneous injection. Tilmicosin has been shown to be fatal in pigs, non-human primates and potentially fatal in horses and humans. It may cause skin irritation.

Management of Overdose/Toxicity—Withdraw the drug and give prompt supportive and symptomatic treatment.

Contraindications—Known hypersensitivity to tilmicosin.

Precautions—Do not administer tilmicosin intravenously. Do not allow horses or other equines access to feeds containing tilmicosin. Safe use in pregnant animals or in animals to be used for breeding purposes has not been demonstrated. Avoid contact with skin and eyes.

Drug Interactions—Epinephrine may enhance mortality due to tilmicosin.

Pharmaceutical Formulations—The drug is available in three dosage forms, namely, sterile solution containing 300 mg tilmicosin base/ml for injection, oral solution containing 250 mg tilmicosin activity for inclusion in the drinking water of chickens and granules containing 100 g tilmicosin for inclusion in animal feeding stuffs.

TOLAZOLINE

Synonyms—Benzazoline.

Proprietary Names—Priscoline® (human preparation); Tolazine® (veterinary preparation).

Chemical Class—Imidazolines.

Pharmacological Class—α-adrenergic receptor blocker.

Source—Synthetic.

Stability and Storage—Tolazoline is soluble 1 in 0.5 of water and 1 in 2 of ethanol. Store formulations between 15-30⁰C in light-resistant containers. Tolazoline is compatible with IV fluids.

Pharmacological Actions—Tolazoline relaxes vascular smooth muscles, causes vasodilatation and reduced peripheral resistance.

Mechanism of Action—Tolazoline blocks the actions of alpha-adrenergic agonists reversibly.

Tolazoline hydrochloride

Indications—To reverse the effects of xylazine.

Dosages—

Horse, dog, cat	4 mg/kg at 1 ml/sec IV rate
Cattle, sheep, goat	2-4 mg/kg.

Route(s) of Administration—Intravenous.

Onset of Action—Within 5 minutes.

Peak Effect—30 minutes.

Duration of Action—Tolazoline has short duration of action.

Distribution—Tolazoline is widely distributed. It attains highest concentrations in the liver and kidneys.

Plasma Half-Life—1 hour in horses and 3-10 hours in neonates. Half-life increases in patients with renal impairment.

Withdrawal Period—30 days (slaughter).

Route(s) of Excretion—Urine (mainly as unchanged drug). Excretion rate is rapid.

Toxicity and Adverse Effects—Tolazoline causes transient tachycardia, sweating, congested mucous membranes, piloerection, clear lacrimal and nasal discharges, apprehension, licking and flipping of lips, and muscle fasciculations. Overdose may cause increased gastrointestinal motility and ventricular arrhythmia which may lead to death.

Management of Overdose/Toxicity—Xylazine reduces the effects of tolazoline overdose. Ephedrine reduces tolazoline-induced hypotension.

Contraindications—Shock; stress; debility; hypovolemia; sympathetic blockage; cardiac disease; cerebrovascular disease; hypersensitivity to tolazoline or related compounds.

Precautions—Humans having conditions that are contraindications for the use of tolazoline should handle the drug with caution. Reduce the dose in animals with renal impairment.

Drug Interactions—Tolazoline decreases the vasopressor effects of norepinephrine and epinephrine when the drugs are used concurrently. This action is followed by a rebound increase in blood pressure. Tolazoline exhibits disulfiram-like action when used with ethanol.

Pharmaceutical Formulations—The drug is available as tolazoline hydrochloride in 100 mg/ml (Tolazine®) or 25 mg/ml (Priscoline®) solution for injection.

TOLTRAZURIL

Toltrazuril

Proprietary Names—Baycox®.

Chemical Class—Triazinetrione derivative; Symmetrical triazinetriones.

Pharmacological Class—Anticoccidial drug.

Source—Synthetic.

Solubility, Stability and Storage—Following dilution in drinking water toltrazuril is stable for 24 hours. Do not store toltrazuril above 25°C. Dilutions which are more concentrated than 1:1,000 (1 ml Baycox 2.5% to 1 litre drinking water) may result in precipitation.

Pharmacological Actions—Toltrazuril has broad spectrum anticoccidial and antiprotozoal properties. It is coccdiocidal, potent and active against developing first and second generation schizonts and gamates of pathogenic *Eimeria* species of various birds (chicken, geese, ducks, others) and mammals (cattle, sheep, goats, pigs, others). It is also active against parasites of fish (microsporidia, myxozoa, monogeneans), and bees (*Nosema* species). Toltrazuril exhibits a long residual activity and may protect chickens against infection for at least 2 weeks.

Mechanism of Action. Toltrazuril inhibits nuclear division and mitochondrial activity. It damages the wall-forming bodies in macrogamates and causes severe vacuolisation by inflation of the endoplasmic reticulum in all intracellular developmental stages of *Eimeria*.

Indications—Treatment and control of coccidiosis in various animal species. Toltrazuril may be medicated intermittently instead of conventional continuous medication. It may allow development of immunity.

Dosages—

Chicken: 7 mg toltrazuril per kg bodyweight per day given for 2 consecutive days. This corresponds to 28 ml Baycox 2.5% solution (equivalent to 700 mg toltrazuril) per 100 kg of bodyweight per day for 2 consecutive days.

Other animals: 5-20 mg/kg.

Route(s) of Administration—Per os.

Absorption—Toltrazuril is slowly but extensively absorbed from the GIT. Peak plasma concentration is attained within 120 hours. In poultry, toltrazuril is absorbed at a rate of 50% or more.

Distribution—Toltrazuril attains high concentration in the liver, kidney muscle and fat.

Metabolism—Toltrazuril is degraded to toltrazuril sulfone which is persistent and mobile in groundwater.

Plasma Half-life—154 hours.

Residue Limit—2 mcg/kg (Acceptable Daily Intake).

Withdrawal Period—19 days.

Route(s) of Excretion. Urine and feces.

Toxicity and Adverse Effects. Toltrazuril is well tolerated in birds, mammals and other animals.

Contraindications. Known hypersensitivity to toltrazuril.

Precautions. Toltrazuril is not recommended for the prevention of coccidioses in broiler chickens because of long withdrawal period. Do not use toltrazuril in layers.

Drug Interactions. There is cross resistance between toltrazuril and diclazuril.

Pharmaceutical Formulations. Available as 2.5% water soluble liquid for mixing with drinking water.

TRIMETHOPRIM

Proprietary Names—

Proprietary Name	Constituents Other Than Trimethoprim
Proloprim*	None
Triampex*	None
Bimotrim*	Sulfadoxine

Borgal*	Sulfadoxine
Potensulf*	Sulfadoxine
Trimidox*	Sulfadoxine
Tribrissen*	Sulfadiazine
Tucoprim*	Sulfadiazine
Uniprim*	Sulfadiazine
Bimotric Co*	Sulfadiazine
Trimazine*	Sulfadiazine
Cotrim*	Sulfadiazine
Diatrim*	Sulfadiazine
Vetcoprim*	Sulfadiazine
Aquarim*	Sulfadiazine
T.S. Sol*	Sulfamethoxazole
Triprim*	Sulfamethazine
Trisulmix*	Sulfadimethoxine
Sultiject*	Sulfadimethoxine

Chemical Class—2,4-diaminopyrimidine.

Pharmacological Class—Antimicrobial drug; Dihydrofolate reductase inhibitor.

Source—Synthetic.

Solubility, Stability and Storage—Trimethoprim is slightly soluble in water; soluble in benzyl alcohol; sparingly soluble in chloroform and in methanol; slightly soluble in alcohol and in acetone; practically insoluble in ether. Store trimethoprim products at room temperature.

Trimethoprim

Pharmacological Actions. Trimethoprim has bacteriostatic action against many Gram-positive cocci, including *Staphylococcus aureus, S. saprophyticus, Streptococcus pyogenes, S. pneumoniae,* and *S. faecalis*. Some Gram positive bacilli such as *Corynebacterium diphtheriae* and *Listeria monocytogenes* are susceptible. Other organisms known to be susceptible to trimethoprim include some strains of *Neisseria meningitides* and *N. gonorrhoeae*; some Gram-negative aerobic bacilli like *E. coli, Proteus mirabilis, Haemophilus influenzae, Klebsiella, Enterobacter, Serratia, Salmonella* and *Shigella* species; certain pathogenic protozoa like *Pneumocystis carinii*; *Toxoplasma* and *Plasmodium* species are susceptible. Trimethoprim produces bactericidal effect when combined with a sulfonamide.

Mechanism of Action—Trimethoprim blocks the action of bacterial dihydrofolate reductase which converts dihydrofolic acid to tetrahydrofolic acid. Because the conversion of dihydrofolic acid to tetrahydrofolic acid is blocked, folate cannot be produced, thus preventing the reactions necessary for the synthesis of certain amino acids (such as glycine, methionine), purines, thymidine, and ultimately, DNA, RNA and protein.

Indications—Treatment of a wide variety of infections in all animal species commonly in combination with sulfonamides.

Dosages—5 mg/kg body weight twice a day.

Route(s) of Administration—Per os.

Absorption—Trimethoprim is rapidly and completely absorbed from the GIT. Peak plasma concentration is attained within 1-4 hours. Absorption is delayed in a fed horse. Trimethoprim is not as well absorbed from oral route in sheep and dogs.

Bioavailability—~ 100% (human); 90 to 92% (pig); 41% (Quail). Bioavailability of oral trimethoprim is greatly reduced in ruminating calves as compared to preruminating calves.

Distribution—Vd = 1.8 ± 0.2 L/kg (human; values are higher in neonates and lower in children); 1.67-2.36 L/kg (calves); 1.68 L/kg (horses); 1.8 L/kg (pigs). Trimethoprim is widely distributed in body tissues and fluids including CSF. It concentrates in prostrate and vaginal fluids; attains high levels in bronchial, seminal fluid, synovial fluids, saliva, sputum, bone, and aqueous humor. It crosses the placenta readily. Trimethoprim is distributed into milk; its concentrations in milk could be 1.3 to 3.5 times the plasma concentration measured at the same time in goats, cows, and pigs.

Plasma Protein Binding—Trimethoprim binding to plasma protein is independent of plasma concentration. Some values are humans, 44%; cows, 57%; goats, 48%; horses, 50%; pigs, 33 to 54%.

Metabolism—Trimethoprim is extensively metabolized in many species, including cows, goats, and pigs.

Plasma Half-Life—11 ± 1.4 hours in humans (longer in uremia; shorter in children and cystic fibrosis); 3.35-5.92 hours (pigs); 1.18 hours (cattle; higher in calves); 0.63 hours (broiler).

Clearance—2.2 ± 0.6 ml/min/kg (humans; lower in uremia; higher in children and cystic fibrosis); 6.6 mL/min/kg (ruminating calves); 8.49 mL/min/kg (horses); 9.1 mL/min/kg (pigs).

Route(s) of Excretion—Urine with 69 ± 17% as unchanged drug.

Dialysis Status—20-50% dialyzable.

Toxicity and Adverse Effects—The most common adverse effects are pruritus, maculopapular and morbilliform skin rash. Gastrointestinal effects such as epigastric distress, nausea, vomiting and glossitis are common. Hematologic reactions like thrombocytopenia, leukopenia, neutropenia, megaloblastic anemia, methemoglobinemia may occur following large doses, prolonged therapy or in folate deficient cases. It produces fetal abnormalities in rats that received large doses.

Management of Overdose/Toxicology—Treat symptomatically.

Contraindications—Hypersensitivity to trimethoprim, or any component; pregnancy; megaloblastic anemia due to folate deficiency; creatinine clearance below 15 ml/min.

Precautions—Intrauterine administration of trimethoprim formulations is not recommended. Concurrent use of other folic acid antagonists with trimethoprim or use of trimethoprim between courses of other folic acid antagonists is not recommended because of the possibility of an increased risk of megaloblastic anemia.

Drug Interactions—A trimethoprim and sulfonamide combination administered to a detomidine-anesthetized horse may cause arrhythmias, hypotension, and death due apparently to potentiation of cardiac changes caused by detomidine. Trimethoprim increases the effect or toxicity of phenytoin. Concurrent use of bone marrow depressants with sulfonamides or aminopyrimidines may increase the leukopenic and/or thrombocytopenic effects. Concurrent use of trimethoprim with cyclosporine may increase the metabolism of cyclosporine, resulting in reduced cyclosporine plasma concentrations. Trimethoprim may inhibit warfarin metabolism and consequently potentiate its activity.

Pharmaceutical Formulations—Trimethoprim in combination with sulfadoxine, silfadiazine, sulfadimethoxine and sulfamethoxazole in tablets, boluses, oral suspensions, oral solutions and wettable powder are available for animal use. Formulations are available in various strengths e.g.

- 5 mg trimethoprim/25 mg sulfadiazine
- 20 mg trimethoprim/100 mg sulfadiazine
- 80 mg trimethoprim/400 mg sulfadiazine
- 160 mg trimethoprim/800 mg sulfadiazine.
- 80 mg trimethoprim/400 mg sulfamethoxazole

Trimethoprim is available singly in 100 mg and 200 mg tablets.

TRIPELENNAMINE

Triplennelamine

Synonyms—Pyribenzamine.

Proprietary Names—PBZ˚; Pelamine˚.

Chemical Class—Ethylenediamine derivative.

Pharmacological Class—Antihistamine; Histamine H_1-receptor antagonist; Antipruritic drug; First generation antihistamine.

Source—Synthetic.

Solubility, Stability and Storage—One gram of tripelennamine is soluble in 1 ml of water or 6 ml of alcohol. Tripelennamine slowly darken upon exposure to light. Store tripelennamine injection at room temperature and protect from light; avoid freezing or excessive heat. Tablets should also be stored at room temperature in tight containers.

Pharmacological Actions—Tripelennamine antagonizes histamine actions in the respiratory tract, intestines, blood vessels and skin. When compared to other antihistamines, tripelennamine has minimal anticholinergic properties and is only moderately sedating.

Mechanism of Action—Tripelennamine competes with histamine at the H_1 receptor sites and prevent the actions of histamine.

Indications—To reduce or prevent the effects of histamine released during allergic reactions in cattle, horses, dogs and cats. The drug is effective in controlling allergic skin conditions, hives, bee stings, and itchy skin. Tripelennamine has been used as a CNS stimulant in "Downer cows" when slowly injected intravenously.

Dosages—

    Horses: 1.1 mg/kg every 6-12 hours.

    Guinea pig: 5 mg/kg.

Route(s) of Administration—Oral and intramuscular routes are popular.

Metabolism—Tripelennamine is metabolized in the liver by hydroxylation and glucuronidation.

Withdrawal Period—Four days before slaughter of cattle and 24 hours before milking.

Route(s) of Excretion—Urine.

Toxicity and Adverse Effects—Tripelennamine causes CNS depression, incoordination and GI disturbances. It may cause transient hyperexcitability, nervousness and muscle tremors in horses if administered intravenously. Overdose may cause CNS excitation, seizures and ataxia.

Management of Overdose/Toxicity. Give symptomatic and supportive treatment. Phenytoin given intravenously may be used in the treatment of seizures caused by tripelennamine overdose.

Contraindications—Known hypersensitivity to tripelennamine; intravenous administration in horses.

Precautions—Extra caution should be used in horses with respiratory problems due to excess mucus.

Drug Interactions—Increased sedation can occur if tripelennamine is combined with other CNS depressant drugs. Antihistamines may partially counteract the anti-coagulation effects of heparin or warfarin.

Pharmaceutical Formulations—It is available as tripelennamine hydrochloride in 20 mg/ml solution for injection; 25 mg and 50 mg tablets; 100 mg extended-release tablets; 37.5 mg (equivalent to 25 mg HCl) per 5 ml elixir.

TUBOCURARINE

Tubocurarine

Synonyms—d-tubocurarine.

Proprietary Names—Curarine*; Jexin*; Tubarine*.

Chemical Class—Cyclic benzylisoquinoline.

Pharmacological Class—Competitive neuromuscular blocker; Non-depolarizing neuromuscular blocker; Muscle relaxant.

Source—Natural; pure alkaloid extract from the stems of *Chondrodendron tomentosum*.

Solubility, Stability and Storage—Tubocurarine is soluble 1 in 20 of water; soluble in ethanol and methanol. Tubocurarine formulations should be refrigerated. The drug is incompatible with barbiturates.

Pharmacological Actions. Tubocurarine causes skeletal muscle paralysis which begins usually in the eyes and spreads to the face, neck, limbs, trunk and finally to the intercostal muscles and the diaphragm. The tail is usually affected at the same time with the head and neck. It does not block muscle contraction arising from direct stimulation of the muscle cell. Tubocurarine also has some ganglion-blocking action and hence may produce a fall in blood pressure. It releases histamine which could be responsible for bronchospasm and increased bronchial secretions observed following its administration.

Mechanism of Action. Tubocurarine competes with acetylcholine (Ach) for the nicotinic receptors at the motor-endplate. It does not activate the receptors but prevent access of Ach molecules to the receptors. Thus, Ach-induced end plate potential are reduced to subthreshold levels or abolished. Consequently, impulse transmission is blocked and the muscle becomes paralysed without preceding stimulation.

Indications—To induce skeletal muscle relaxation as an adjunct to anesthesia; to control convulsions and trauma during tetanus and status epilepticus; also to immobilization non domestic animals.

Dosages.

Dog, cat.	0.4 mg/kg.
Goat	0.3 mg/kg
Sheep	0.4 mg/kg
Guinea pig	0.1-0.2 mg/kg
Mouse	1 mg/kg
NHP	0.09 mg/kg
Rat	0.4 mg/kg
Rabbit	0.4 mg/kg
Pig.	0.2-0.3mg/kg.

Route(s) of Administration. Intravenous and intramuscular (for immobilization).

Absorption—Tubocurarine is poorly absorbed from the GIT.

Onset of Action—4 to 6 minutes.

Peak Action—4 minutes.

Duration of Action—30 to 60 minutes.

Distribution—Vd = 0.22 to 0.39L/kg. Tubocurarine penetrates cells poorly hence it is distributed primarily in the extracellular space but it concentrates at the myoneural junctional regions. Its short duration of action is due to redistribution.

Plasma Protein Binding—About 33 to 50%.

Metabolism—Tubocurarine is minimally metabolized.

Plasma Half-life—2 to 4 hours.

Plasma Clearance—About 2 (mL/min/kg).

Route(s) of Excretion—Urine (with 33-75% as unchanged drug) and bile (with ~10% as unchanged drug).

Dialysis Status. Tubocurarine is nondialyzable.

Toxicity and Adverse Effects. The drug induces hypotension if injected rapidly in dogs.

Management of Overdose/Toxicity—Action of tubocurarine is reversed by anticholinesterase e.g. neostigmine (0.022mg/kg). Atropine (0.04mg/kg) should be administered prior to or in conjunction with neostigmine to circumvent the muscarinic effect of neostigmine.

Contraindications—Hypersensitivity to tubocurarine.

Precautions—Tubocurarine has cumulative tendency; the dose should be reduced if repeated injection is necessary. Due to narrow safety margin of neuromuscular blocking drugs, aminoglycoside antibiotics should be administered with caution in a subject recovering from surgery in which muscle relaxants have been used. Administer tubocurarine to effect.

Drug Interactions—The concurrent use of more than one competitive neuromuscular blocker results in additive effect. Some general anaesthetic agents (e.g. ether, halothane, methoxyflurane, pentobarbital) depress impulse transmission at the somatic myoneural junction. Hence, these agents may synergize with competitive neuromuscular blockers. Magnesium sulphate, ketamine, verapamil, quinidine and furosemide enhance the blocking action of tubocurarine. Aminoglycoside antibiotics are potential neuromuscular blockers; hence, their actions are synergistic with those of other neuromuscular blockers. Tubocurarine reduces the arrhythmogenic action of epinephrine.

Pharmaceutical Formulations—The drug is available as tubocurarine chloride in 3 mg/ml solution for injection.

TYLOSIN

Tylosin

Proprietary Names—Tylamix*; Tylan*; Tyluvet*.

Chemical Class—Macrolide.

Pharmacological Class—Macrolide antibiotic; narrow spectrum antibiotic.

Source—Natural; isolated from a strain of *Streptomyces fradiae*.

Solubility, Stability and Storage—Tylosin is slightly soluble in water. It is soluble in lower alcohols. Tylosin tartrate is soluble 1 in 10 of water, slightly soluble in ethanol, very slightly soluble in chloroform and practically insoluble in ether.

Pharmacological Actions—Tylosin is primarily bacteriostatic to Gram-positive organisms which are generally susceptible to the macrolide antibiotics. It is highly active against *Mycoplasma* species. Some Gram-negative organisms and spirochaetes are susceptible.

Mechanism of Action—Tylosin inhibits protein synthesis by binding reversibly to the 23s rRNA on the 50s ribosomal subunit of susceptible organisms and blocking aminoacyl translocation reaction and elongation of peptide chain.

Indications—Treatment and prevention of chronic respiratory disease in chickens, infectious sinusitis in turkeys and pig dysentery caused by *Treponema hyodysenteriae*. Tylosin is effective in erysipelas, pneumonia and dysentery caused by *Vibrio coli* in pigs, upper respiratory tract infections, cellulites, otitis, metritis, leptospirosis, secondary bacterial infections associated with viral infection in dogs and cats. It is effective in infections associated with surgical procedures or injuries as well as colitis in pets.

Dosages—

Bird	10-40 mg/kg IM 3 to 3 times daily or 0.5 g/liter of drinking water.	
Bovine	18 mg/kg /day IM not to exceed 5 days	
Dog, cat.	0.5-2 mg/kg IM every12-24 hours (do not mix with any other solution) or 20-40 mg/kg /day PO divided every 6-8 hours.	
Mouse	0.2-0.8 mg/100 g IM twice daily or 10 mg/kg SC twice daily or 10 mg/100 g BW PO for 21 days.	
NHP	10 mg/kg IM twice daily.	
Rat	10 mg/kg SC twice daily or 5 g/l in drinking water mixed with dextrose; give 100 ml treated water to each rat daily or 10 mg/100 g PO for 21 days.	
Rabbit	10 mg/kg IM, SC, PO bid	
Reptile	25 mg/kg IM, PO once a day for 7 days	
Pig	8.8 mg/kg BW IM q12h not to exceed 3 days or 2-10 mg/kg BW IM once a day	

Route(s) of Administration—Per os, intramuscular and intravenous routes are popular.

Absorption—Tylosin tartrate is readily absorbed while tylosin phosphate has limited absorption from the intestine. Peak plasma concentration is attained within 1-2 hours.

Plasma Half-Life—4 to 5 hours.

Residue Limit—0.2 ppm in edible tissues.

Withdrawal Period—The values before slaughter are chicken, 3 days following parenteral treatment or 24 hours following oral administration; turkey, 5 days; pig, 21 days. The period before milk is certified consumable is 96 hours.

Route(s) of Excretion—Urine and bile.

Toxicity and Adverse Effects—Tylosin may cause mild reaction characterized by edema of rectal mucosa, partial anal protrusion (rosebudding), erythema and pruritus in pigs. Pain and local reaction may occur at IM site.

Management of Toxicity/Overdose—Give symptomatic treatment.

Contraindications—Laying birds; known hypersensitivity to tylosin.

Precautions—Avoid direct contact with skin. Use tylosin cautiously in patients taking digoxin for heart failure.

Drug Interactions—Tylosin can increase digoxin blood levels.

Pharmaceutical Formulations—Tylosin is available as the base, tartrate and phosphate salts in solution for injection and powder for dispensing in drinking water or feed. Fixed dose combinations with other antibacterial drugs such as doxycycline (Kepro-TyloDox˚) and sulfisoxazole (Tylosin plus˚) are also available.

URSODIOL

Synonyms—Ursodeoxycholic acid.

Proprietary Names—Actigall˚.

Chemical Class—Cholesterol derivative.

Pharmacological Class—Choleretic; Bile acid.

Source—Naturally obtained from the Chinese black bear but it is now synthesized.

Pharmacological Actions—Ursodiol improves the flow of bile to the gall bladder from the liver and from the gall bladder into the intestine. Thus, it facilitates the removal of toxic bile acids (as well as other toxins excreted in bile) from the body. Ursodiol has immunomodulatory, cytoprotective, and membrane stabilizing effects on hepatic cells. It suppresses cholesterol synthesis, secretion and intestinal absorption.

Indications—Treatment of chronic hepatitis, acute hepatic failure or toxic injury, congenital abnormalities including primary portal vein hypoplasia, and juvenile fibrosing liver disease in dogs. It may be used in cats to treat chronic hepatitis, and congenital portosystemic shunts.

Dosages—Ursodiol should be given with food. Refer to the package insert for specific doses.

Route(s) of Administration—Per os.

Absorption—Ursodiol is well absorbed oral site.

Distribution—It is not known if ursodiol is excreted in breast milk.

Toxicity and Adverse Effects—No serious side effects have been reported in dogs and cats. Occasionally, ursodiol causes nausea and diarrhea. It can lower blood cholesterol levels. Chronic use in cats may deplete the levels of taurine, an essential amino acid, thus necessitating dietary supplementation. Ursodiol is toxic to rabbits, baboons, and rhesus monkeys. Overdose causes increase in severity of GI signs, particularly diarrhea.

Management of Overdose/Toxicity—Gastric emptying, activated charcoal and oral administration of an aluminum containing antacid may be indicated.

Contraindications—Biliary obstruction, fistula, and other complications associated with gallstones, or pancreatitis.

Drug Interactions. Aluminum containing antacids may bind ursodiol if both compounds are administered concurrently.

Pharmaceutical Formulations. Ursodiol is available in 300 mg capsules.

VECURONIUM

Proprietary Names—Norcuron˙.

Chemical Class—Ammonio Steroid.

Pharmacological Class—Competitive neuromuscular blocker; Non depolarizing neuromuscular blocker; Intermediate-acting competitive neuromuscular blocker.

Source—Synthetic.

Solubility, Stability and Storage—Vecuronium has solubilities of 9 and 23 mg/mL in water and in alcohol respectively. Store vecuronium powder for injection at room temperature. Protect the formulation from light. Vecuronium bromide solution following reconstitution is only stable for 1-5 days at room temperature. It is unstable in alkaline solutions. Do not mix in the same syringe or administer through the same needle with alkaline solution. Use the reconstituted solution within 24 hours or discard after that. Vecuronium bromide is physically and chemically compatible with normal saline, 5% dextrose and lactated Ringer's solution. Any of these fluids may be used for reconstitution.

Pharmacological Actions—Vecuronium causes skeletal muscle paralysis. Unlike tubocurarine, vecuronium has no ganglion blocking effects and it rarely releases histamine.

Mechanism of Action—Vecuronium competes with acetylcholine (Ach) for the nicotinic receptors at the motor-endplate. It does not activate the receptors but prevent access of Ach molecules to the receptors. Thus, Ach-induced end plate potential are reduced to subthreshold levels or abolished. Consequently, impulse transmission is blocked and the muscle becomes paralysed without preceding stimulation.

Indications—To induce skeletal muscle relaxation as an adjunct to anesthesia; to facilitate endotracheal intubation; to relax skeletal muscle during mechanical ventilation.

Dosages—0.1 mg/kg.

Route(s) of Administration—Intravenous.

Absorption—Poorly absorbed from the GIT.

Onset of Action—1.5 minutes (dose dependent).

Peak Action—3 to 5 minutes.

Duration of Action—30 min (dose dependent).

Distribution—Vd = 0.19-0.25 L/kg in humans.

Metabolism—Vecuronium is partially metabolized in the liver.

Plasma Half-life—58 to 80 min in humans (higher in renal failure).

Clearance—3.0 to 5.2 (ml/min/kg).

Route(s) of Excretion—Urine and bile.

Dialysis Status—Nondialyzable.

Toxicity and Adverse Effects—Vecuronium is well tolerated. Overdose causes prolonged skeletal muscle weakness and apnea.

Management of Overdose/Toxicity—Vecuronium effects can be reversed by anticholinesterase agents e.g. neostigmine (0.022 mg/kg). Atropine (0.04 mg/kg) should be administered prior to or in conjunction with neostigmine to circumvent the muscarinic effect of neostigmine.

Contraindications—Hypersensitivity to vecuronium.

Precautions—Use vecuronium cautiously in animals with myasthenia gravis. Reduce the dose in animals with hepatic or biliary diseases.

Drug Interactions—The concurrent use of vecuronium and another competitive neuromuscular blocker results in additive effect. Some general anaesthetic agents (e.g. halothane, enflurane and isoflurane) synergize with the neuromuscular blocking action of vecuronium. Verapamil, quinidine, furosemide, magnesium sulphate, local anaesthetics, and immuno-depressants enhance its blocking action. Aminoglycoside antibiotics are potential neuro-muscular blockers. Hence, their actions are synergistic with those of other neuromuscular blockers. Cholinesterase inhibitors reverse the action of competitive neuromuscular blockers.

Pharmaceutical Formulations—Available as vecuronium bromide in 10 mg and 20 mg powder for reconstitution to injectable solution.

VINBLASTINE

Synonyms—Vincaleukoblastine; VLB.

Proprietary Names—Alkaban-AQ®; Velban®; Velsar®.

Chemical Class—Alkaloid.

Pharmacological Class. Antineoplastic drug; Anticancer agent; Antimitotic agent; Spindle poison.

Source—Natural; obtained from the periwinkle plant (*Vinca rosea*).

Solubility, Stability and Storage—Vinblastine is freely soluble in water, soluble in methanol and slightly soluble in ethanol. Protect vinblastine products from light. The powder for injection may remain viable for 1-3 months at room temperature. However, it is recommended that the product be stored in the refrigerator. Reconstituted solution for injection may be viable for one month if refrigerated. Do not mix vinblastine with doxorubicin or heparin in the same syringe.

Pharmacological Actions—Vinblastine has antiproliferative action by inhibiting cell replication at the M phase. It is strongly myelosuppressive and has moderate (30-60%) emetogenic potential.

Vinblastine

Mechanism of Action—Vinblastine binds to and cause dissolution of tubulin, an important protein in microtubules. This prevents the assembly of mitotic spindles and failure of chromosomes to move apart during mitosis. Therefore, mitosis is blocked. Microtubules are also important as conduits for the transport of solutes and neurotransmitters, maintenance of cell integrity and secretion of hormones (e.g. insulin and thyroxin). The effect of vinca alkaloids on these later functions may be responsible for their adverse effects.

Indications—Treatment of lymphomas, carcinomas, mastocytomas and splenic tumors in small animals.

Dosages—2-3 mg/m^2.

Route(s) of Administration—Intravenous. Intrathecal administration has been shown to cause death in humans.

Absorption—Absorption from the GIT is not reliable.

Distribution—Vd = 27.3 L/kg. Vinblastine binds to tissue proteins; penetrates the CNS less than vincristine in spite of its higher lipid solubility.

Plasma Protein Binding—99%.

Metabolism—Vinblastine is extensively metabolized in the liver to an active desacetylvinblastine.

Plasma Half-life—Biphasic; 0.164 hours (initial) and 25 hours (terminal).

Route(s) of Excretion—Bile and urine (with 1% as unchanged drug).

Toxicity and Adverse Effects—Severe bone marrow depression characterized by leukopenia and throbocytopenia is the dose-limiting toxicity. Gastroenterocolitis, constipation, stomatitis, inappropriate ADH secretion, alopecia, jaw and muscle pain have all been reported. Peripheral neurotoxicity may be observed at high doses. Vinblastine causes severe tissue irritation. The drug may be teratogenic and embryotoxic.

Management of Overdose/Toxicity—Give symptomatic and supportive therapy. Restrict fluid intake.

Contraindications—Hypersensitivity to vinblastine; pre-existing bone marrow depression or infection.

Precautions—Vinblastine has vesicant properties, therefore, subcutaneous extravasation must be avoided. A different needle other than that used for withdrawing should be used to administer the drug. Handle vinblastine formulations with care. It is recommended that gloves and protective clothing be worn. Wash exposed body parts copiously with soap and water. Inject hyaluronidase subcutaneously and apply heat to the site of extravasation.

Drug Interactions—Concomitant administration of vinblastine and phenytoin may decrease the plasma level of the latter. Bronchospasm may occur if co-administered with or within 8 days of mitomycin-C administration.

Pharmaceutical Formulations—Available as vinblastine sulfate in 1 mg/ml solution for injection.

VINCRISTINE

Synonyms—Leucocristine; VCR; LCR.

Proprietary Names—Oncovin®; Vincasar® PFS.

Chemical Class—Alkaloid.

Pharmacological Class—Antineoplastic drug; Anticancer agent; Antimitotic agent; Spindle poison.

Source—Natural; obtained from the periwinkle plant (*Vinca rosea or Catharanthus roseus*).

Stability and Storage—Keep vincristine products refrigerated although the solution for injection may be stable for one month at room temperature.

Pharmacological Actions—Vincristine has antiproliferative action by inhibiting cell replication at the M phase. It is strongly myelosuppressive and has low (10%) emetogenic potential.

Mechanism of Action—Same as for vinblastine.

Indications—Adjunctive treatment of lymphoid and hematopoietic neoplasm in dogs and cats. Treatment of transmissible venereal neoplasm and immune-mediated thrombocytopenia in dogs.

Dosages—0.5-0.75 mg/m² every week.

Route(s) of Administration—Intravenous. Intrathecal administration has been shown to cause death in humans.

Absorption—Absorption from the GIT is poor.

Distribution—Vincristine distributes rapidly from blood to tissues. It binds to tissue proteins. It penetrates the CNS poorly.

Plasma Protein Binding—75%.

Metabolism—Vincristine is extensively metabolized in the liver.

Plasma Half-life—Biphasic; initial or alpha phase is 13 minutes in dogs while the terminal or beta phase is 75 minutes in dogs or 24 hours in humans.

Clearance—Cleared rapidly from blood.

Route(s) of Excretion—Bile and urine (with 1% as unchanged drug).

Toxicity and Adverse Effects—Neurotoxicity characterized by sensory impairment, paresthesia and paralytic ileus resulting in constipation are prominent adverse effects. Increased liver enzymes, inappropriate ADH secretion, alopecia, jaw and muscle pain, seizures in small animals have also been reported. Overdose causes bone marrow depression, central and peripheral neuronal shrinkage. Seizure, leukopenia and general debility has been reported in cats after overdose. Vincristine causes tissue irritation that can lead to necrosis and sloughing.

Management of Overdose/Toxicity—Give supportive and symptomatic therapy. Restrict fluid intake.

Contraindications—Hypersensitivity to vincristine; pre-existing bone marrow depression or infection.

Precautions—Observe the same precaution as with vinblastine.

Drug Interactions—Same with vinblastine. Additive neurotoxic effect occurs if administered with asparaginase.

Pharmaceutical Formulations. Available as vincristine sulfate in 1 mg/ml solution for injection.

WARFARIN

Proprietary Names—Coumadin*.

Chemical Class—Coumarin derivative.

Pharmacological Class—Anticoagulant.

Source—Synthetic.

Solubility, Stability and Storage—Warfarin is very soluble in water and freely soluble in alcohol. Warfarin sodium is discolored by light; its preparations should be protected from light and stored at controlled room temperature.

Pharmacological Actions—Warfarin alters the synthesis of blood coagulation factors II (prothrombin), VII (proconvertin), IX (Christmas factor or plasma thromboplastin component) and X (Stuart-Prower factor) in the liver. It inhibits thrombus formation when stasis is induced and may prevent extension of existing thrombi. The effect of warfarin is usually delayed until depletion of circulating functional vitamin K-dependent coagulation factors occurs.

Mechanism of Action—Warfarin acts indirectly by interfering with the action of vitamin K_1 in the synthesis of the coagulation factors II, VII, IX, and X. Sufficient amounts of vitamin K_1 can override this effect.

Indications—Long-term treatment (or prevention of recurrence) of thrombotic conditions, usually in cats, dogs or horses.

Dosages—Horse, 30-75 mg/450 kg body weight.

Route(s) of Administration—Per os and intravenous.

Absorption—Warfarin is rapidly and completely absorbed from the GIT in humans. Oral absorption is dissolution-rate controlled and may vary from one commercially available tablet to another. The rate, but not the extent of absorption of the drug is decreased by the presence of food in the GI tract. Peak plasma concentrations of warfarin usually are attained within 90 minutes. Warfarin is absorbed from percutaneous site. Severe toxicity has occurred from repeated skin contact with rodenticides containing the drug.

Effective Concentration—Plasma warfarin concentrations are not necessarily related to antithrombogenic effects and are not useful determinants of anticoagulant dosage requirements.

Onset of Action—Synthesis of vitamin K-dependent coagulation factors occurs within 24 hours but antithrombogenic effects may not occur until 2-7 days.

Distribution—Warfarin is distributed to the liver, lungs, spleen, and kidneys. It crosses the placenta; fetal plasma drug concentrations may be equal to maternal plasma concentrations.

Plasma Protein Binding—99% in humans. There are wide species variations; horses have a higher free (unbound) fraction of the drug than do rats, sheep or pig.

Metabolism—Warfarin is metabolized in the liver to inactive products.

Plasma Half-life—40 hours in humans (range: 20-60 hours); plasma half-life of warfarin is independent of dose and show considerable individual and species variation.

Route(s) of Excretion—Urine and bile.

Toxicity and Adverse Effects—Warfarin may cause hemorrhage, which may manifest as anemia, thrombocytopenia, weakness, hematomas and ecchymoses, epistaxis, hematemesis, and hematuria. The signs of toxicity may not be apparent for 2-5 days after treatment. Acute overdose may result in life-threatening hemorrhage. In dogs and cats, single doses of 5-50 mg/kg have been associated with toxicity. Cumulative toxic doses of warfarin have been reported as 1-5 mg/kg for 5-15 days in dogs and 1 mg/kg for 7 days in cats. Warfarin can cause congenital malformations.

Management of Overdose/Toxicity—Initiate general antidotal therapy. Administer vitamin K_1.

Contraindications—Pregnancy; patients with pre-existent hemorrhagic tendencies or diseases; patients undergoing or contemplating eye or CNS surgery or surgery of large open surfaces; patients with active bleeding from the digestive, respiratory or genitourinary tract; known hypersensitivity to coumarin compounds.

Drug Interactions—In humans, concurrent administration of numerous drugs or dietary or herbal supplements has been reported to affect patient response to coumarin-derivative anticoagulants.

Pharmaceutical Formulations—The drug is available as warfarin sodium in 1-, 2-, 2.5-, 3-, 4-, 5-, 6-, 7.5—and 10-mg tablets and in lyophilized powder for reconstition to injectable solution.

XYLAZINE

Proprietary Names—Rompun®; Gemini®; Agrar xylazine®; Chanazine®; AnaSed®; Sedazine®.

Pharmacological Class—α_2-Adrenergic agonist; sedative; analgesic; muscle relaxant.

Source—Synthetic.

Solubility, Stability and Storage—Xylazine hydrochloride is readily soluble in water, ethanol and methanol.

Pharmacological Actions—Xylazine causes CNS depression and sedation in most animal species. It possesses several actions of morphine but it does not cause CNS stimulation in cats, horses and cattle. It produces analgesia which is superior to those produced by butorphanol, meperidine and pentazocine. Xylazine causes emesis in cats and occasionally in dogs. It causes muscle relaxation and depresses thermoregulatory mechanisms. Its action on the circulatory system is variable. In many species, a short-lived arterial hypertension is followed by a longer period of hypotension and bradycardia. Xylazine causes hypersalivation in cattle. Ruminants are extremely sensitive to the action of xylazine, as they require 1/10th the dose for horses.

Xylazine

Mechanism of Action—Xylazine acts on central and peripheral α_2—adrenergic receptors to decrease sympathetic discharge and release of norepinephrine. α_2-adrenergic receptors in the CNS are found on neurons that control blood pressure. The stimulation of these receptors also modulates pain perception.

Indications—To produce sedation accompanied by analgesia; preanesthetic medication before local or general anesthesia; sometimes to induce vomition in cats following ingestion of poison. Xylazine has been used in combination with etorphine to demobilize wild animals.

Dosages—

Dog, cat.	1.1 mg/kg IV or 1.1 to 2.2 mg/kg IM or SC.
Cattle	0.05-0.15 mg/kg IV or 0.10-0.33 mg/kg IM.
Horse	1.1 mg/kg IV or 2.2 mg/kg IM.
Sheep, goat.	0.05-0.10 mg/kg IV or 0.10-0.22 mg/kg IM
Pig	10 mg/kg IM.
Rabbit	3-5 mg/kg IM.
Rat	3-8 mg/kg IM.
NHP	1-2 mg/kg IM.
Mouse	4-8 mg/kg IM.
Guinea pig	3-5 mg/kg IM.

Route(s) of Administration—Parenteral routes are appropriate.

Absorption—Xylazine is rapidly absorbed from IM site.

Bioavailability—40 to 48% (horse); 17-73% (sheep); 52-90% (dog).

Onset of Action—1 to 2 minutes (horse) following IV; 10-15 minutes in dogs and cats following IM or SC injections or 3-5 minutes (IV).

Peak Action—Sedation peaks at 3-10 minutes in horses following IV; 10-15 minutes in dogs following IM & SC, and 3-5 minutes (IV).

Duration of Action—Dose dependent; the actions produced may last for different durations of time. Analgesia produced may last for 10-15 minutes in dogs but sedation may last for 1-2 hours. Complete recovery occurs in 2-4 hours (dogs and cats) or 2-3 hours (horses). In cattle, some associated effects of xylazine are long lasting; e.g. polyuria (5 hours), hyperthermia (18 hours), hypothermia (24 hours), appearance of diarrhea (12-24 hours). A high dose may cause prostration in a cow for as long as 36 hours.

Distribution—Vd = 1.9-2.7L/kg (dog, horse, sheep, cow).

Metabolism—Xylazine is rapidly and extensively metabolized to several by-products.

Plasma Half-Life—50 minutes (horse), 36.5 minutes (cattle), 23 minutes (sheep), 30 minutes (dog).

Withdrawal Period—3 days (meat) and 48 hours (milk).

Route(s) of Excretion—Urine (with 1% as unchanged drug in cattle).

Toxicity and Adverse Effects—Xylazine causes emesis in cats and occasionally in dogs. It also causes muscle tremors, bradycardia, reduced respiratory rate in cats, dogs and horses. Salivation, ruminal atony, hypothermia, bradycardia and bloat have been reported in cattle. Bloat arising from aerophagia during xylazine treatment has also been reported in dogs. Xylazine has been implicated in premature parturition in cattle. Increased urination has also been observed in cats. Overdose may cause cardiac arrhythmia, hypotension, and severe respiratory and CNS depression.

Management of Overdose/Toxicity—Atropine pretreatment may prevent the salivation and bradycardia. α-Adrenergic blocking agents such as yohimbine or tolazoline can be used to reverse the toxicity of xylazine. The respiratory depression can be reversed by doxapram.

Contraindications—Dehydrated cattle; concurrent administration of epinephrine; ventricular arrhythmia; restraint for radiography (gas filled stomach makes interpretation of radiology more difficult); last month of pregnancy.

Precautions—Use xylazine cautiously in animals with compromised cardiopulmonary function, in combination with neuroleptics or tranquilizers (reduce dose of tranquilizers), seizure disorder, hepatic and renal dysfunction.

Drug Interactions—Other CNS depressants such as barbiturates, narcotics, anesthetics etc. will produce additive effects when used in concurrently with xylazine. The doses of such agents must be reduced.

Pharmaceutical Formulations—The drug is available as xylazine hydrochloride in solution for injection.

YOHIMBINE

Yohimbine

Proprietary Names—Yobine®; Antagonil®.

Chemical Class—Indolealkylamine alkaloid; Rauwolfia alkaloid.

Pharmacological Class—α_2-Adrenergic antagonist; 5-HT receptor antagonist.

Source—Natural; obtained from the bark of the *Pausinystalia yohimbe* tree, and *Rauwolfia* root.

Solubility, Stability and Storage—Yohimbine is sparingly soluble in water but soluble in ethanol. Store products at room temperature; protect from light and heat.

Pharmacological Actions—Yohimbine produces actions opposite those of clonidine. Its central actions cause increases in blood pressure, heart rate and motor activities. Yohimbine enhances sexual activity and has been of benefit to some human patients with psychogenic erectile dysfunction.

Mechanism of Action—Yohimbine selectively and competitively blocks α_2-adrenergic receptors. It also blocks 5-HT receptors.

Indications—Reversal of xylazine effect in many animal species. It has also been used as antiemetic in dogs and cats.

Dosages—

Dog, cat.	0.1 mg/kg IV (for xylazine reversal); 0.25-0.5 mg/kg SC or IM (for antiemetic action).
Rabbits and other rodents.	0.2 mg/kg IV or IP
Cattle	0.125 mg/kg IV
Horse	0.075 mg/kg IV
Wild herbivores	0.2-0.3 mg/kg IV or IM

Route(s) of Administration—Parenteral routes are appropriate.

Onset of Action—3 minutes.

Distribution—Vd = 2-58 L/kg (horses); 4.5 L/kg (dogs); 5 L/kg (steers). Yohimbine is widely distributed; it enters the CNS readily.

Metabolism—Unknown.

Plasma Half-Life (hours)—Established values are 0.5-1 in steer, 0.5-1.5 in horses and 1.5-2 in dogs.

Clearance—(ml/min/kg)—70 in steers, 35 in horses and 30 in dogs.

Toxicity and Adverse Effects—Small animals appear to be more prone to adverse effects of yohimbine than large ones. The drug causes tremor due to increased motor activity. Central effects such as transient apprehension and excitement have been reported. Yohimbine also causes salivation, increased respiration and hyperemic mucous membranes. Overdose may cause tremors and seizures.

Management of Overdose/Toxicity—Give symptomatic and supportive therapy.

Contraindications—Hypersensitivity to yohimbine; renal impairment.

Precautions—Use yohimbine cautiously in seizure cases.

Drug Interactions—Other α_2-adrenoceptor antagonists may give additive effect.

Pharmaceutical Formulations—The drug is available as yohimbine hydrochloride in 2 mg/ml and 5 mg/ml sterile solutions for injection.

Bibliography

Abbah JG, Eghianruwa KI, Ola-Davies EO, Abu HH. Comparative effects of aqueous extracts of Ocimum basilicum and loperamide on intestinal transit in rats. Nig J Exp Appl Bio. 2006;7:141–4.

Abdallah JG, Schrier RW, Edelstein C, Jennings SD, Wyse B, Ellison DH. Loop diuretic infusion increases thiazide-sensitive Na(+)/Cl(-)-cotransporter abundance: role of aldosterone. J Am Soc Nephrol. 2001;12:1335-41.

Adamantos S, Valtolina C. Amitraz toxicity: Standards of Care. Emergency and critical care medicine. 2009;11:8-11

Ajuwon KO, Eghianruwa KI. Veterinarians' drug prescriptions; To what extent do pet owners comply? Trop Vet. 2001; 20:83-8.

Akande M, Eghianruwa KI, Onakpa MM. Effects of phenobarbitone and chloramphenicol pretreatment on ketamine and chloral hydrate anaesthesia in rats. Nig Vet J. 2009;30:19-25.

Alada ARA, Fagbohun TD, Oyebola DDO. Effect of adrenaline on glucose uptake by the canine large bowel. Afr J Biomed Res. 2001;4:123–6.

Aliu, Y, Asuzu, UI, Lawal TW, Eghianruwa KI, Maddo DG. Nigerian Veterinary Formulary – Handbook of Essential Veterinary Drugs, Biologics and Pesticide Chemicals. I[st] ed. Abuja: Veterinary Council of Nigeria; 2007.

Amitraz (Internet). Retrieved December 10, 2012 from Wikipaedia at http://en.wikipedia.org/wiki/Amitraz.

Andes D, Craig WA. Animal model pharmacokinetics and pharmacodynamics: a critical review. Int J Antimicro Ag. 2002;19:261–8.

Andres M, Pena A, Derick S, Raufaste D, Trojnar J, Wisniewski, K, Trueba M, Serradeil-le Gal C, Guillon G. Comparative pharmacology of bovine, human and rat vasopressin receptor isoforms. Eur J Pharmacol. 2004;501:59–69.

Anthelmintics for Animal Use (Internet). Retrieved January 23, 2012 from http://www.scribd.com/doc/29272635/Anthelmintics-for-Animal-Use.

Appel LJ. The verdict from ALLHAT—thiazide diuretics are the preferred initial therapy for hypertension. JAMA. 2002;288:3039-42.

Awadzi K, Hero M, Opoku NO, Büttner DW, Coventry PA, Prime MA, Orme ML, Edwards G. The chemotherapy of onchocerciasis XVII. A clinical evaluation of albendazole in patients with onchocerciasis; effects of food and pretreatment with ivermectin on drug response and pharmacokinetics. Trop Med Parasitol. 1994;45:203-8.

Azoulay-Dupuis E, Bedos JP, Vallée E, Hardy DJ, Swanson RN, Pocidalo JJ. Antipneumococcal activity of ciprofloxacin, ofloxacin, and temafloxacin in an experimental mouse pneumonia model at various stages of the disease. J Infect Dis. 1991;163:319-24.

Ballard S, Shults T, Kownacki AA, Blake JW, Tobin T. The pharmacokinetics, pharmacological responses and behavioral effects of acepromazine in the horse. J Vet Pharmacol Thera. 1982;5:21–31.

Baneth G, Shaw SE. Chemotherapy of canine leishmaniosis. Vet Parasitol. 2002;106:315-24.

Barberis C, Mouillac B, Durroux T. Structural bases of vasopressin/oxytocin receptor function. J Endocrinol. 1998;156:223–9.

Batts TW, Spangenburg EE, Ward CW, Lees SJ, Williams JH. Effects of acute epinephrine treatment on skeletal muscle sarcoplasmic reticulum Ca2+ATPase. Basic Appl Myol. 2007;17:229–35.

Benson GJ, Thurmon JC. Intravenous anesthesia. Vet Clin North Am Equine Pract. 1990;6:513-28.

Braide VB, Eghianruwa KI. Isometamedium residues in goat tissues after parenteral administration. Res Vet Sci.1980;29:111-3.

Brajtburg J, Bolard J. Carrier effects on biological activity of amphotericin. Clin Microbiol Rev. 1996;9:512–31.

Callréus T, Höglund P. Pharmacokinetics and antidiuretic effect of intravenous administration of desmopressin in orally overhydrated male volunteers. Pharmacol Toxicol. 1998;83:259–62.

Carpenter JW, editor. Exotic animal formulary. 4th ed. New York: Elsevier; 2013.

Chávez B, Espinosa-Cantellano M, Cedillo Rivera R, Ramírez A, Martínez-Palomo A. Effects of albendazole on Entamoeba histolytica and Giardia lamblia trophozoites. Arch Med Res. 1992;23:63-7.

Chiang CM, Flynn GL, Weiner ND, Szpunar GJ. Bioavailability assessment of topical delivery systems: Effect of intersubject variability on relative in-vitro deliveries of minoxidil and hydrocortisone from solution and ointment formulations. Int J Pharma. 1989;50:21–6.

Chyka PA, Seger D, Krenzelok EP, Vale JA Position paper: Single-dose activated charcoal; American Academy of Clinical Toxicology; European Association of Poisons Centres and Clinical Toxicologists. Clin Toxicol (Phila). 2005;43:61-87.

Clarke's analysis of drugs and poisons (Internet). Available from https://www.medicinescomplete.com.

Cynthia M. Kahn CM, Line S, editors. The Merck Veterinary Manual. 9th ed. Whitehouse station, NJ: Merck and Co., Inc; 2005.

Dada YO, Lamidi MT, Eghianruwa KI, Adepoju FO. Effects of oral administration of the latex of Calotropis procera on weights, hematology and plasma biochemistry in rats. Trop Vet. 2002;20:218–25.

Damia G, D'Incalci M. Mechanisms of resistance to alkylating agents. Cytotechnology. 1998;27:165–73.

Daugschies A, Agneessens J, Goossens L, Mengel H, Veys P. The effect of a metaphylactic treatment with diclazuril (Vecoxan) on the oocyst excretion and growth performance of calves exposed to a natural Eimeria infection. Vet Parasitol. 2007;149:199-206.

Diao X, Jensen J, Hansen AD. Toxicity of the anthelmintic abamectin to four species of soil invertebrates. Environ Pollut. 2007;148:514-9.

DrugBank database. Available from http://www.drugbank.ca.

Duarte JD, Cooper-DeHoff RM. Mechanisms for blood pressure lowering and metabolic effects of thiazide and thiazide-like diuretics. Expert Rev Cardiovasc Ther. 2010;8:793-802.

Eghianruwa KI Anika SM. Effects of selenium and tocopherol supplementation on the efficacy of diminazene aceturate in reversing T. brucei–induced anemia in rats. Vet arhiv. 2011;81:647-56.

Eghianruwa KI, Adaudi AO, Lawal T, Anaga AO, Adeyemi S. O. Nigerian Veterinary Formulary – Handbook of Essential Veterinary Drugs, Biologics and Pesticide Chemicals. 2nd ed. Abuja: Veterinary Council of Nigeria; 2013.

Eghianruwa KI, Anika SM, Akpavie SO. Efficacy of diminazene with and without ascorbic acid supplementation in T. brucei infected rats. Trop Vet. 2009;27:20-36.

Eghianruwa KI, Anika SM. Effects of dimethyl sulphoxide and ascorbic acid pretreatment on prepatent period, parasitemia, hematology and tissue pathology in rats infected with T. brucei. Trop Vet. 2010;28:13-20.

Eghianruwa KI, Anika SM. Effects of DMSO on diminazene efficacy in experimental murine T. brucei infection. Int J Anim Vet Adv. 2012;4: 93-8.

Eghianruwa KI, Anika SM. Efficacy of diminazene aceturate with and without levamisole or dimethyl sulfoxide in reducing organ weight and parasitemia in T. congolense infected rats. Int J Anim Vet Adv. 2012;4: 06-11.

Eghianruwa KI, Eyre P. The receptors mediating vascular responses to autonomic agonists in isolated perfused bovine external ear. Trop Vet. 1990;8:219–25.

Eghianruwa KI, Eyre P. The isolated perfused bovine ear, a model for pharmacological study of cutaneous vasculature and anaphylaxis. Vet Res Comm. 1991;15:117-25.

Eghianruwa, K. I. and Eyre, P. Failure of disodium cromoglycate to inhibit active cutaneous anaphylaxis in the calf. Farmaci and Terapia. 1991;8:58-61.

Eghianruwa KI, Eyre P. The vascular responses of isolated perfused bovine external ear to exogenous histamine and 5-HT (serotonin). Vet Res Comm. 1992;16:345-54.

Eghianruwa KI, Eyre P. The Schultz-Dale reaction in isolated perfused calf ear and its inhibition by isoproterenol. Res Vet Sci. 1994;57:159–62.

Eghianruwa KI, Obidike RI. Effects of antioxidants on the efficacy of diminazene aceturate treatment of experimental murine *Trypanosoma congolense* infection. Ani Prod Res Adv. 2011;7:134–40.

Eghianruwa KI, Odiaka PCG, Ogunpolu J. A preliminary comparative efficacy study of isometamedium following oral and intramuscular administration in mice experimentally infected with T. congolense. Sahel J Vet Med. 2004; 3:33–7.

Eghianruwa KI, Ogunleye OA, Saba AB, Famakinde SA, Ola-Davies EO, Abu HH. Influence of atropine and loperamide on reduced intestinal transit induced by *Calotropis procera* latex in rats. Afr J Biomed Res. 2006;9:125–8.

Eghianruwa KI, Utho EM. Compliance with veterinary drug prescriptions by selected livestock and poultry owners in southwestern Nigerian cities of Ibadan, Abeokuta and Lagos- A survey. Sahel J Vet Med. 2004;3:25-32.

Eghianruwa KI. Effect of supplemental antioxidants, vitamin C and DMSO on weight gain and survivability in T. brucei infected and diminazene treated rats. Vet arhiv. 2012;82:519-29.

Eghianruwa KI. Prior administration of diminazene may not sensitize guinea pigs to subsequent treatment with isometamedium. Trop Vet. 1994;12:130-3.

Eghianruwa, KI. Dictionary of Pharmacology and Toxicology. Lagos: Stirling-Horden; 2002.

Elviss NC, Williams LK, Jørgensen F, Chisholm SA, Lawson AJ, Swift C, Owen RJ, Griggs DJ, Johnson MM, Humphrey TJ, Piddock LJV. Amoxicillin therapy of poultry flocks: effect upon the selection of amoxicillin-resistant commensal Campylobacter spp. J Antimicrob Chemother. 2009;64:702-11.

Food and Drug Administration (Internet). USA Animal Drugs @ FDA. Available from http://www.fda.gov/AnimalVeterinary/

Green R, Grierson R, Sitar DS, Tenenbein MJ. How long after drug ingestion is activated charcoal still effective? Toxicol Clin Toxicol. 200;39:601-5.

Grossman M.R. Amitraz toxicosis associated with ingestion of an acaricide collar in a dog. J Am Vet Med Assoc. 1993;203:55-7.

Gulati K, Ray A, Vijayan VK. Free radicals and theophylline neurotoxicity : an experimental study. Cell Mol Biol (Noisy-le-grand). 2007;53:42-52.

Hanberger H. Pharmacodynamic effects of antibiotics. Studies on bacterial morphology, initial killing, postantibiotic effect and effective regrowth time. Scand J Infect Dis Suppl. 1992;81:1-52.

Hassanpour H, Bahadoran S, Koosha S, Askari E, Homai S. Effect of Diclazuril, Semduramicin, Salinomycin and Maduramycin as Preventive Anticoccidial Drugs on Chicken Intestinal Morphology. Global Veterinaria 2010;5:01-05.

Hedner T, Edgar B, Edvinsson L, Hedner J, Persson B, Pettersson, A. Yohimbine pharmacokinetics and interaction with the sympathetic nervous system in normal volunteers. Eur J Clin Pharmacol. 1992;43:651–6.

Higgs GA, Salmon JA, Henderson B, VANE JR. Pharmacokinetics of aspirin and salicylate in relation to inhibition of arachidonate cyclooxygenase and antiinflammatory activity (inflammation/thromboxane/prostaglandins). Proc. Natl. Acad. Sci. USA. 1987;84:1417-1420.

Huang KL, Shieh JP, Chu CC, Cheng KI, Wang JJ, Lin MT, Yeh MY. Prolonged analgesic effect of amitriptyline base on thermal hyperalgesia in an animal model of neuropathic pain. Eur J Pharmacol. 2013;702:20-24.

Hughes R, Chapple DJ. The pharmacology of atracurium: a new competitive neuromuscular blocking agent. Br. J. Anaesth. 1981;53: 31-44.

Hugnet C, Buronrosse F, Pineau X, Cadoré JL, Lorgue G, Berny PJ. Toxicity and kinetics of amitraz in dogs. Am J Vet Res. 1996;57:1506-10.

Hunter JM. Muscle relaxants in renal disease. Acta Anaesthesiol Scand Suppl. 1994;102:2-5.

Ishida Y, Kurosaka Y, Murakami Y, Otani T, Yamaguchi K. Therapeutic effect of oral levofloxacin, ciprofloxacin, and ampicillin on experimental murine pneumonia caused by penicillin intermediate Streptococcus pneumoniae for which the minimum inhibitory concentrations of the quinolones are similar. Chemother. 1999;45:183-91.

Joukar S, Sheibani M, Joukar F. Cardiovascular effect of nifedipine in morphine dependent rats: hemodynamic, histopathological, and biochemical evidence. Croat Med J. 2012;53:343–9.

Kehe K, Balszuweit F, Steinritz D, Thiermann H. Molecular toxicology of sulfur mustard-induced cutaneous inflammation and blistering. Toxicol. 2009;263:12–9.

Keshmiri M, Baharvahdat H, Fattahi SH, Davachi B, Dabiri RH, Baradaran H, Rajabzadeh F. Albendazole versus placebo in treatment of echinococcosis. Trans R Soc Trop Med Hyg. 2001;95:190-4.

Kim KS, Chun YS, Chon SU, Suh JK. Neuromuscular interaction between cisatracurium and mivacurium, atracurium, vecuronium or rocuronium administered in combination. Anaesthesia. 1998;53:872-8.

Kobel W, Sumner DD, Campbell JB, Hudson DB, Johnson JL. Protective effect of activated charcoal in cattle poisoned with atrazine. Vet Hum Toxicol. 1985;27:185-8.

Koplovitz I, Menton R, Matthews C, Shutz M, Nails C, Kelly S. Dose-response effects of atropine and Hi-6 Treatment of organophosphorus poisoning in guinea pigs. Drug Chem Toxicol. 1995;18:119-36.The effects of topical (gel) astemizole and terfenadine on wound healing

The effects of topical (gel) astemizole and terfenadine on wound healing

Koutinas AF, Saridomichelakis MN, Mylonakis ME, Leontides L, Polizopoulou Z, Billinis C, Argyriadis D, Diakou N, Papadopoulos O. A randomised, blinded, placebo-controlled clinical trial with allopurinol in canine leishmaniosis. Vet Parasitol. 2001;98:247-61.

Krautwald-Junghanns ME, Zebisch R, Schmidt V. Relevance and treatment of coccidiosis in domestic pigeons (Columba livia forma domestica) with particular emphasis on toltrazuril. J Avian Med Surg. 2009;23:1-5.

Laragh JH. The Mode of Action and Use of Chlorothiazide and Related Compounds (Internet). Circulation.1962; 26:121-132. Retrieved June 10, 2012 from http://circ.ahajournals.org/content/26/1/121.

Lasota JA, Dybas RA. Abamectin as a pesticide for agricultural use. Acta Leiden. 1990; 59:217-225.

Laurence DR, Bennett PN, Brown MJ. Clinical Pharmacology. 8th ed. London: Churchill Livingstone; 1997.

Lee JA. Complications and controversies of decontamination: activated charcoal—to use or not to use, in Proceedings. Am Coll Vet Intern Med Conf, 2010.

Lemke LA. 2007. Anticholinergics and Sedatives. In: Tranquilli WJ, Thurmon JC, Grimm KA, editors. Lumb and Jones' Veterinary Anaesthesia and Analgesia 4th ed. Hoboken: Wiley-Blackwell; p. 203-239.

Lester GD, Merritt AM, Neuwirth L, Vetro-Widenhouse T, Steible C, Rice B. Effect of alpha 2-adrenergic, cholinergic, and nonsteroidal anti-inflammatory drugs on myoelectric activity of ileum, cecum, and right ventral colon and on cecal emptying of radiolabeled markers in clinically normal ponies. Am J Vet Res. 1998;59:320-7.

Lundblad LK, Rinaldi LM, Poynter ME, Riesenfeld EP, Wu M, Aimi S, Barone LM, Bates JH, Irvin CG. Detrimental effects of albuterol on airway responsiveness requires airway inflammation and is independent of β-receptor affinity in murine models of asthma. Respir Res. 2011;12: 12-27.

Maier G, Rubino C, Hsu R, Grasela T, Baumgartner RA. Population pharmacokinetics of (R)-albuterol and (S)-albuterol in pediatric patients aged 4-11 years with asthma. Pulm Pharmacol Ther. 2007;20:534-42.

McCleane G. Antidepressants as analgesics. CNS Drugs. 2008; 22:139-56.

McMurphy RM, Davidson HJ, Hodgson DS. Effects of atracurium on intraocular pressure, eye position, and blood pressure in eucapnic and hypocapnic isoflurane-anesthetized dogs. Am J Vet Res. 2004;65:179-82.

Mellinghoff H. Modern muscle relaxants and their clinical application Anaesthesist. 1994;43:270-82.

Miller AB, Nelson RW, Kirk CA, Neal L, Feldman EC. Effect of glipizide on serum insulin and glucose concentrations in healthy cats. Res Vet Sci. 1992;52:177-81.

Mingeot-Leclercq M, Tulkens PM. Aminoglycosides: Nephrotoxicity. Antimicrob. Agents Chemother. 1999;43:1003-12.

Moen MD, Lyseng-Williamson KA, Scott LJ. Liposomal amphotericin B: a review of its use as empirical therapy in febrile neutropenia and in the treatment of invasive fungal infections. Drugs. 2009;69:361-92.

Mokra D, Drgova A, Mokry J, Bulikova J, Pullmann R, Durdik P, Petraskova M, Calkovska A. Combination of budesonide and aminophylline diminished acute lung injury in animal model of meconium aspiration syndrome. J Physiol Pharmacol. 2008;59 Suppl 6:461-71.

Molinari G, Soloneski S, Larramendy ML. New ventures in the genotoxic and cytotoxic effects of macrocyclic lactones, abamectin and ivermectin. Cytogenet Genome Res. 2010;128:37-45.

Morgan MR, Gaynor JS, Monnet E. The effects of sodium ampicillin, sodium cefazolin, and sodium cefoxitin on blood pressures and heart rates in healthy, anesthetized dogs. J Am Anim Hosp Assoc. 2000;36:111-4.

Morrisa DL, Taylora DH. Echinococcus granulosus: development of resistance to albendazole in an animal model. J Helminthol. 1990;64:171-4.

Muir WW 3rd, Lerche P, Robertson JT, Hubbell JA, Beard W, Miller T, Badgley B, Bothwell V. Comparison of four drug combinations for total intravenous anesthesia of horses undergoing surgical removal of an abdominal testis. J Am Vet Med Assoc. 2000;217:869-73.

Mundt HC, Bangoura B, Mengel H, Keidel J, Daugschies A. Control of clinical coccidiosis of calves due to Eimeria bovis and Eimeria zuernii with toltrazuril under field conditions. Parasitol Res. 2005;97 Suppl 1:S134-42.

National Agency for Food and Drug Administration and Control (NAFDAC) (Internet). Abuja, Nigeria. Registered products. Retrieved from http://realsgroup.com/products/nafdac-registered-products.html.

Neuvonen PJ, Olkkola KT. Oral activated charcoal in the treatment of intoxications. Role of single and repeated doses. Med Toxicol Adverse Drug Exp. 1988;3:33-58.

Nicholson A, Ilkiw JE. Neuromuscular and cardiovascular effects of atracurium in isoflurane-anesthetized chickens. Am J Vet Res. 1992;53:2337-42.

Nicoli S, Santi P. Assay of amikacin in the skin by high-performance liquid chromatography. J Pharm Biomed Anal. 2006;41:994–7.

Obemeasor RE, Eghianruwa KI, Akintola AA. The use and misuse of nematocides in Ibadan area of Nigeria, misuse effects on therapeutic efficacy in small ruminants - a survey. Rev Elev Med Vet Pays Trop. 1997;50: 217-20.

Odenholt-Tornqvist I, LOWDIN E, CARS O. Postantibiotic Sub-MIC Effects of Vancomycin, Roxithromycin, Sparfloxacin, and Amikacin Antimicrob. Agents Chemother. 1992;36:1852-8.

Ogun OO, Eghianruwa KI. A preliminary study of the absorption of isometamedium chloride (Samorin) by the stomach and small intestine of rat. J Chemother. 1993;5:107-9.

O'Kell AL, Grant DC, Panciera DL, Troy GC, Weinstein NM. Effects of oral prednisone administration with or without ultralow-dose acetylsalicylic acid on coagulation parameters in healthy dogs. Am J Vet Res. 2012;73:1569-76.

Olson ME, Vizzutti D, Morck DW, Cox AK. The parasympatholytic effects of atropine sulfate and glycopyrrolate in rats and rabbits. Can J Vet Res. 1994; 58(4):254–8.

Parameshappa B, Rao NV, Gouda TS, Sen S, Chakraborty R, Md Ali Basha MdA, Reddy, SA, Kumar SMS. A study on drug-drug interaction between anti-hypertensive drug (propranolol) and anti-diabetic drug (glipizide). Ann Biol Res. 2010;1:35-40.

Peter R., de Bruin C., Odendaal D., Thompson P.N. The use of a pour-on and spray dip containing Amitraz to control ticks (Acari: Ixodidae) on cattle. J S Afr Vet Assoc. 2006;77:66-9.

Petruska JM, Beattie JG, Stuart BO, Pai S, Walters KM, Banks CM, Lulham GW, Mirro EJ. Cardiovascular effects after inhalation of large doses of albuterol dry powder in rats, monkeys, and dogs: a species comparison. Fundam Appl Toxicol. 1997;40:52-62.

Pfeiffer JB, Mevissen M, Steiner A, Portier CJ, Meylan M. In vitro effects of bethanechol on specimens of intestinal smooth muscle obtained from the duodenum and jejunum of healthy dairy cows. Am J Vet Res. 2007;68:313-22.

Plevraki K, Koutinas AF, Kaldrymidou H, Roumpies N, Papazoglou LG, Saridomichelakis MN, Savvas I, Leondides L. Effects of allopurinol treatment on the progression of chronic nephritis in Canine leishmaniosis (Leishmania infantum). J Vet Intern Med. 2006;20:228-33.

Plumb DC. Veterinary Drug Handbook. 7th ed. NJ, USA: Wiley-Blackwell; 2011.

Rainer TH, Robertson CE. Adrenaline, cardiac arrest, and evidence based medicine. J Accid Emerg Med. 1996;13:234–37.

Ray A, Gulati K, Anand S, Vijayan VK. Pharmacological studies on mechanisms of aminophylline-induced seizures in rats. Indian J Exp Biol. 2005;43:849-53.

Reinero CR, Delgado C, Spinka C, DeClue AE, Dhand R. Enantiomer-specific effects of albuterol on airway inflammation in healthy and asthmatic cats. Int Arch Allergy Immunol. 2009;150:43-50.

Richardson JA, Allen C. ASPCA Tips to Manage a Poison Emergency. ASPCA Animal Poison Control Center (cited 2012 Jan 21). Available from http://www.vspn.org/Library/Misc/VSPN_M01158.htm

Ringger NC, Lester GD, Neuwirth L, Merritt AM, Vetro T, Harrison J. Effect of bethanechol or erythromycin on gastric emptying in horses. Am J Vet Res. 1996;5712:1771-5.

Riviere JE, Mark G. Papich MG, editors. Veterinary pharmacology and therapeutics. 9th ed. Hoboken, NJ: Wiley-Blackwell; 2009.

Ruediger K, Schulze M. Post-farrowing stress management in sows by administration of azaperone: Effects on piglets performance J Anim Sci. 2012;90:2331-6.

Ruff MD, Garcia R, Chute MB, Tamas T. Effect of amprolium on production, sporulation, and infectivity of Eimeria oocysts. Avian Dis. 1993;37:988-92.

Samuelson J. Why Metronidazole Is Active against both Bacteria and Parasites Antimicrob Agents Chemother. 1999; 43:1533.

Sano T, Nishimura R, Mochizuki M, Sasaki N. Effects of midazolam-butorphanol, acepromazine-butorphanol and medetomidine on an induction dose of propofol and their compatibility in dogs. J Vet Med Sci. 2003;65:1141-3.

Saridomichelakis MN, Mylonakis ME, Leontides LS, Billinis C, Koutinas AF, Galatos AD, Gouletsou P, Diakou A, Kontos VI. Periodic administration of allopurinol is not effective for the prevention of canine leishmaniosis (Leishmania infantum) in the endemic areas. Vet Parasitol. 2005;130:199-205.

Schaffer SW, Warner BA, Wilson GL. Effects of chronic glipizide treatment on the NIDD heart. Horm Metab Res. 1993;25:348-52.

Schmidt-Oechtering GU, Alef M, Röcken M. Anesthesia of horses with xylazine and ketamine. 2. Anesthesia in adult horses. Tierarztl Prax. 1990;18:47-52.

Seidman MD, Shivapuja BG, Quirk WS The protective effects of allopurinol and superoxide dismutase on noise-induced cochlear damage. Otolaryngol Head Neck Surg. 1993;109:1052-6.

Shalaby HA. Anthelmintics Resistance; How to Overcome it? Iran J Parasitol. 2013;8:18–32.

Sica DA, Carter B, Cushman W, Hamm L. Thiazide and loop diuretics. J Clin Hypertens (Greenwich). 2011;13:639-643.

Sinclair MD. A review of the physiological effects of alpha2-agonists related to the clinical use of medetomidine in small animal practice. Can Vet J. 2003;44:885-97.

Singh S, McDonell WN, Young SS, Dyson DH. Cardiopulmonary and gastrointestinal motility effects of xylazine/ketamine-induced anesthesia in horses previously treated with glycopyrrolate. Am J Vet Res. 1996; 57(12):1762-70.

Srikanth D, Shenoy RR, Rao CM. The effects if topical (gel) astemizole and terfenadine on wound healing. The effects of topical (gel) astemizole and terfenadine on wound healing Indian J Pharmacol. 2008;40:170–4.

Steiner A, Roussel AJ, Martig J. Effect of bethanechol, neostigmine, metoclopramide, and propranolol on myoelectric activity of the ileocecocolic area in cows. Am J Vet Res. 1995;56:1081-6.

Stepanenko SI. Effect of ampicillin and rifampicin on biochemical and immunological processes in the organs of immunized animals. Antibiotiki. 1980;25:664-9.

Susan KM, Plumb DC. The Elephant Formulary. Elephant Care International; c2003-05. Available from http://www.elephantcare.org/

Swan GE. The pharmacology of halogenated salicylanilides and their anthelmintic use in animals. J S Afr Vet Assoc. 1999;70:61-70.

Talukder MH, Hikasa Y. Diuretic effects of medetomidine compared with xylazine in healthy dogs. Can J Vet Res. 2009;73:224-36.

Taylor DH, Morris DL, Reffin D, Richards KS. Comparison of albendazole, mebendazole and praziquantel chemotherapy of Echinococcus multilocularis in a gerbil model. Gut 1989;30:1401-1405.

The American Society of Health-System Pharmacists (ASHP) (Internet). Drug information. Available from https://www.medicinescomplete.com.

The National Office of Animal Health (NOAH) (Internet). Compendium of Data Sheets for Animal Medicines. Available from http://www.noahcompendium.co.uk.

Thummel KE, Shen DD, Isoherranen N. Design and Optimization of dosage regimens; pharmacokinetic data. In: Laurence L. Brunton LL, Chabner BA, Knollmann BC, editors. Goodman and Gilman's The Pharmacological basis of Therapeutics. 12th ed. New York: McGraw-Hill; 2011. p. 1891–1990.

Tobias KM, Marioni-Henry K, Wagner R. A Retrospective Study on the Use of Acepromazine Maleate in Dogs With Seizures. J Am Ani Hosp Ass. 2006;42:283-9.

Tricarico D, Barbieri M, Camerino DC. Acetazolamide opens the muscular K Ca^{2++} channel: A novel mechanism of action that may explain the therapeutic effect of the drug in hypokalemic periodic paralysis. Ann Neurol. 2000;48:304–12.

University of Pennsylvania Medical Center (2004, June 7). Adrenaline Packs A Powerful Punch In The Use Of Antidepressants. Science Daily. Retrieved January 4, 2013, from http://www.sciencedaily.com /releases/2004/06/040604031830.htm.

Wang X, Wang B, Fan Z, Shi X, Ke Z.-J, Luo J. Thiamine deficiency induces endoplasmic reticulum stress in neurons. Neurosci. 2007; 144(3, 9):1045–56.

Williams JC. Efficacy of albendazole, levamisole and fenbendazole against gastrointestinal nematodes of cattle, with emphasis on inhibited early fourth stage Ostertagia ostertagi larvae. Vet Parasitol. 1991;40:59-71.

Wrzos HF, Tandon T, Ouyang A. Mechanisms mediating cholinergic antral circular smooth muscle contraction in rats. World J Gastroenterol. 2004;10:3292-8.

Xylazine (Internet). Retrieved June 12, 2011 from http://www.inchem.org/documents/jecfa/jecmono/v38je03.htm

Yamashita K, Muir WW 3rd, Tsubakishita S, Abrahamsen E, Lerch P, Izumisawa Y, Kotani T. Infusion of guaifenesin, ketamine, and medetomidine in combination with inhalation of sevoflurane versus inhalation of sevoflurane alone for anesthesia of horses. J Am Vet Med Assoc. 2002;221:1150-5.

Yoneda I, Goto H, Nishizawa M, Unruh GK, Arakawa K. Effect of atracurium, vecuronium, pancuronium and tubocurarine on renal sympathetic nerve activity in baroreceptor denervated dogs. Br J Anaesth. 1994;72:679-82.